Spinal Cord Injury
Patient Education Manual

Aspen Reference Group

Sara Nell Di Lima
Managing Editor

Christina S. Schust
Research Editor

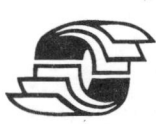

AN ASPEN PUBLICATION
Aspen Publishers, Inc.
Gaithersburg, Maryland
1998

To the best of our knowledge, the patient information sheets, forms, and practitioner guidelines reflect currently accepted practice; nevertheless, they cannot be considered absolute and universal recommendations for the care of patients. All recommendations must be considered in light of each patient's condition and care.

The authors and the publisher disclaim responsibility for any adverse effects resulting directly or indirectly from the use of the materials, from any undetected errors, and from the reader's misunderstanding of the text.

The authors and the publisher exerted every effort to ensure that any suggestions or recommendations set forth in this text were in accord with current regulations, recommendations, and practice at the time of publication. The authors do not endorse the use of any commercial product mentioned in the text.

Library of Congress Cataloging-in-Publication Data

Spinal cord injury patient education resource manual / Aspen Reference Group; Sara Nell Di Lima, managing editor; Una Hildebrandt, editor; Christina S. Schust, editor.
   p.   cm.
Includes bibliographical references and index.

1. Spinal cord—Wounds and injuries—Patients—Rehabilitation—Handbooks, manuals, etc. 2. Patient education—Handbooks, manuals, etc. I. Di Lima, Sara. II. Hildebrandt, Una. III. Schust, Christina S. IV. Aspen Reference Group (Aspen Publishers)
RD594.3.S6692   1996
617.4'82044—dc20

96-11459
CIP

Editorial Resources: Ruth Bloom
Printing and Manufacturing: Terri Miner

Copyright © 1996, 1997, 1998 by Aspen Publishers, Inc.

All rights reserved. No part of this publication may be reproduced; stored in or introduced into a retrieval system now known or to be invented; transmitted in any form or by any means (electronic, mechanical, recording, or otherwise); or used for advertising or promotional purposes, general distribution, creating new collective works, or for resale, without prior written permission of the copyright owner and publisher. An exception to this policy is the reproduction of forms, handouts, policies, or procedures contained herein solely for use within the site-of-purchase facility. Submit written permission requests to: Aspen Publishers, Inc., Permissions Department, 200 Orchard Ridge Drive, Suite 200, Gaithersburg, Maryland 20878.

Orders: (800) 638-8437
Customer Service: (800) 234-1660

About Aspen Publishers • For more than 35 years, Aspen has been a leading professional publisher in a variety of disciplines. Aspen's vast information resources are available in both print and electronic formats. We are committed to providing the highest quality information available in the most appropriate format for our customers. Visit Aspen's Internet site for more information resources, directories, articles, and a searchable version of Aspen's full catalog, including the most recent publications: **http://www.aspenpub.com**
Aspen Publishers, Inc. • The hallmark of quality in publishing
Member of the worldwide Wolters Kluwer group

Library of Congress Catalog Card Number: 96-11459
ISBN: 0-8342-1064-9

Printed in the United States of America

1 2 3 4 5

Contents

For a detailed listing of chapter contents, please see the first page of each chapter.

Editorial Board	v
Introduction	vii
Acknowledgments	ix
Chapter 1—Introduction to Spinal Cord Injury	1
Chapter 2—Circulatory System	27
Chapter 3—Respiratory System	43
Chapter 4—Neuromusculoskeletal System	65
Chapter 5—Bladder and Bowel Management	111
Chapter 6—Skin Care	173
Chapter 7—Sexuality and Reproduction	209
Chapter 8—Psychosocial Adjustment	257
Chapter 9—Pain Management	311
Chapter 10—Medications	333
Chapter 11—Independent Living Strategies	351
Chapter 12—Home Modification and Assistive Technology	385
Chapter 13—Maintaining Optimal Health	451
Appendix	471
Index	483

Editorial Board

Mindy Aisen, MD
Associate Professor of Clinical Neurology
Cornell University
Chief SCI, Burke Rehabilitation Hospital
White Plains, New York

Vivian Beyda, DrPH
Director, Research and Education
Eastern Paralyzed Veterans Association
Jackson Heights, New York

Geno Bonetti
Director of Business Development
HealthSouth Rehabilitation Hospital of Greater Pittsburgh
Monroeville, Pennsylvania

Debra L. Burdsall, MPH, OTR
Community Liaison
Spinal Cord Injury Project
Santa Clara Valley Medical Center
San Jose, California

Janeen Earwood, PT
Spinal Cord Injury Program Manager
Rehabilitation Hospital of Indiana
Indianapolis, Indiana

Cynthia Kraft Fine, RN, MSN, CRRN
Program Director, Spinal Cord Injury Program
Magee Rehabilitation Hospital
Philadelphia, Pennsylvania

Kenneth A. Gerhart, RPT, MS
Director of Training, Rehabilitation Research and Training
Center on Aging with Spinal Cord Injury
Craig Hospital
Englewood, Colorado

Kathryn M. Gillespie, RN, CRRN
Director of Nursing
HealthSouth Treasure Coast Rehabilitation Hospital
Vero Beach, Florida

Irmo Marini, PhD, CRC
Program Coordinator and Assistant Professor
Arkansas State University
Jonesboro, Arkansas

Sara James Migliarese, MS, PT, NCS
Neurologic Certified Specialist
John C. Whitaker Regional Rehabilitation Center
Forsyth Memorial Hospital
Winston–Salem, North Carolina

Grace Nolde-Lopez, RN, MS, CRRN
Clinical Nurse Specialist
Craig Hospital
Englewood, Colorado

Ricardo Oliver
Rehabilitation Team Director
Accessible Alternatives, Inc.
Orlando, Florida

Lucille M. O'Neil, PT
Assistant Director of Physical Therapy
Children's Hospital
Richmond, Virginia

Marca L. Sipski, MD
Director of Medical Systems Development
Kessler Institute for Rehabilitation
West Orange, New Jersey
Associate Professor of Clinical PM&R
UMDNJ–New Jersey Medical School
Newark, New Jersey

Jay V. Subbarao, MD, MS
Clinical Professor
Chief, Division of PMR
Loyola University Medical Center
ACOS/Rehabilitation
Director, Comprehensive Rehabilitative Services
Hines VA Hospital
Hines, Illinois

Karen Teague, MS, RN, CNA
Director of Nursing
Medical Surgical Hospital
Mississippi State Hospital
Whitfield, Mississippi

Elisabeth Wall-Smith, RN, MS, CS, CRRN
Advanced Practice Nurse
Rusk Rehabilitation Center
Columbia, Missouri

Kelly B. Wascher, RN, MS, CRRN
Rehabilitation Clinical Nurse Specialist
St. Joseph Healthcare System
Albuquerque, New Mexico

Angela Wu, MLS
Eastern Paralyzed Veterans Association
Director, Library and Information Services
Jackson Heights, New York

Introduction

The impact of spinal cord injury (SCI) on the individual remains one of the most compelling and challenging in the field of rehabilitation. Persons with SCI often require considerable motivation and reeducation to regain a satisfying quality of life and ensure community reintegration. Crucial to rehabilitation is the communal effort of an interdisciplinary team whose members work together to meet the specific needs of both the individual and the family. Physicians, therapists, social workers, and psychologists have the specialized knowledge needed to address the unique problems of the patient, and must work together to develop a customized patient education program.

The amount of relearning involved in rehabilitation is often overwhelming to the person with SCI, as well as to the family and the members of the interdisciplinary team. Adding to this pressure is the trend toward shorter lengths of stay in hospitals and rehabilitation facilities. Based on this premise, the *Spinal Cord Injury Patient Education Manual* was developed to present materials, geared primarily for the patient, that cover the diverse components of SCI rehabilitation.

Here, in a single comprehensive and practical resource, you will find step-by-step patient instructions, definitions, charts, figures, checklists, assessment forms, timetables, and support resources designed for distribution to patients by members of the SCI rehabilitation team. Beginning with basic information on SCI, the manual explores its effects on the patient's body systems, psychological and social well-being, and independent living after discharge. Issues vital to the person with SCI, including bladder and bowel management, sexuality and reproduction, personal attendant services, home modification, and assistive devices, are thoroughly addressed.

The contents of the manual represent a compilation of the best patient education materials available throughout the United States. They were gathered from hospitals, clinics, health organizations, and practices and through an extensive review of both professional and lay literature. We also turned to our Editorial Board members for their input on the most relevant topics and timeliest materials. The resulting volume contains items useful to every practitioner who treats individuals with SCI.

The subdivided chapters allow for quick and easy reference and a detailed table of contents begins each chapter. Large print and numerous illustrations make the patient information sheets accessible to nearly all individuals. An appendix lists resources for both patient and practitioner, and a complete index makes locating and cross-referencing specific items nearly effortless.

As you extract and adapt materials from the manual, you may customize improvements to particular items. All materials selected for publication include a complete source line crediting the contributor. In this way, we hope to ensure the usefulness of the *Spinal Cord Injury Patient Education Manual* so that it remains a valuable part of your SCI rehabilitation program.

Una Hildebrandt
Christina S. Schust
Editors, Aspen Reference Group

Acknowledgments

Developing a publication as comprehensive as the *Spinal Cord Injury Patient Education Manual* demands enormous care and effort. Shaping the focus of the manual, identifying the contributors, collecting and evaluating materials, and striving to maintain a practical, easy-to-use format are among the many time-consuming, challenging tasks facing the Aspen editor.

Foremost among the people who help fulfill these responsibilities are the Editorial Board members. By answering queries, suggesting contacts, contributing materials, and reviewing the manuscript, they are vital to the development process. We particularly appreciate the generous and enthusiastic cooperation of the following Board members: Cynthia Kraft Fine, Kenneth Gerhart, Irmo Marini, Sara James Migliarese, Marca Sipski, Elisabeth Wall-Smith, Kelly Wascher, and Angela Wu. We also thank Mindy Aisen, Vivian Beyda, Geno Bonetti, Debra Burdsall, Janeen Earwood, Kathryn Gillespie, Grace Nolde-Lopez, Ricardo Oliver, Lucille O'Neil, Carolyn Schmaltz, Jay Subbarao, and Karen Teague.

In addition to those resources provided by our Editorial Board, the *Spinal Cord Injury Patient Education Manual* features contributions from a wide range of individuals and organizations. We extend our sincerest thanks to all those who shared their materials with us. Special appreciation goes to Frank Martin, Access to Independence, Inc.; American Association of SCI Psychologists and Social Workers; American Spinal Injury Association (ASIA); Shirley McCluer, Arkansas Spinal Cord Commission; Peter Lawless, Social Service Programs, Health and Welfare Canada; Jane Gay, Iowa Program for Assistive Technology; FES Information Center; Jim McAleer, National Spinal Cord Injury Association (NSCIA); Northwest Regional Spinal Cord System; Sue Murphy, SCI Project at Santa Clara Valley Medical Center; Donna Schachtel, Shepherd Center; Linda Lindsey, UAB–Spain Rehabilitation Center; Catherine Flanagan, University of Rochester–Strong Memorial Hospital; Virginia SCI System; and Jo Ann Ford, SARDI Project, Wright State University.

Finally, this project never would have progressed from a "bare bones" idea to a finished product without the unflagging support of Rosemarie Cooper, Administrative Assistant; the attention and skill of Marsha Davies, Managing Editor, Editorial Resources; the cooperation of Terri Miner, Production Coordinator; the insight of Stephen M. Zollo, Senior Acquisitions Editor; the support of Kenneth E. Lawrence, Director, Research Publishing; and, last but not least, the insight and guidance of Sara Nell Di Lima, Managing Editor, and Sandra Painter, Senior Editor, Aspen Reference Group.

Una Hildebrandt
Christina S. Schust

Introduction to Spinal Cord Injury

> Most materials in the *Spinal Cord Injury Patient Education Resource Manual* are intended for the health care professional to share with the patient. Materials that are intended solely for the professional are labeled "Exhibit" in the table of contents.

General Information

What Is Spinal Cord Injury? (level: basic) 3
Understanding Your Spinal Cord Injury (level: advanced) 8
Clinical Syndromes (Exhibit) 14

Classification

International Standards for Neurological and Functional Classification of Spinal Cord Injury (Exhibit) 14

Standard Neurological Classification of Spinal Cord Injury (Exhibit) 19
Spinal Cord Injury/Functional Chart 20

Rehabilitation

Selecting a Rehabilitation Center for Spinal Cord Injury 23
The Members of the Rehabilitation Team 25

GENERAL INFORMATION

What Is Spinal Cord Injury?

Any damage to the spinal cord is a very complex injury. Each injury is different, and injuries can affect the body in many different ways. This is a brief summary of the changes that take place after a spinal cord injury. It tells how the spinal cord works and what can happen to the body following a spinal cord injury.

THE NORMAL SPINAL CORD

The **spinal cord** is a part of your nervous system. It is the largest nerve in the body. Nerves are cordlike structures made up of many **nerve fibers**. The spinal cord has many spinal nerve fibers. Nerve fibers carry messages between the brain and different parts of the body. The messages may be for motion, telling a body part to move. Other nerve fibers bring messages of feeling or sensation back to the brain from the body, such as heat, cold, or pain. The body also has an autonomic nervous system. It controls the involuntary activities of the body, such as blood pressure, body temperature, and sweating.

These nerve fibers make up the communication systems of the body. The spinal cord can be compared to a telephone cable. It connects the main office (the brain) to many individual offices

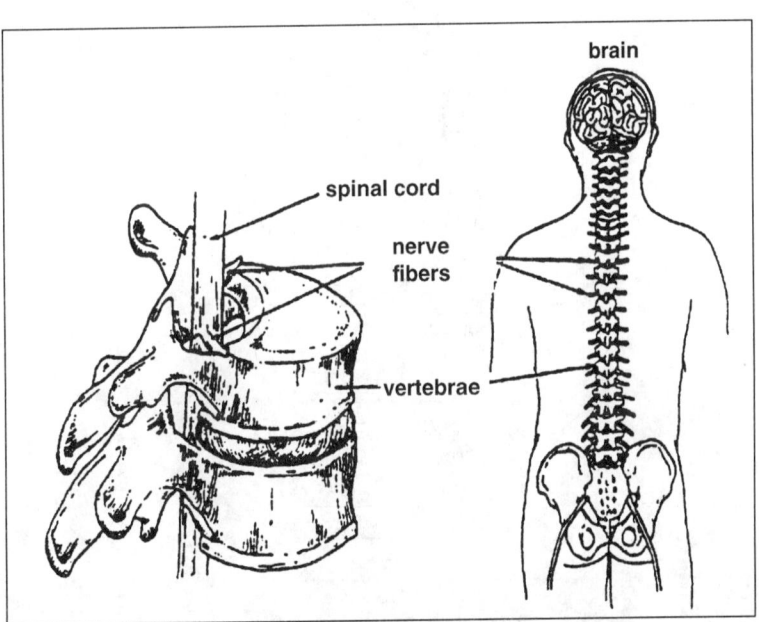

The **spinal cord** goes through the center of the stacked **vertebrae**. These bones protect the spinal cord. The **nerve fibers** branch out from the spinal cord to other parts of the body.

continues

continued

(parts of the body) by telephone lines (nerve fibers). The spinal cord is the pathway that messages use to travel between the brain and the other parts of the body.

Because the spinal cord is such an important part of our nervous system, it is surrounded and protected by bones called **vertebrae**. The vertebrae, or backbones, are stacked on top of each other. This is called the **vertebral column** or the spinal column. The vertebral column is the number one support for the body. The spinal cord actually runs through the middle of the vertebrae.

The spinal cord is about 18 inches long. It extends from the base of the brain, down the middle of the back, to about the waist. The bundle of nerve fibers that make up the spinal cord itself are **upper motor neurons** (UMNs). Spinal nerves branch off the spinal cord all the way up and down the neck and back. These nerves, **lower motor neurons** (LMNs), exit between each two vertebrae and go out to all parts of the body. The spinal cord ends near the waistline. From this point, the lower spinal nerve fibers continue down through the spinal canal to the sacrum or tailbone.

The spinal column is divided into four sections. The top portion is called the **cervical** area. It has seven cervical vertebrae. The next section, the **thoracic**, includes the chest area and has

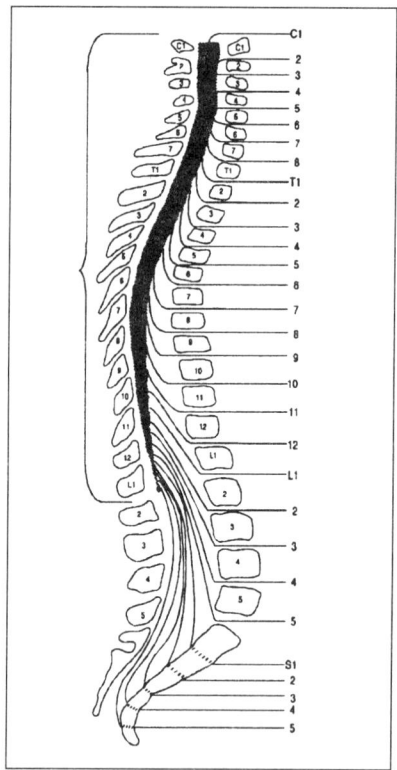

The **spinal cord** ends in the back area near the waistline. The nerves within the spinal cord are **upper motor neurons** (UMNs). **Nerves** descend from the end of the spinal cord down through the vertebral column, exiting at each level. **Spinal nerves** branch out between each two **vertebrae**. These are **lower motor neurons** (LMNs).

continues

continued

12 thoracic vertebrae. The lower back section is called the **lumbar** area. There are five lumbar vertebrae. The bottom section has five **sacral** vertebrae and is called the sacral area. The bones in the sacral section are actually fused together into one bone.

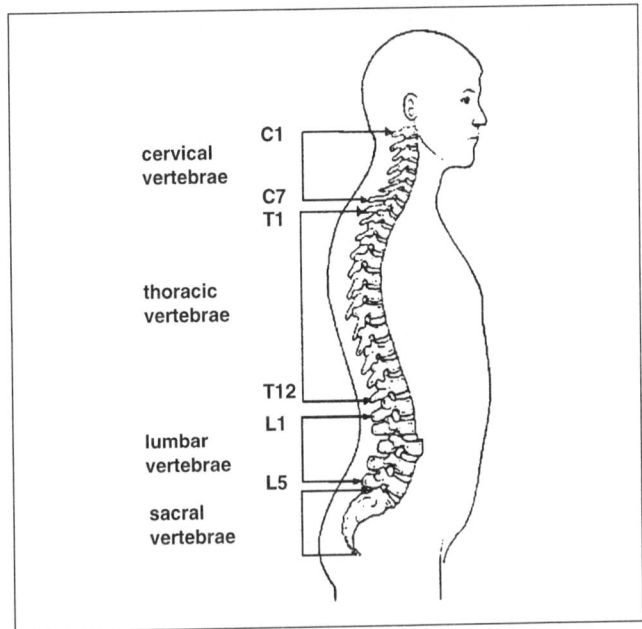

The **vertebrae** are numbered and named according to their location in the vertebral column.

THE SPINAL CORD AFTER AN INJURY

A spinal cord injury can occur either from an injury or from a disease to the vertebral column or the spinal cord. In most spinal cord injuries, the backbone pinches the spinal cord. The spinal cord may become bruised or swollen. The injury may actually tear the spinal cord and/or its nerve fibers. An infection or a disease can cause similar results.

After a spinal cord injury, all the nerves above the level of injury keep working like they always have. Below the level of injury, the spinal cord nerves cannot send messages between the brain and parts of the body like they did before the injury.

The doctor examines the individual to understand what type of damage has been done to the spinal cord. An X-ray shows where the damage occurred to the vertebrae. The doctor does a "pin prick" test to see what feeling the person has all over his or her body (sensory level). The doctor also asks, "what parts of the body can you move?" (motor level). The exams that the doctor does are important because they tell the doctor what nerves and muscles are working.

Each spinal cord injury is different. A person's injury is described by its **type** and **level**.

continues

continued

COMPLETE OR INCOMPLETE INJURY

The **type** of spinal cord injury is classified by the doctor as **complete** or **incomplete**. The complete injury is like cutting off all telephone service to a building. No messages can reach the offices. An incomplete injury is like stopping telephone service to some offices in a building. Some messages can get through to some offices, while others cannot. The amount and type of message that can pass between the brain and the parts of the body will depend on how many nerves are not damaged.

Some people with an incomplete injury may have a lot of feeling but little movement. Others may have some movement and very little feeling. Incomplete spinal injuries will differ from one person to another because different nerve fibers are damaged in each person's spinal cord.

LEVEL OF INJURY

The **level of injury** is determined after the doctor does the different tests. The level is the lowest point on the spinal cord below which there is a decrease or absence of feeling (sensory level) *and* movement (motor level).

The higher the spinal cord injury is on the vertebral column, or the closer it is to the brain, the more loss of function (feeling and movement) there is. Fewer parts and systems of the body work normally with a higher level of injury.

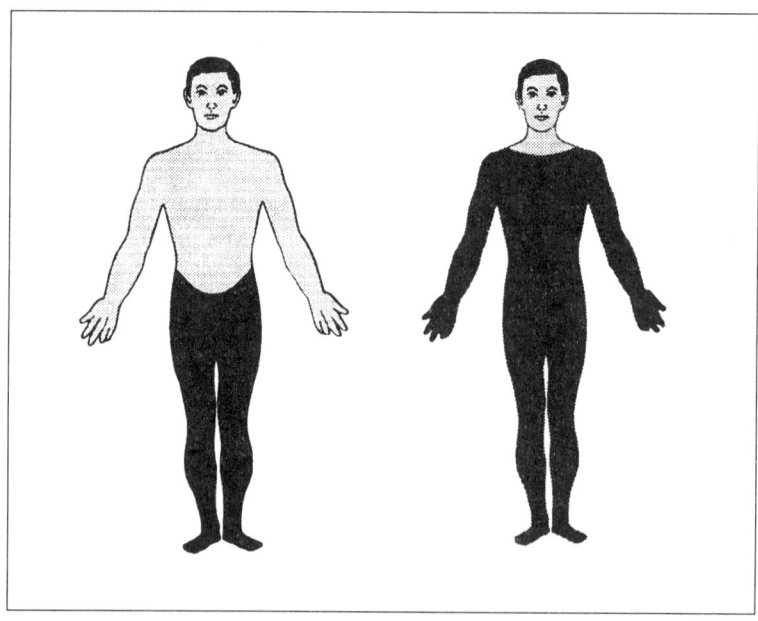

The shaded area shows those parts of the body that do not work in the same way after a spinal cord injury.

The dark shading shows the areas of the body affected by a T11 level injury to the lower spinal cord. This person has **paraplegia**.

The dark shading shows the areas of the body affected by a C3 level injury to the neck. This person has **tetraplegia**.

continues

continued

For example, an injury at the T8 level means the individual has a decrease or loss of feeling and movement below the eighth thoracic spinal cord segment. A person with a C5 level of injury has a decrease or loss of feeling and movement below the 5th cervical spinal cord segment. Someone with a T8 level of injury would have more feeling and movement than someone with a C5 level of injury. Remember that the amount of feeling and movement also depends on whether the injury is complete or incomplete.

A person is said to have **paraplegia** if the person has lost feeling and is not able to move the lower parts of his or her body. The injury is in the thoracic, lumbar, or sacral area.

A person with **tetraplegia** (formerly called quadriplegia) has lost movement and feeling in both the upper and lower parts of his or her body. This injury is in the cervical area.

CHANGES AFTER THE INITIAL INJURY

Sometimes the spinal cord is only bruised or swollen after the initial injury. As the swelling goes down, the nerves may begin to work again. There are no tests at this time to tell how many nerves, if any, will begin to work again. The longer there is no improvement, the less likely it is that there will be improvement. If a little recovery in function does occur, there is considerably more hope. This is no guarantee that more function will return.

Some individuals have involuntary movements, such as twitching or shaking. These movements are called spasms. Spasms are not a sign of recovery. A spasm occurs when a wrong message from the nerve causes the muscle to move. The individual often cannot control this movement.

In addition to movement and feeling, a spinal cord injury affects other body functions. The lungs, bowel, and bladder may not work the same as before the injury. There may also be changes in sexual function. During rehabilitation, the medical team teaches the individual with spinal cord injury new ways to manage his or her bodily functions.

Source: Developed by Linda Lindsey, Medical RRTC in Secondary Complications in SCI, Department of Rehabilitation Medicine, University of Alabama at Birmingham—Spain Rehabilitation Center, Birmingham, Alabama, © 1994. Supported in part by a grant (#Hi33B30025) from the National Institute on Disability and Rehabilitation Research, U.S. Department of Education. Opinions expressed in this document are not necessarily those of the granting agency.

Understanding Your Spinal Cord Injury

Understanding the physiological effects of a spinal cord injury requires a basic knowledge of the anatomy and physiology of the spinal cord. Knowledge of the pathologic anatomy and physiology of a spinal cord injury (SCI) is also needed. Following this brief summary is a list of additional resources.

ANATOMY AND PHYSIOLOGY

The **spinal cord** is the largest nerve in the body. Nerves are cordlike structures made up of **nerve fibers**. Nerve fibers are responsible for the communication systems of the body, which include sensory, motor, and autonomic functions. The nerve fibers within the spinal cord carry messages between the brain and the rest of the body.

Because the spinal cord is such an important part of the nervous system, it is surrounded by protective bone segments, together called the **vertebral column**.

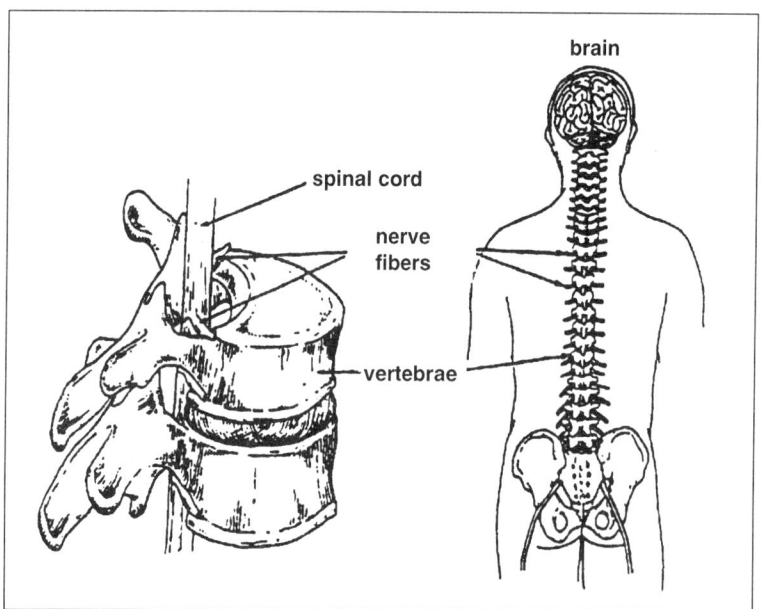

The **spinal cord** runs through the stacked **vertebrae** that make up the **vertebral column**. These bones protect the spinal cord. The **nerve fibers** branch out from the spinal cord to other parts of the body.

The vertebral column, also referred to as the spinal column, is made up of seven **cervical** vertebrae, 12 **thoracic** vertebrae, five **lumbar** vertebrae, and five **sacral** vertebrae. The sacral vertebrae are actually fused together into one bone.

continues

continued

The number of cervical spinal nerves (eight) differs in number from the cervical vertebrae (seven). The number of vertebral segments and spinal nerves are equal in the thoracic, lumbar, and sacral regions.

As the body grows, the vertebral column grows more in length than the spinal cord. The spinal cord usually ends at the level between the L1 and L2 vertebrae. From this point, the nerve roots branch out from the spinal cord, descending inside the spinal canal before leaving the vertebral column at their corresponding vertebrae. This causes a discrepancy between the location of the

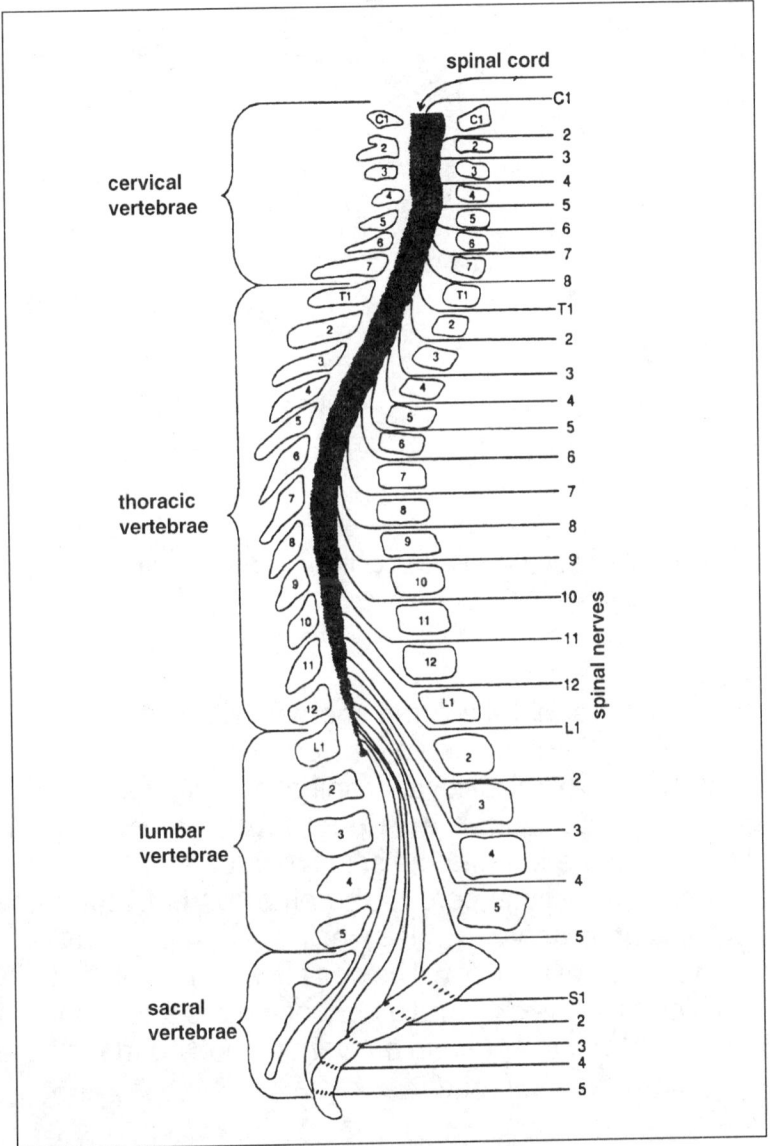

The vertebrae are numbered and named according to their location in the spinal column. The spinal nerves are numbered and indicate their corresponding vertebrae.

continues

continued

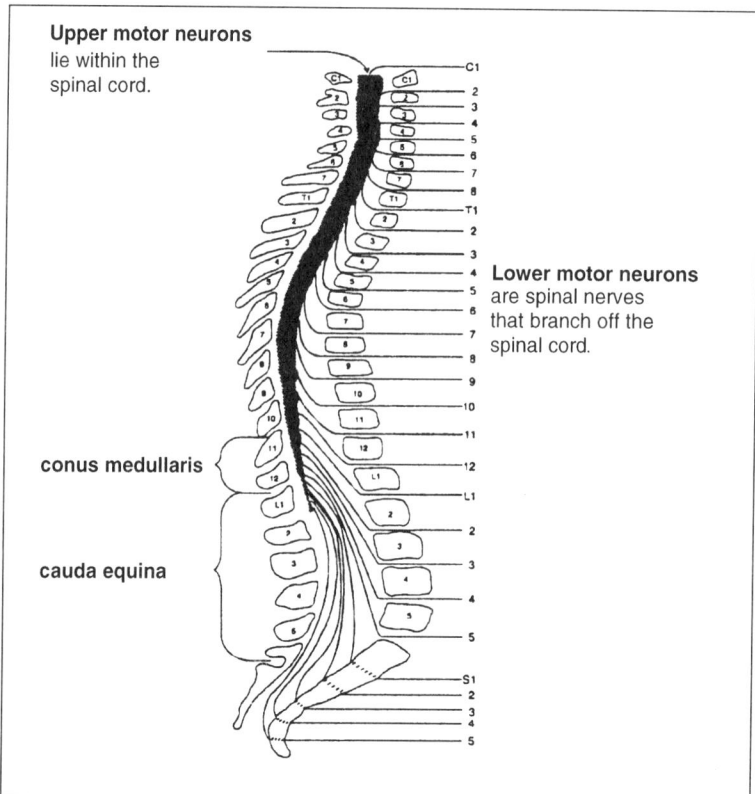

The **spinal cord** ends between L1 and L2. The **nerves** continue to descend in the spinal column, exiting between the vertebrae and through the sacrum.

spinal cord segments and the vertebral column segments, particularly in the lower part of the spinal system. For this reason, there is often a discrepancy between the skeletal or bony level of vertebral fracture and the neurological level of spinal cord injury.

The nerves that lie within the spinal cord are **upper motor neurons** (UMNs). They carry the messages back and forth from the brain to the spinal nerves along the spinal tract. The spinal nerves that branch out from the spinal cord to the other parts of the body are **lower motor neurons** (LMNs). These spinal nerves (LMNs) exit and enter at each vertebral level and communicate with specific areas of the body. The **sensory** portion of the LMN carries messages to the brain about sensation from the skin and other body parts and organs. The **motor portion** of the LMN sends messages from the brain to the various body parts to initiate actions such as muscle movement.

continues

continued

WHAT HAPPENS AFTER A SPINAL CORD INJURY?

The term **spinal cord injury** refers to any injury of the neural (pertaining to nerves) elements within the spinal canal. SCI can occur from trauma or disease to the vertebral column or the spinal cord itself. Most spinal cord injuries are the result of trauma to the vertebral column. Such trauma can cause a fracture of bone or tearing of ligaments with displacement of the bony column. This causes a pinching of the spinal cord. The vertebral trauma may cause contusion with hemorrhage and swelling of the spinal cord, or it may cause a tearing of the spinal cord and/or its nerve roots.

The damage from the spinal cord injury affects the sending and receiving of messages from the brain to the body's systems that control sensory, motor, and autonomic function below the level of injury. Messages from the body below the level of injury can no longer get to the brain. The brain cannot send messages to the body below the level of injury.

It is important to distinguish between injuries that occur in the spinal cord proper and those that occur to the **conus medullaris** or to the **cauda equina**.

A spinal cord injury with preservation of segments of spinal cord below the level of injury usually produces an upper motor neuron (UMN) type of injury or **spastic paralysis**. The intrinsic reflexes are now uninhibited and become hyperreflexic and lead to increased muscle tone, spasms, and spasticity.

A conus medullaris injury, without preservation of spinal cord segments below the lesion, or a cauda equina injury produces a lower motor neuron (LMN) type of injury or **flaccid paralysis**. With this type of injury, the stimuli cannot reach the spinal cord; therefore, the reflexes and muscle tone remain decreased or absent (flaccid).

CLASSIFICATION

A complete exam to determine the neurological level evaluates both the sensory and motor levels affected by the spinal cord injury. The recommended neurological assessment follows the classifications published in the *International Standards for Neurological and Functional Classification of Spinal Cord Injury*, revised 1992, endorsed by the American Spinal Injury Association and the International Medical Society of Paraplegia.

The **neurologic level of injury** is defined as "the most caudal (lowest) segment of the spinal cord with normal sensory and/or motor function on both sides of the body."

The physician examines the 28 **dermatomes** (the nerve roots that receive sensory information from the skin areas) for sensitivity to pin prick and light touch. The motor levels are tested in the 10 paired **myotomes** (groups of muscles).

The **sensory and motor levels** need to be evaluated for both the right and left sides of the body. It is not unusual to have a discrepancy between the lowest normal motor level and the lowest normal sensory level. The physician uses this evaluation to classify the injury as **complete** or **incomplete** and assign a **level of injury**.

continues

continued

Another way that the level of spinal cord injury can be categorized is **tetraplegia** and **paraplegia**. **Tetraplegia**, previously called quadriplegia, refers to injuries of the cervical region of the spinal cord. **Paraplegia** refers to injuries that occur in the thoracic, lumbar, or sacral segments.

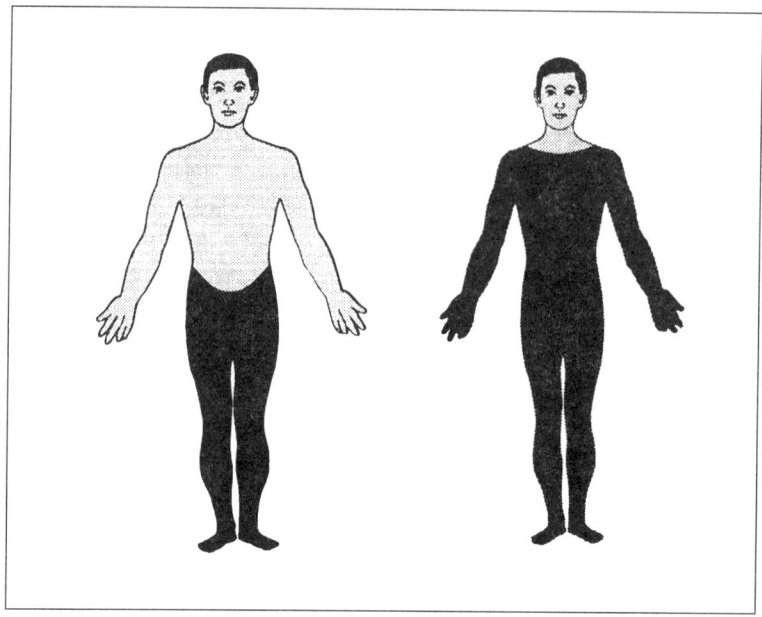

The shaded area shows those parts of the body that do not work in the same way after a spinal cord injury.

The dark shading shows the area of the body affected by a T11 level injury to the lower spinal cord. This person has **paraplegia**.

The dark shading shows the areas of the body affected by a C3 level injury to the neck. This person has **tetraplegia**.

When a spinal cord injury is graded as **incomplete**, it means the cord has been partially damaged. An incomplete injury results in partial preservation of sensation and/or motor function below the neurologic level of injury and includes the lowest sacral segment. A **complete** injury indicates a complete blockage of nerve messages. With a complete injury there is no sensation or motor function in the lowest sacral segment.

The nerve rootlets leave the spinal cord continually and then aggregate into nerve roots. In a spinal cord injury, only fractions of the rootlets going to a nerve root level may be damaged. Therefore, the nerve root, which is equivalent to a spinal segment, may be only partially damaged.

Also included in the neurological assessment is the classification of **clinical syndromes**. The syndromes include central cord syndrome, Brown-Sequard syndrome, anterior cord syndrome,

continues

continued

conus medullaris syndrome, and cauda equina syndrome. A mixed or unclassified syndrome is sometimes found.

A recently added classification used in the evaluation process is the **functional independence measure** (FIM). The FIM is a method for monitoring and evaluating progress associated with treatment. It measures daily life activities in the areas of self-care, sphincter control, mobility, locomotion, communication, and social cognition. Activities such as eating, toileting, and dressing are rated on a scale that measures dependence/independence.

With an accurate and complete examination to determine the neurologic level of injury, future rehabilitation goals can be established and a rehabilitation program can be developed around realistic goals.

Notes:

Source: Developed by Linda Lindsey, Medical RRTC in Secondary Complications in SCI, Department of Rehabilitation Medicine, University of Alabama at Birmingham—Spain Rehabilitation Center, Birmingham, Alabama, © 1994. Supported in part by a grant (#Hi33B30025) from the National Institute on Disability and Rehabilitation Research, U.S. Department of Education. Opinions expressed in this document are not necessarily those of the granting agency.

Exhibit
CLINICAL SYNDROMES

Central Cord Syndrome
A lesion, occurring almost exclusively in the cervical region, that produces sacral sensory sparing and greater weakness in the upper limbs than in the lower limbs.

Brown-Sequard Syndrome
A lesion that produces relatively greater ipsilateral proprioceptive and motor loss and contralateral loss of sensitivity to pin prick and temperature.

Anterior Cord Syndrome
A lesion that produces variable loss of motor function and of sensitivity to pin prick and temperature, while preserving proprioception.

Conus Medullaris Syndrome
Injury of the sacral cord (conus) and lumbar nerve roots within the neural canal, which usually results in an areflexic bladder, bowel, and lower limbs, with lesions as at B in the figure at right. Sacral segments may occasionally show preserved reflexes, e.g., bulbocavernosus and micturition reflexes, with lesions as at A.

Cauda Equina Syndrome
Injury to the lumbosacral nerve roots within the neural canal resulting in areflexic bladder, bowel, and lower limbs, with lesions as at C in the figure at right.

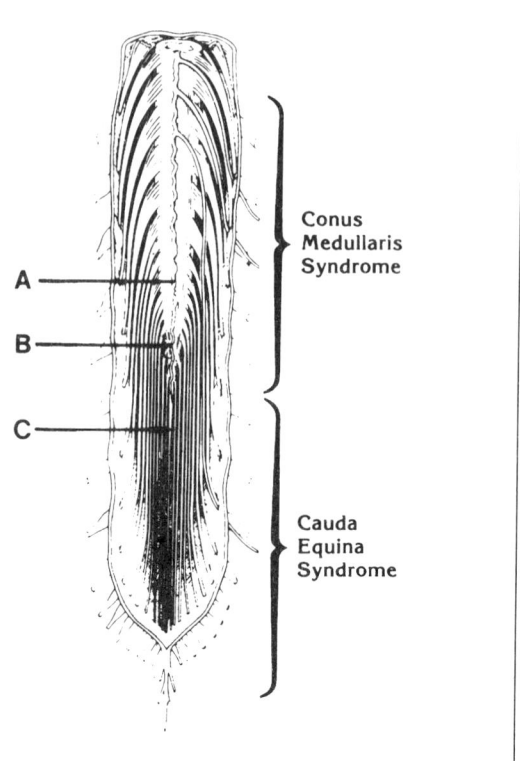

Source: American Spinal Injury Association, International Medical Society of Paraplegia. Supported by the American Paraplegia Association.

CLASSIFICATION

Exhibit
INTERNATIONAL STANDARDS FOR NEUROLOGICAL AND FUNCTIONAL CLASSIFICATION OF SPINAL CORD INJURY

NEUROLOGICAL EXAMINATION

Introduction

The neurological examination has two components (sensory and motor), which are separately described below. Further, the neurological examination has both required as well as optional, though recommended, elements. The required elements are used in determining the sensory/motor/neurological levels, in generating scores to characterize sensory/motor functioning and in determining completeness of the injury. The optional measures, though not used in scoring, may add to a specific patient's clinical description.

When the Patient Is Not Fully Testable

When a key sensory point or key muscle is not testable for any reason, the examiner should record "NT" instead of a numeric score. In such cases, sensory and motor scores for the affected side of the body, as well as total sensory and motor scores, cannot be generated with respect to the injury *at that point in treatment*. Further, when associated injuries, e.g., traumatic brain injury, brachial plexus injury, limb fracture, etc., interfere with completion of the neurological examination, the neurological level should still be determined as accurately as possible. However, obtaining the sensory/motor scores and impairment grades should be deferred to later examinations.

continues

continued

Sensory Examination: Required Elements

The required portion of the sensory examination is completed through the testing of a key point in each of the 28 dermatomes on the right and on the left sides of the body.

At each of these key points, two aspects of sensation are examined: sensitivity to pin prick and to light touch. Appreciation of pin prick and of light touch at each of the key points is separately scored on a three-point scale:

0 = absent
1 = impaired (partial or altered appreciation, including hyperaesthesia)
2 = normal
NT = not testable

The testing for pin sensation is usually performed with a disposable safety pin; light touch is tested with cotton. In testing for pin appreciation, the inability to distinguish between dull and sharp sensation is graded as 0.

The following key points are to be tested bilaterally for sensitivity (see Figure 1). Asterisks indicate that the point is at the mid-clavicular line:

C2–Occipital protuberance
C3–Supraclavicular fossa
C4–Top of the acromioclavicular joint
C5–Lateral side of the antecubital fossa
C6–Thumb
C7–Middle finger
C8–Little finger
T1–Medial (ulnar) side of the antecubital fossa
T2–Apex of the axilla
T3–Third intercostal space (IS)*
T4–Fourth IS (nipple line)*
T5–Fifth IS (midway between T4 and T6)*
T6–Sixth IS (level of xiphisternum)*
T7–Seventh IS (midway between T6 and T8)*
T8–Eighth IS (midway between T6 and T10)*
T9–Ninth IS (midway between T8 and T10)*
T10–Tenth IS (umbilicus)*
T11–Eleventh IS (midway between T10 and T12)*
T12–Inguinal ligament at midpoint
L1–Half the distance between T12 and L2
L2–Mid-anterior thigh
L3–Medial femoral condyle
L4–Medial malleolus
L5–Dorsum of the foot at the third metatarsal phalangeal joint
S1–Lateral heel
S2–Popliteal fossa in the midline
S3–Ischial tuberosity
S4–5–Perianal area (taken as one level)

In addition to bilateral testing of these key points, the external anal sphincter should be tested through insertion of the examiner's finger; perceived sensation should be graded as being present or absent (i.e., enter Yes or No on the patient's summary chart). This information is needed in determining completeness/incompleteness of injury.

Sensory Examination: Optional Elements

For purposes of SCI evaluation, the following aspects of sensory function are defined as optional (though they are strongly recommended): position sense and awareness of deep pressure/deep pain. If these are examined, it is recommended that they be graded using the sensory scale provided herein (absent, impaired, normal). It is also suggested that only one joint be tested for each extremity; the index finger and the great toe of the right and left sides are recommended.

Motor Examination: Required Elements

The required portion of the motor examination is completed through the testing of a key muscle (one on the right and one on the left side of the body) in the 10 paired myotomes. Each key muscle should be examined in a rostral-caudal sequence.

The strength of each muscle is graded on a six-point scale:

0 = total paralysis
1 = palpable or visible contraction
2 = active movement, full range of motion (ROM) with gravity eliminated
3 = active movement, full ROM against gravity
4 = active movement, full ROM against moderate resistance
5 = (normal) active movement, full ROM against full resistance
NT = not testable

The following muscles are to be examined (bilaterally) and graded using the scale defined above. These muscles were chosen because of their consistency for being innervated by the segments indicated and their ease of testing in the clinical situation, where testing in any position other than the supine position may be contraindicated.

C5–Elbow flexors (biceps brachialis)
C6–Wrist extensors (extensor carpi radialis longus and brevis)
C7–Elbow extensors (triceps)
C8–Finger flexors (flexor digitorum profundus) to the middle finger
T1–Small finger abductors (abductor digiti minimi)
L2–Hip flexors (iliopsoas)
L3–Knee extensors (quadriceps)

continues

continued

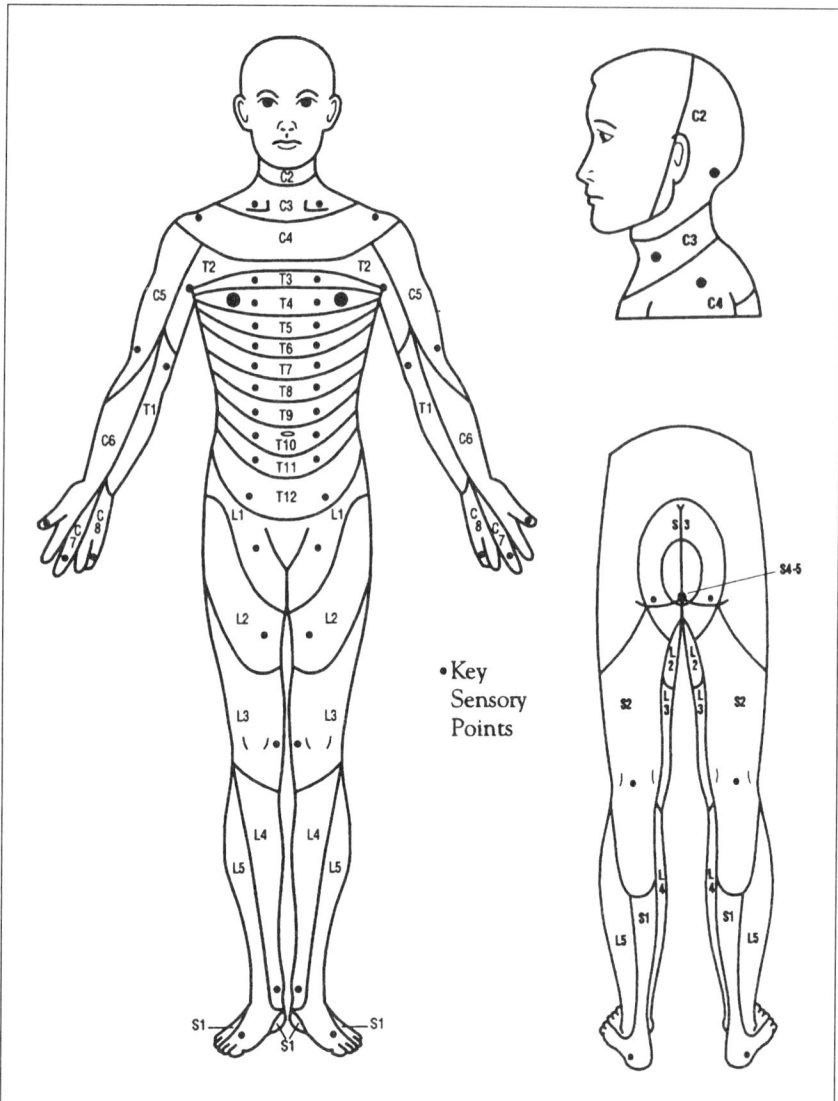

Figure 1

L4–Ankle dorsiflexors (tibialis anterior)
L5–Long toe extensors (extensor hallucis longus)
S1–Ankle plantarflexors (gastrocnemius, soleus)

In addition to bilateral testing of these muscles, the external anal sphincter should be tested on the basis of contractions around the examiner's finger and graded as being present or absent (i.e., enter Yes or No on the patient's summary sheet). This latter information is used solely for determining the completeness of injury.

Motor Examination: Optional Elements

For purposes of SCI evaluation, it is recommended that other muscles be evaluated, but their scores are not used in determining the motor score, motor level, or completeness. As warranted, it is suggested that the following muscles be tested: (1) diaphragm, (2) deltoid, and (3) lateral hamstrings. Their strength is to be rated as absent, weak, or normal.

continues

SENSORY AND MOTOR SCORES/LEVELS

Sensory Scores and Sensory Level

Required testing generates four sensory modalities *per dermatome*: R-pin prick, R-light touch, L-pin prick, L-light touch. As is indicated on the summary chart enclosed, these scores are then summed across dermatomes and sides of body to generate two summary sensory scores: Pin Prick and Light Touch Score. The sensory scores provide a means of numerically documenting changes in sensory function.

Further, through the required sensory examination the sensory components for determining neurological level (i.e., the sensory level), zone of partial preservation, and impairment grade are obtained.

Motor Scores and Motor Level

The required motor testing generates two motor grades *per paired myotome*: right and left. These scores are then summed across myotomes and sides of body to generate a single summary motor score. The motor score provides a means of numerically documenting changes in motor function.

Further, through the required motor examination, the motor components for determining neurological level (i.e., the motor level), zone of partial preservation, and impairment grade are obtained.

Motor Level Determination: Further Considerations

Just as each segmental nerve (root) innervates more than one muscle, most muscles are innervated by more than one nerve segment. Therefore, the assigning of one muscle or one muscle group (i.e., the key muscle) to represent a single spinal nerve segment is a simplification, used with the understanding that in any muscle the presence of innervation by one segment and the absence of innervation by the other segment will result in a weakened muscle.

By convention, if a muscle has at least a grade of 3, it is considered to have intact innervation by the more rostral of the innervating segments. In determining the motor level, the next most rostral key muscle must test as 4 or 5, since it is assumed that the muscle will have both of its two innervating segments intact. For example, if no activity is found in the C7 key muscle and the C6 muscle is graded as 3, then the motor level for the tested side of the body is C6, providing the C5 muscle is graded at least 4.

The examiner's judgment is relied upon to determine whether a muscle that is graded at least 4 is fully innervated. This is necessary because a number of factors may, in some patients, inhibit a full effort during clinical testing at varying times postinjury. Examples include pain, position of the patient, hypertonicity, and disuse. A grade 4 should not be considered normal if the examiner feels none of these inhibiting factors is present and the patient is exerting a full effort, yet only produces a grade 4 in that muscle.

In short, the motor level (the lowest normal motor segment, which may differ by side of body) is defined by the lowest key muscle that has a grade of at least 3, providing the key muscles represented by segments above that level are judged to be normal (4 or 5).

ASIA IMPAIRMENT SCALE (modified from Frankel)

The following scale is used in grading the degree of impairment:

A = Complete. No sensory or motor function is preserved in the sacral segments S4–S5.

B = Incomplete. Sensory but not motor function is preserved below the neurological level and extends through the sacral segments S4–S5.

C = Incomplete. Motor function is preserved below the neurological level, and the majority of key muscles below the neurological level have a muscle grade less than 3.

D = Incomplete. Motor function is preserved below the neurological level, and the majority of key muscles below the neurological level have a muscle grade greater than or equal to 3.

E = Normal. Sensory and motor function is normal.

FUNCTIONAL INDEPENDENCE MEASURE

To fully describe the impact of SCI on the individual and to monitor/evaluate progress associated with treatment, a standard measure of daily-life activities is necessary. The functional independence measure (FIM) is one approach to functional assessment that has become widely used in the United States and is gaining acceptance internationally.

The FIM focuses on six areas of functioning: self-care, sphincter control, mobility, locomotion, communication, and social cognition. Within each area, two or more specific activities/items are evaluated, with a total of 18 items. For example, six activity items (eating, grooming, bathing, dressing-upper body, dressing-lower body, and toileting) constitute the self-care area.

Each of the 18 items is evaluated in terms of independence of functioning, using a seven-point scale:

Independent (no human assistance is required):

7 = Complete independence: The activity is typically performed safely, without modification, assistive devices or aids, and within reasonable time.

6 = Modified independence: The activity requires an assistive device and/or more than reasonable time and/or is not performed safely.

Dependent (human supervision or physical assistance is required):

continues

continued

> 5 = Supervision or setup: No physical assistance is needed, but cuing, coaxing, or setup is required.
> 4 = Minimal contact assistance: Subject requires no more than touching and expends 75 percent or more of the effort required in the activity.
> 3 = Moderate assistance: Subject requires more than touching and expends 50 percent to 75 percent of the effort required in the activity.
> 2 = Maximal assistance: Subject expends 25 percent to 50 percent of the effort required in the activity.
> 1 = Total assistance: Subject expends 0 percent to 25 percent of the effort required in the activity.
>
> Thus, the FIM total score (summed across all items) estimates the cost of disability in terms of safety issues and of dependence on others and on technological devices. The profile of area scores and item scores pinpoints the specific aspects of daily living that have been most affected by SCI.
>
> In using the FIM with individuals who have experienced SCI, it should be kept in mind that the FIM was developed for the disabled population in general. It samples those areas of activity that have been found to be affected by impairment among diverse disability groups. Although basic issues of reliability and validity of the FIM have been explored by the developers, its validity as an instrument for precisely gauging changed functioning with all SCI subpopulations has yet to be demonstrated empirically. For example, it is not yet clear that the self-care items sensitively gauge changes in self-care functioning experienced by persons with tetraplegia during the course of rehabilitation. Further, the reliability estimates for the communication and social cognition areas have been found to be lower than for other areas assessed. Despite these caveats, the use of the FIM is recommended, as it is relatively simple to use, reflects functional issues of importance to SCI, and guidelines for its use have been carefully developed.
>
> Source: The American Spinal Injury Association, International Medical Society of Paraplegia. Supported by the American Paraplegia Association.

Notes:

Exhibit
STANDARD NEUROLOGICAL CLASSIFICATION OF SPINAL CORD INJURY

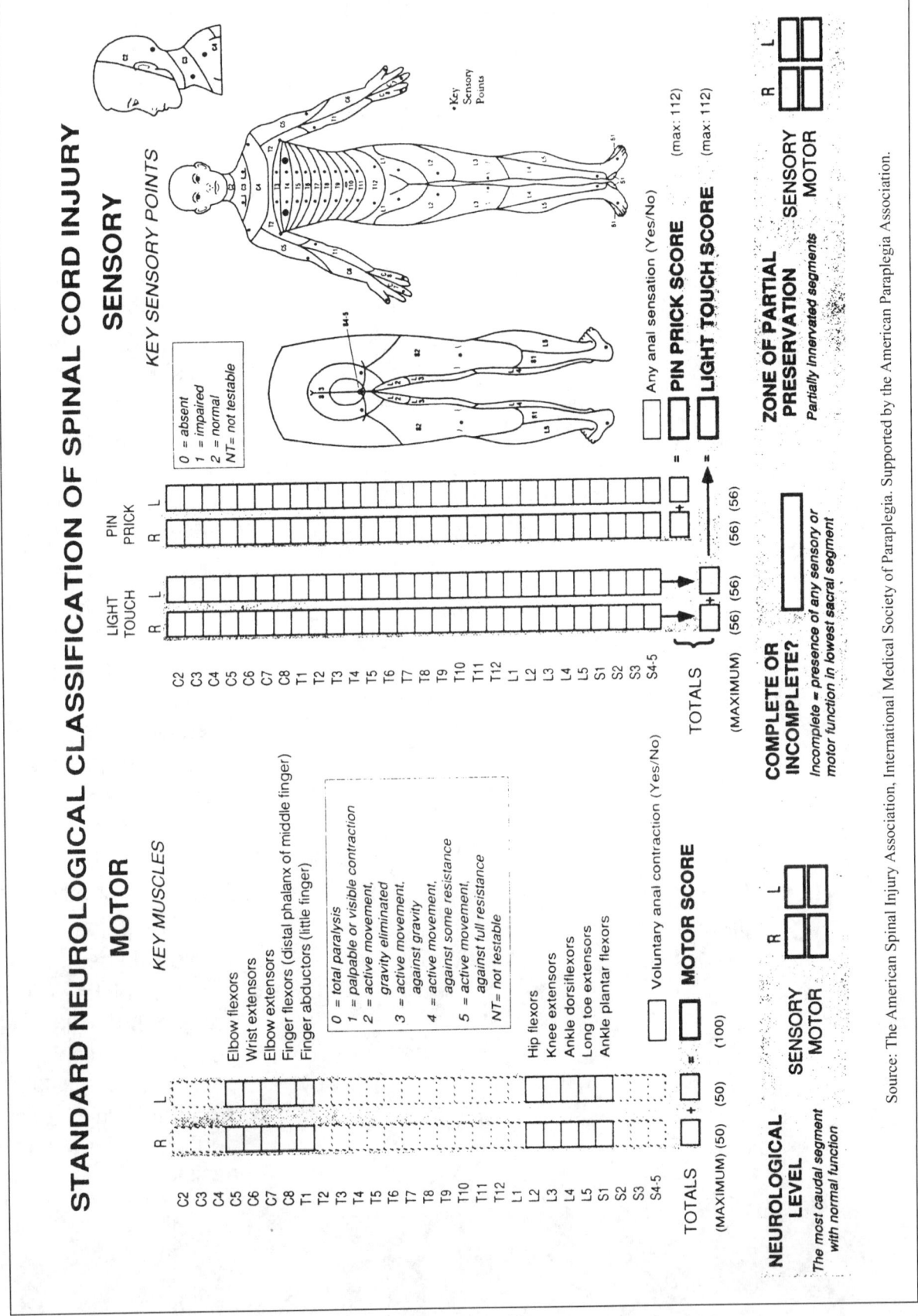

Source: The American Spinal Injury Association, International Medical Society of Paraplegia. Supported by the American Paraplegia Association.

Spinal Cord Injury/Functional Chart

Use this chart as a general guideline, keeping in mind that everyone is unique. Goals should be set based on the person's own unique abilities and recovery.

Spinal Cord Level/ Spinal Nerve	Spinal Nerve Connected to Muscle	What Can the Muscles Do?	Possible Goals
C3 to C4	1. Neck (*sternocleid-mastoid*) 2. Shoulder (trapezius) 3. Diaphragm	1. Fair neck control 2. Shrug shoulders	1. Control electric wheelchair with sip and puff (mouth) or chin control 2. Type with adaptive equipment
C5	*Has above plus:* 1. Shoulder (deltoid) 2. Arm (biceps) 3. Forearm	1. Good neck control 2. Fair to good shoulder control 3. Arm bends at elbow 4. Forearm rotates up	1. Dress upper body (time consuming) 2. Feed self with equipment 3. Comb hair, brush teeth, wash face 4. Turn self in bed with arm slings 5. Push wheelchair with handrim projections 6. Operate electric wheelchair
C6	*Has above plus:* 1. Wrist 2. Forearm (all) 3. Some chest	1. Good shoulder control 2. Bend wrist up 3. Turn hand down 4. Weak trunk	1. Dress upper body 2. Dress lower body (time consuming) 3. Turn self in bed 4. Push wheelchair with handrim projections 5. Feed self with splints (hand or tenodesis splints) 6. Transfer from wheelchair to bed, car, toilet with little or no assistance

continues

continued

Spinal Cord Level/ Spinal Nerve	Spinal Nerve Connected to Muscle	What Can the Muscles Do?	Possible Goals
			7. Able to do bowel/bladder program with adaptive equipment
			8. May be able to drive
C7	*Has above plus*: 1. All arm (*triceps*) 2. More chest 3. Some finger	1. Good arm control 2. Some hand function 3. Better chest control	1. Independent in transfer to bed, car, and toilet 2. Independent in dressing 3. Propel wheelchair without handrim projections 4. Independent with feeding 5. Independent with bathing and other self-care activities 6. Able to drive
C8 to T4	*Has above plus*: 1. Hand 2. Some chest 3. All arm 4. Some trunk/back	1. T1: All arm and hand 2. Better trunk control	1. Independent in all transfers, including floor 2. Push wheelchair without handrim projections 3. Push wheelchair up and down curb 4. Independent with homemaking activities 5. Independent with bowel/bladder program
T5 to T12	*Has above plus*: 1. All chest 2. All breathing (*intercostals*)	1. All upper body 2. Fair to good trunk control	1. Independent with wheelchair 2. Able to do all of above easier 3. T12: Walk with walker and long leg braces (difficult)
L1 to L5	*Has above plus*:	1. Bend hips	1. Independent in all activities

continues

continued

Spinal Cord Level/ Spinal Nerve	Spinal Nerve Connected to Muscle	What Can the Muscles Do?	Possible Goals
	1. All lower back 2. Some leg (*quadriceps*)	2. Straighten knees	2. Walking with short leg braces and crutches (easier) 3. Independent with bowel and bladder program
S1 to S5	*Has above plus*: 1. All knee 2. All ankle 3. Bowel 4. Bladder	1. Straighten hip 2. Bend knee 3. Good ankle control 4. Point toe	1. Able to walk if able to push off ground (may need adaptive equipment) 2. Independent in all activities Bowel/bladder and sexual functioning may still be impaired.

Source: Kelly B. Wascher, ed., *Patient Education and Discharge Planning Manual for Rehabilitation*, St. Joseph Rehabilitation Hospital and Outpatient Center, Aspen Publishers, Inc., © 1995.

REHABILITATION

Selecting a Rehabilitation Center for Spinal Cord Injury

The following guidelines may be helpful in evaluating rehabilitation facilities for the treatment of a new spinal cord injury (SCI). Whenever possible, it is advisable to visit any center that you are considering and ask to see the program in action.

Accreditation

Is the center CARF accredited for SCI? The Commission on Accreditation of Rehabilitation Facilities (CARF) offers several types of accreditation, so it is important to be specific. Accreditation for general rehabilitation (or other non-SCI programs) is good, but does not indicate any special expertise in the care of SCI. A center that is accredited for spinal cord injury has met a series of standards that are considered important in the care of patients with SCI.

The CARF requirements for SCI are listed below. If a center is not accredited, it may be helpful to ask which of these services are available.

How Many Patients with SCI Are Treated?

CARF recommends a minimum of 30 new SCI admissions per year to maintain a viable SCI program.

Provision for Peer Interaction of Patients

How many patients with SCI are currently in the hospital? Patients need to interact with the medical staff, but they also benefit from interaction with other patients with SCI. Is there a designated area (beds) within the nursing unit where these patients are assigned?

Specialized SCI Rehabilitation Team

The rehabilitation team should have training and experience in the unique needs of patients with SCI and should consist of at least a rehabilitation nurse, physical therapist, occupational therapist, social worker, physician, respiratory therapist, and recreational therapist. Each of these should have special training or experience with SCI because it is significantly different from other disabilities.

Attending Physician

Does the physician who will be in charge of the rehabilitation program have special interest and competence in the care of SCI? Is there 24-hour physician coverage seven days per week?

Bladder Management

Is there an organized program for urological examination (including urodynamics) and bladder management? Is it under the direction of a urologist (or other qualified physician) with special interest and competence in the care of SCI?

Equipment

Is there access to a supply of specialized wheelchairs, cushions, and other equipment

continues

continued

that can be used for trial until individual needs can be determined?

Patient and Family Education

Is there a formally organized program (with mandatory attendance) for education of the patient and family about the unique medical problems of SCI, including:

- bladder management and prevention of complications
- bowel management
- skin care and prevention of pressure sores
- autonomic dysreflexia
- sexuality and fertility
- instruction in medications and drug abuse
- nutrition
- equipment care and community resources for availability and repair

Sexual Counseling

Since most patients with SCI are young adults and SCI has a significant effect on sexual function, accurate information is essential.

Medical Consultation

Are specialists available for consultation (if needed) in specialties such as neurosurgery, orthopaedics, urology, plastic surgery, internal medicine, pulmonary medicine, general surgery, and pediatrics?

Acute Care Hospital

Is there immediate access and safe transport to acute hospital services in the event of medical emergencies?

Community Integration Services

Is there an organized program to help patients adapt to activities outside the hospital? This includes supervised community excursions and provisions for overnight therapeutic home visits prior to discharge (as appropriate).

Other Services

The following services should be provided by the rehabilitation center staff or through consultation arrangements:

- psychological evaluation and counseling
- vocational counseling
- driver's training
- special education for school-age children
- orthotics (braces and splints)

Follow-Up

Is there an organized program for long-term follow-up to maintain and/or improve health status after discharge? The SCI program should provide follow-up care for patients remaining in the geographic service area. A specific written plan should be provided for each patient on discharge.

Courtesy of Shirley McCluer, MD, Medical Director, Arkansas Spinal Cord Commission, Little Rock, Arkansas, March 1993.

The Members of the Rehabilitation Team

The Physiatrist. A medical doctor who specializes in physical medicine and rehabilitation whose primary responsibility is for the medical care of the patient. He or she initiates the rehab program and coordinates the work of the professional health care team by directing therapy services and ordering medication, braces, wheelchair, etc.

Physical Therapist (PT). The physical therapist is concerned with teaching patients to do as much for themselves as possible. This involves evaluating patients' needs and then initiating exercises to increase muscle strength and joint movement. Patients are taught bed mobility, transfers, and how to operate a wheelchair. If the injury allows, the physical therapist may also teach patients to walk again, using whatever equipment is necessary.

Occupational Therapist (OT). The occupational therapist, through evaluation and treatment, provides patients with an opportunity to reach their maximum level of physical and psychosocial function so that they can live independently. Occupational therapists teach patients how to perform activities of daily living (ADLs) such as dressing, bathing, feeding, personal hygiene, and other activities. Exercise programs are developed to improve muscle strength and endurance of the upper extremities and trunk musculature. The OT may conduct evaluations to help the family make the home physically more accessible as part of this program.

Speech and Language Pathologist (SP). The speech pathologist evaluates patients for communication problems and initiates therapy as needed. Patients may indicate or demonstrate difficulty expressing what they want and need. Muscle weakness may have resulted in some slurred speech. The speech pathologist works with patients to improve their communication skills. Patients with tetraplegia may need assistive communication devices and items that assist in tasks such as turning lights on and off, operating a television, etc.

Psychologist. The psychologist evaluates intellect, personality functions, and emotional adjustment, as needed. Each new patient is screened to determine special needs. Factors important in understanding each patient may include cognitive processes, such as thinking, perception, and memory; the experience and expression of emotions; and methods of coping. The psychologist works very closely with the other members of the team to develop a plan of care and is involved in counseling for the patient and the family.

Recreational Therapist. Through involvement and participation in therapeutic recreational programs, the patient will become more socially involved with others, develop and use physical and intellectual abilities, learn new skills, and/or modify old ones. Programs and outings are provided, such as bowling and swimming. Taking time to play is an important part of good mental health.

Respiratory Therapist (RT). A respiratory therapist is available to assess the breathing status of patients. Treatment is provided by the respiratory staff as deemed necessary by the physician.

continues

continued

Respiratory therapists provide the family and the patient with education regarding patients' respiratory needs.

Social Worker. The social worker is a patient and family advocate to ensure family input into the patient's treatment program, and also keeps the family informed of the patient's progress and sets up family conferences and teaching sessions. The social worker also provides educational material concerning the individual's disability and provides supportive counseling as needed. The social worker assists the patient and family in their discharge planning by making appropriate community referrals and helping to obtain special equipment. Assistance in understanding financial resources, community services, and follow-up issues will also be provided by the social worker. Vocational referrals and sexual counseling are also available through the social worker.

Rehabilitation Nurse. The rehabilitation nurse, along with other team members, provides 24-hour care to persons with spinal cord injury. The nurse will see that the doctor's orders are carried out. A record is kept to keep the physician informed of all phases of the patient's care and treatment. The rehabilitation nurse works with the patient on self-care, including bowel/bladder programs and maintenance of healthy skin.

Dietitian. The dietitian plays an integral role in the care of the patient with spinal cord injury. A thorough nutritional assessment is conducted upon admission to determine each patient's unique needs. Common to many patients with spinal cord injury is the potential for rapid weight gain or loss and skin breakdown. Overall, the dietitian monitors each patient's nutritional status, ensures that the patient's nutritional needs are met, and assists patients and families in choosing a healthy lifetime diet. The dietitian also monitors the patient's medications for any food-drug interactions.

Case Manager. A case manager may be assigned to each patient on admission. He or she provides clinical coordination for all services provided to the patient. The case manager also acts as a liaison between the professional team, the patient and family, and third-party insurers.

Courtesy of HealthSouth Corporation, Birmingham, Alabama.

2
Circulatory System

> Most materials in the *Spinal Cord Injury Patient Education Resource Manual* are intended for the health care professional to share with the patient. Materials that are intended solely for the professional are labeled "Exhibit" in the table of contents.

General Information

Arteries and Veins of the Body	29
How Does Circulation Work?	30
Keeping the Circulatory System Healthy	31
When Something Goes Wrong	32

Complications

Postural Hypotension	33
Edema	34
Deep Vein Thrombosis (DVT)	36
Pulmonary Embolism	39
Temperature Regulation	40

GENERAL INFORMATION

Arteries and Veins of the Body

A vast web of blood vessels supplies all areas of the body with blood. The arteries (shown as solid black in illustration) carry fresh, oxygen-rich blood. The veins (shown as gray) carry used, oxygen-poor blood. The pumping heart keeps the blood moving through the vessels. Blood in the heart can travel to the big toe and back in less than 60 seconds.

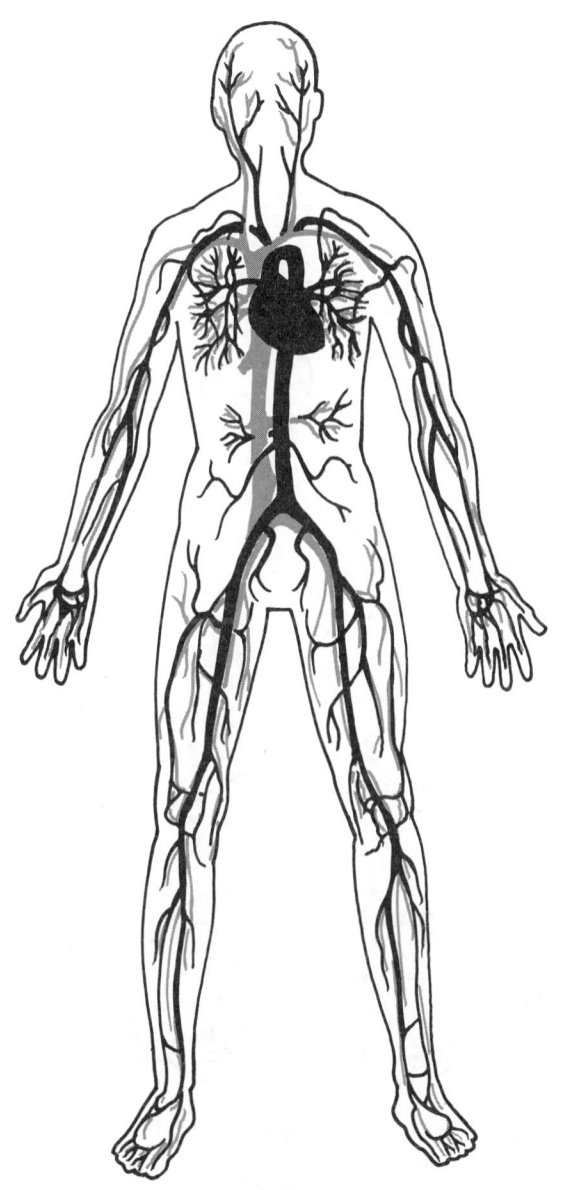

Source: Office of Information, National Heart, Lung, and Blood Institute, DHEW Publication No. (NIH) 78-1058.

How Does Circulation Work?

Blood circulation is like a circle. It is continuous:
1. The heart pumps blood with oxygen through arteries.
2. The body gets the blood.
3. Through the capillaries:
   - Oxygen and nutrients go **to** cells.
   - Waste is picked up **from** cells.
4. Blood with waste goes back to the heart through veins.
5. The heart sends this blood to the lungs.
6. The lungs give oxygen to the blood.
7. The blood goes back to the heart.
8. The cycle begins again.

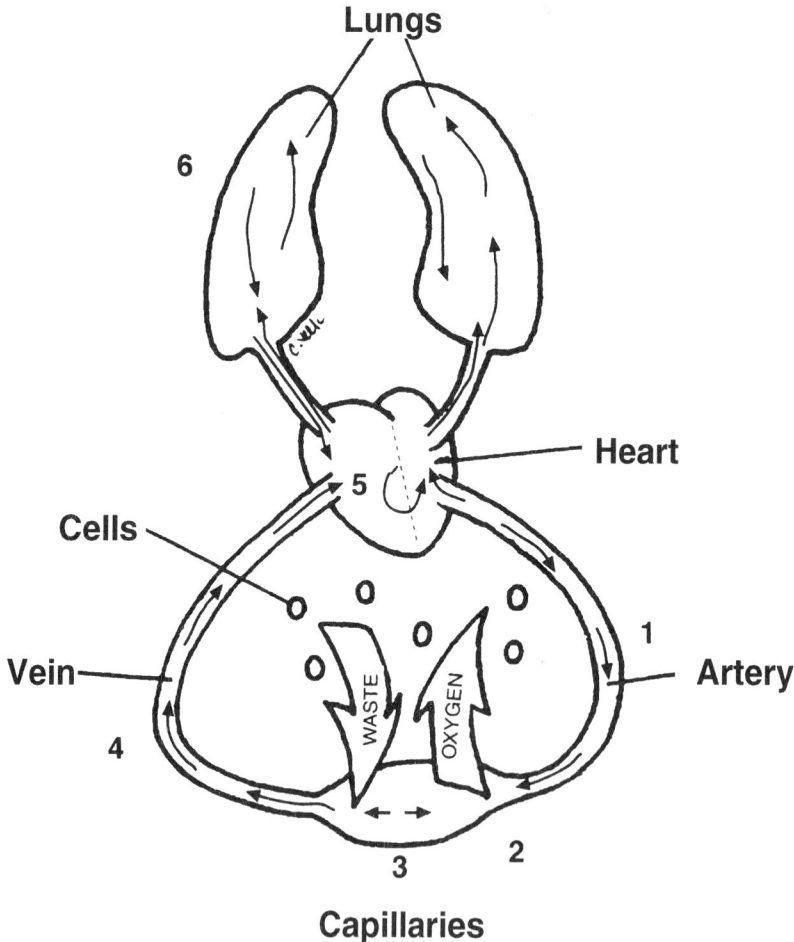

Source: Kelly B. Wascher, ed., *Patient Education and Discharge Planning Manual for Rehabilitation*, St. Joseph Rehabilitation Hospital and Outpatient Center, Aspen Publishers, Inc., © 1995.

Keeping the Circulatory System Healthy

You can do several things to help keep your blood circulating in the best way possible:

- **Diet**: Eat a well-balanced diet, and avoid the use of extra salt.

- **Exercise and Rest:** While daily range of motion exercise and self-care activities improve the circulation to paralyzed parts of the body, rest periods are equally important. When resting, try to lie down and elevate your legs. Even if you are at work, try to elevate your feet and legs when you rest. This will help the blood to return to your heart.

- **Weight Shifts:** Shifting your weight regularly promotes circulation to all skin areas, and changes of position help decrease chances of edema in your feet and ankles. Avoid leg positions that decrease or restrict circulation to your lower legs. These include crossing your legs or letting your legs dangle from a shower chair or toilet seat.

- **Breathing Exercises:** Do your breathing exercises regularly. Remember that the amount of blood the heart pumps increases with deep breathing.

- **Equipment:** Elastic support stockings (antiembolic hose) and an abdominal binder can assist blood flow back to the heart. Be sure to use them if and as directed, and be sure they fit properly.

Notes:

Source: John C. Whitaker Rehabilitation Medicine Centers of Forsyth Memorial Hospital, Winston-Salem, North Carolina.

When Something Goes Wrong

CIRCULATORY PROBLEMS[*]

Any illness or injury that results in paralysis can have an effect on the way the body's circulatory system works. The movement of blood is more difficult in the paralyzed parts.

All along the system of veins that carry blood from everywhere in the body back to the heart, there are one-way valves that keep the blood from flowing back in the wrong direction. If the skeletal muscles in the legs, for instance, are affected by paralysis, these valves in the veins do not work as well. Blood does not flow to the heart as quickly and may even accumulate, or "pool," especially in the feet and ankles.

Remember that after a spinal cord injury, the heart usually continues to function normally. Blood pressure and pulse rates, however, will be lower, because the rate at which blood is pumped through the system will be slower. The problems that develop are in the portions of the system that are away from the heart. They are known as the "peripheral" parts of the system.

WHAT CIRCULATION PROBLEMS CAN ILLNESS/INJURY CAUSE?[**]

Illness/injury can affect the body's ability to circulate blood. This may cause problems including:

- **Postural Hypotension:** Low blood pressure when changing position.
- **Edema:** Swelling of ankles, feet, and hands.
- **Deep Vein Thrombosis (DVT):** Blood clot in leg.
- **Pulmonary Embolism (PE):** Blood clot in lung.

Notes:

---

[*]Source: John C. Whitaker Rehabilitation Medicine Centers of Forsyth Memorial Hospital, Winston-Salem, North Carolina.
[**]Source: Kelly B. Wascher, ed., *Patient Education and Discharge Planning Manual for Rehabilitation*, St. Joseph Rehabilitation Hospital and Outpatient Center, Aspen Publishers, Inc., © 1995.

COMPLICATIONS

Postural Hypotension

WHAT IS POSTURAL HYPOTENSION?

Postural hypotension is a lower-than-normal drop in blood pressure when moving to a sitting or standing position. Postural hypotension happens if illness/injury has affected the circulatory (blood vessel) system.

WHAT CAUSES POSTURAL HYPOTENSION?

Postural hypotension happens when blood vessels cannot respond to position changes as before. (For example, veins and arteries cannot tighten and widen.) This may be caused by:

- Illness affecting the blood vessels
- Injury to the blood vessels
- Prolonged bed rest
- Surgery

WHAT ARE THE SIGNS OF HYPOTENSION?

When changing position (lying to sitting to standing), a person may have the following signs:

- Dizziness
- Lightheadedness
- Nausea
- Drop in blood pressure (of about 20 points)
- Drop in pulse (10–20 points)
- Fainting
- Sweating
- Cool, clammy skin

HOW IS POSTURAL HYPOTENSION PREVENTED?

- Move slowly when changing positions.
- Elevate head of bed prior to transferring to chair.
- If ordered by doctor, support the veins and arteries by wearing:
  - elastic stockings (for veins in legs)
  - abdominal binder (for arteries in stomach)

Source: Kelly B. Wascher, ed., *Patient Education and Discharge Planning Manual for Rehabilitation*, St. Joseph Rehabilitation Hospital and Outpatient Center, Aspen Publishers, Inc., 1995.

Edema

WHAT IS SWELLING?

Swelling is the collection of fluid under the skin. Fluid moves from the blood vessels into the tissues. This is called **edema**.

WHAT CAUSES SWELLING OF ANKLES, FEET, AND HANDS?

There are three major causes of swelling:

Cause	Reason
Gravity	While sitting, feet and legs dangle. Because of gravity: • Blood pools (stays) in the feet, ankles, and legs longer than normal. • Veins must work against gravity to bring the blood back to the heart. • Fluid moves into the tissue of the feet and ankles, causing swelling.
Veins	Illness/injury may affect the veins' ability to pump blood back to the heart: • Valves do not work. • Muscles around veins do not work.
Paralyzed or Weak Muscles	Muscles help veins pump blood back to the heart. If muscles are weak and/or paralyzed: • It takes longer for veins to pump the blood back to the heart. • Blood stays in legs longer. • Fluid moves into tissues, causing swelling.

HOW CAN SWELLING BE PREVENTED?

- **Do** wear support stockings (if prescribed).
- **Do** prop legs and feet on a chair when sitting. Be careful not to cause a blockage behind the knee.
- **Do** prop hands on pillow when sitting.
- **FOR HANDS ONLY: Do** massage hand toward arm. (Start at fingers and rub toward wrist.)
- **Do** use muscles (exercise, walk, range of motion) often.

continues

continued

HOW IS SWELLING TREATED?

- Lie in bed.
- Put feet or hands above level of heart when lying down.
- Prop hands or feet on pillows.

Notes:

Source: Kelly B. Wascher, ed., *Patient Education and Discharge Planning Manual for Rehabilitation*, St. Joseph Rehabilitation Hospital and Outpatient Center, Aspen Publishers, Inc., © 1995.

Deep Vein Thrombosis (DVT)

WHAT IS DEEP VEIN THROMBOSIS?

Deep vein thrombosis (DVT) is a blood clot. A blood clot may develop in the deep veins of the body if the conditions are right.

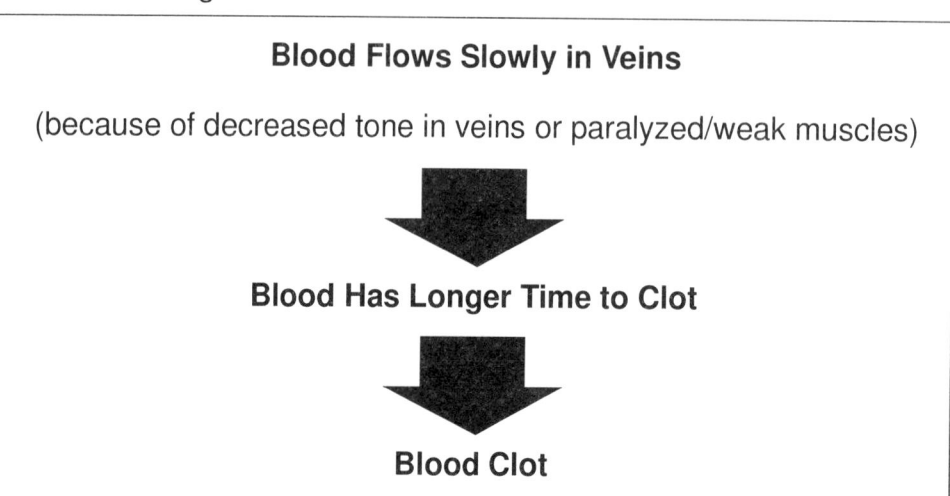

This is where a blood clot may occur:

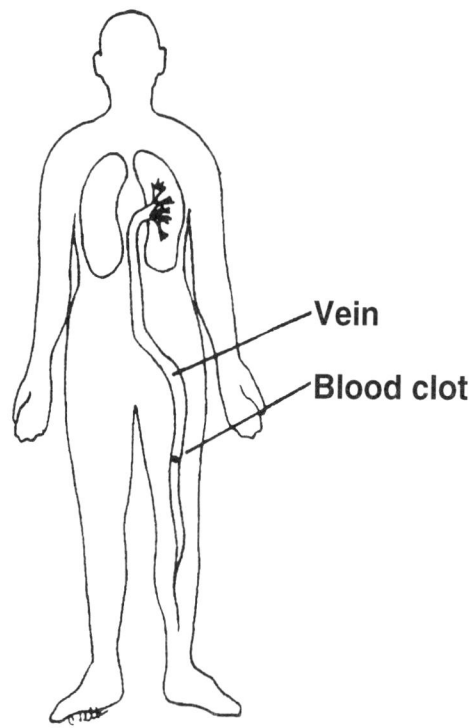

continues

continued

WHAT HAPPENS?

A deep vein thrombosis may be life threatening. The blood clot may:

1. break away from the vein
2. travel to the heart
3. travel to the lung
4. get stuck in the lung causing:
   - breathing problems
   - possible death

WHAT ARE THE RISK FACTORS FOR GETTING DVT?

- Injury
- Surgery
- History of varicose veins or thrombosis (blood clot)
- Decreased muscle tone
- Changes in activity
- Age (over age 40)
- Hormone therapy
- Heart disease
- Tumors
- Infection
- Pregnancy

WHAT ARE THE SIGNS OF A BLOOD CLOT?

- Swelling
- Warm when touched
- Redness over area of the clot
- Pain in affected leg (people with spinal cord injuries may not feel pain)
- Fever
- Increased spasticity

Note: 50 percent of all people with DVT may have NO SIGNS of a blood clot.

WHAT TO DO IF SIGNS OF DVT DEVELOP

1. **Call doctor right away.**
2. **Prop up leg/arm that has a clot.**
3. ***DO NOT* MASSAGE OR EXERCISE AFFECTED LEG.**

continues

continued

Your Doctor May Order Tests (ultrasound, venogram). Follow his or her instructions, which will depend on test results:

BLOOD CLOT PRESENT	NO BLOOD CLOT
1. Bed rest	1. Continue prevention.
2. Prop up leg/arm that has clot.	2. Watch for signs.
3. Medication (Heparin) through vein for 7–10 days.	
4. May take blood thinner medication by mouth for three months or more.	

ALWAYS FOLLOW DOCTOR'S ORDERS.

HOW CAN A DVT BE PREVENTED?

- Wear elastic stockings (Ted hose or antiembolism stockings), if prescribed.
- Practice range of motion—passive or active.
- Walk, if able.
- Change position often.
- Drink plenty of fluids.
- Take medication (such as Heparin or Coumadin), if ordered.
- Look at legs every day for signs of DVT, including:
  - Swelling
  - Redness
  - Pain
  - Any changes

Source: Kelly B. Wascher, ed., *Patient Education and Discharge Planning Manual for Rehabilitation*, St. Joseph Rehabilitation Hospital and Outpatient Center, Aspen Publishers, Inc., © 1995.

Pulmonary Embolism

Pulmonary embolism is the medical term for when a blood clot (known as a *thrombus*) plugs the arteries supplying blood to the lungs. It is a potentially life-threatening condition. A blood clot in the lung is not formed there, but comes from elsewhere in the body. About 95 percent of the time, clots that end up in the lungs develop in the large vein deep inside the muscles of the leg and pelvis.[*]

CAUSES

A clot lodges in the lung preventing oxygen/carbon dioxide exchange. Injury to a vein, blood that is prone to clot excessively, and sluggish blood flow (due to immobilization or prolonged bed rest) all contribute to the formation of a clot.

SIGNS

- Pain in the chest, which may extend to the jaw or shoulder area (if sensation is present)
- Heavy feeling in the chest
- Inability to take a deep breath
- Irritable or anxious feeling
- Fast heartbeat (pulse)
- Complexion pale or face and lips a slightly bluish color
- Red streaks in coughed-up secretions

STEPS TO TAKE

1. **THIS IS A MEDICAL EMERGENCY. CALL YOUR DOCTOR IMMEDIATELY, AND BE PREPARED TO CALL THE PARAMEDICS!**
2. Avoid massaging the legs.
3. Avoid pressure behind the legs.
4. Decrease activity level; stay in bed.
5. Sit up in bed and lean forward (over a table, if possible) to assist in breathing more easily.
6. Remove any tight clothing that may restrict breathing.
7. Use supplemental oxygen if available.

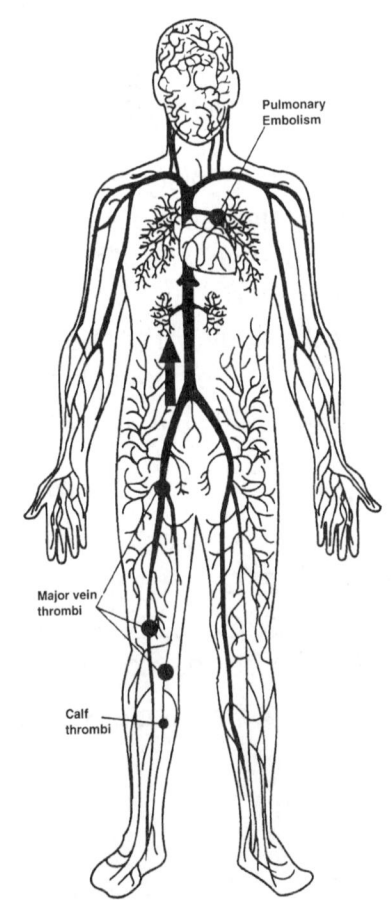

Pulmonary Embolism[*]

[*]Source: Adapted from "Pulmonary Embolism," *FDA Consumer*, U.S. Food and Drug Administration, 1989.
Source: John C. Whitaker Rehabilitation Medicine Centers of Forsyth Memorial Hospital, Winston-Salem, North Carolina.

Temperature Regulation

WHAT IS TEMPERATURE REGULATION?

The body's "thermostat" or temperature regulation center is located in the brain. The spinal cord helps send information to the brain about the outside environment, body organs, and temperature changes in the blood vessels. Temperature regulation may also be called thermoregulation.

The body controls its temperature by:

1. Sweating to cool off.
2. Changing the size of the blood vessels:
   - The blood vessels become smaller when it is cold to increase the blood flow and warm the body.
   - The blood vessels become bigger when it is warm to decrease the blood flow and cool the body.

HOW IS TEMPERATURE REGULATION AFFECTED?

After a spinal cord injury, the body temperature may not be controlled below the level of the injury. How much temperature regulation is affected will depend on the amount of damage to the spinal cord. (A person with a complete spinal cord injury will have more difficulty controlling his or her temperature.)

After injury, the body will not be able to adapt to the environment; the body cannot cool or warm itself as before. So, the body takes on the temperature of the environment. If the environment is hot, the body becomes hot. If the environment is cool, the body becomes cool.

Environment	Problem	Helpful Suggestions
COOL	1. Very cold. 2. Shivering. 3. Goose bumps above the level of spinal cord injury. 4. Skin feels cool to touch.	1. Wear warm clothing, socks, pants, gloves. 2. Use blankets to stay warm. 3. Drink warm fluids. 4. Avoid very cold temperature exposure. 5. Do not use electric blankets, heating pads, or water bottles on areas where you do not have sensation. 6. If your temperature does not change, call your doctor.

continues

continued

Environment	Problem	Helpful Suggestions
HOT	1. Sweating above the level of the spinal cord injury. 2. Overheating (headaches, dizziness, flushing of the skin, stomach sickness). 3. Skin feels warm to touch. 4. May run a fever.	1. Stay out of the sun. 2. Wear hats/shades. 3. Spray self with cool water to cool off. 4. Drink cool fluids. 5. Use a fan or air conditioner. 6. Avoid hot tubs. 7. Watch for decreased urine output.

Notes:

Source: Kelly B. Wascher, ed., *Patient Education and Discharge Planning Manual for Rehabilitation*, St. Joseph Rehabilitation Hospital and Outpatient Center, Aspen Publishers, Inc., © 1995.

3
Respiratory System

> Most materials in the *Spinal Cord Injury Patient Education Manual* are intended for the health care professional to share with the patient. Materials that are intended solely for the professional are labeled "Exhibit" in the table of contents.

General Information

Diagrams of the Lungs	45
How Does Respiration Work?	47
Respiratory Complications	49

Maintaining Respiratory Health

Six Things You Can Do to Take Care of Your Breathing System	51
Chest Physical Therapy	52
Clapping	54
Positions for Postural Drainage	56
Breathing Exercises	58

Smoking and Spinal Cord Injury

Facts about Smoking and Spinal Cord Injury	60

Ventilators

Ventilatory Dysfunction in Spinal Cord Injury (Exhibit)	61
Types of Ventilator Support (Exhibit)	61
Ventilator Weaning and Interventions to Improve Ventilatory Function (Exhibit)	63

GENERAL INFORMATION

Diagrams of the Lungs

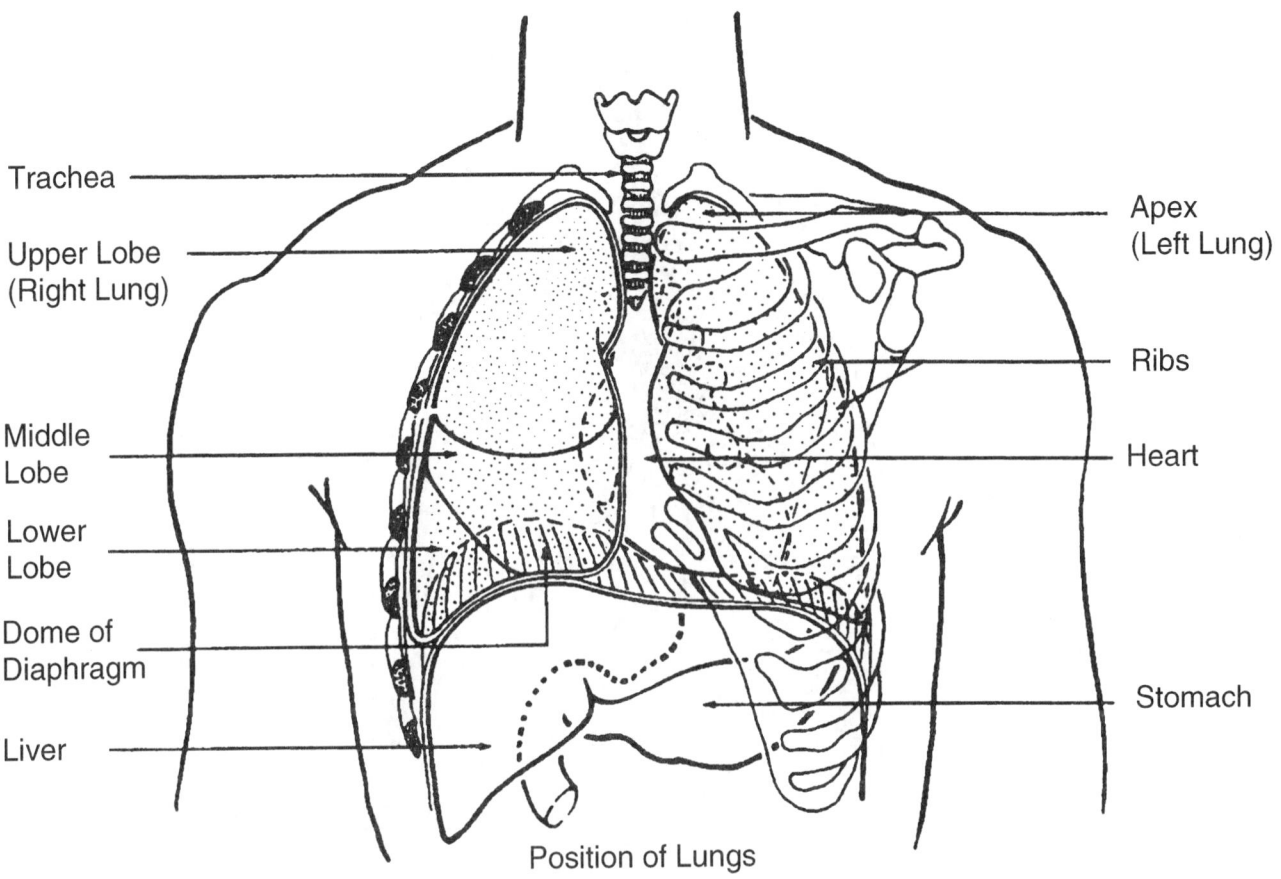

Position of Lungs

continues

continued

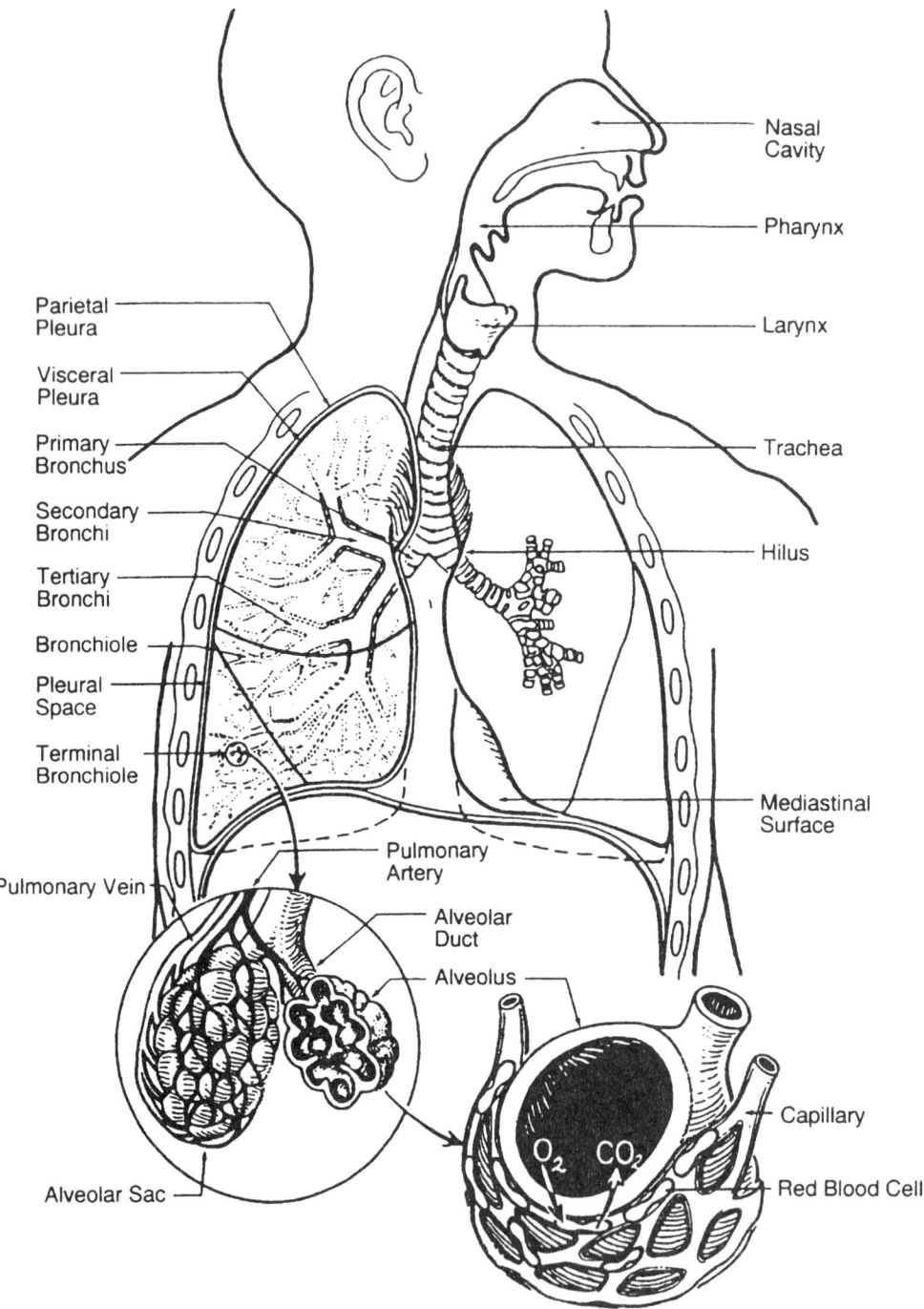

Source: *Cancer of the Lung: Research Report*, U.S. Department of Health and Human Services, Public Health Service, National Institutes of Health, National Cancer Institute, 1989.

How Does Respiration Work?

There is no better example of how one body system is related to and depends on another one than the circulatory and the respiratory systems. It is important that your blood receive oxygen (nourishment) and have carbon dioxide (waste) removed. It is through the respiratory (breathing) system that the oxygen gets into the body in the first place, and it is in areas of this system that the oxygen/carbon dioxide exchange takes place.

RESPIRATORY EQUIPMENT

Your breathing system starts with your nose and your mouth, through which air enters your body from the outside. The air passes next through the air passage in your neck called the "trachea." In your chest, the trachea divides into two parts, called "bronchi," that lead into your two lungs, which are spongy, cone-shaped organs that have a rich blood supply. At the end of each of the bronchi, there are many small air passageways, called "bronchioles," that end in 300 million tiny air sacs, called "alveoli." In these alveoli, the oxygen/carbon dioxide exchange takes place.

THE BREATHING "OPERATORS"

While your circulatory system has the powerful heart muscle to activate it, the respiratory system depends on four different groups of muscles to make it operate:

1. **Neck muscles:** Muscles in the neck, called "accessory muscles," help to expand the upper chest when you take in a breath.
2. **Diaphragm:** The diaphragm is a strong, dome-shaped involuntary muscle that is located across and just above your abdominal cavity. It is the main muscle for inhaling and exhaling air.
3. **Intercostal muscles:** These muscles are located between the ribs and help in moving the chest in and out when you breathe or cough.
4. **Abdominal muscles:** Muscles located in the abdomen are used for deep breathing and coughing.

All the muscles that operate your respiratory system are supplied with nerves ("innervated") through your spinal cord.

BREATHING

Now that we have looked at the parts of the respiratory system, let's see how they all work together in the process of breathing, which simply means the movement of air in and out of the lungs.

continues

continued

When we take air in, it is called "inhalation" or "inspiration." Air enters the nose and mouth, where it is filtered and cleaned, warmed, and moisturized (humidified). As the inhaled air moves down the trachea and into the lungs, the lungs stretch. The diaphragm flattens, and the rib cage inside the chest expands. In the millions of little air sacs (alveoli), the oxygen/carbon dioxide exchange takes place. In this exchange, oxygen leaves the inhaled air and passes into the capillary blood supply. At the same time, carbon dioxide leaves the capillaries and passes into the alveoli.

When air is expelled from the lungs, it is called "exhaling" or "expiration." During this part of the breathing process, the intercostal muscles between the ribs relax, the rib cage moves down and the big diaphragm muscle comes back up to its dome-like shape. Because of all this activity, the resulting pressure changes in the chest, and the air containing the carbon dioxide is pushed up the trachea and out through the nose and throat.

In addition to inhaling and exhaling, the respiratory system is capable of contractions such as coughing and sneezing. The contractions help to keep the system healthy and the passageways clean. When you cough or sneeze, your intercostal and abdominal muscles, as well as your diaphragm, contract strongly, increasing the pressure in your lungs. This forces air and any irritating matter up and out of your body through your nose and mouth. The most common irritants that cause the contractions are thickened mucous secretions. Some mucus in the respiratory system is normal, but every effort should be made to keep it thin enough to be coughed up easily.

SPINAL CORD INJURY AND BREATHING

Remember that the nerves that control the breathing muscles come from the brain through the spinal cord. For this reason, any illness or injury involving those areas of the spine will affect the respiratory system, so the amount of air inhaled and exhaled will be less.

An injury to the spine in the neck or cervical area will result in partial or total loss of respiratory muscles. For example, if the injury is in the C1 to C5 area, not only could the neck muscles be affected, but the functioning of the diaphragm and the intercostal area may be affected temporarily or permanently. If that were to occur, a breathing machine, called a "ventilator," could be required.

If an injury occurs in the thoracic area of the spine (T1 to T12), the result could be the loss of some of the intercostal as well as abdominal muscles. If the loss were to be complete, the diaphragm and neck muscles would be the only ones left to accomplish the breathing process.

Injury to the cord below the T12 level has no effect on the respiratory system or the cough reflex, which is the reflex action center that triggers coughing.

Source: John C. Whitaker Rehabilitation Medicine Centers of Forsyth Memorial Hospital, Winston-Salem, North Carolina.

Respiratory Complications

There are potential problems from spinal cord injury that may occur in the respiratory system.

DECREASED LUNG VOLUMES

Causes

- Change in the function of the respiratory muscles.
- Thickened mucous secretions in the lungs.

Signs

- Shortness of breath.

Steps to Take or How to Prevent

- Do deep breathing exercises daily.
- Wear an abdominal binder if necessary.
- Sit in wheelchair daily.
- Maintain regular turning schedule in bed.
- Perform the manual cough procedure as needed to bring up secretions.
- Do respiratory treatments as ordered by the doctor.

CONGESTION AND/OR PNEUMONIA

Cause

- Thickened secretions in the lungs that are not being coughed up and out.

Signs

- Shortness of breath.
- Excess secretions in the lungs.
- Heavy feeling in the chest.
- Elevated temperature (above normal).
- Irritable and/or anxious feeling.
- Pale complexion.

Steps to Take

- Do manual cough as needed to bring up secretions.
- Do respiratory treatments as ordered by your doctor.

continues

continued

- Contact your doctor if secretions are yellow-green and/or you have a temperature, have shortness of breath, and are unable to bring up secretions adequately.
- Maintain regular turning schedule.
- Do deep breathing exercises as prescribed.

How to Prevent

- Drink two to three quarts of fluid daily.
- Do daily deep breathing exercises.
- Sit in wheelchair daily.
- Maintain regular turning schedule in bed.

Notes:

Source: John C. Whitaker Rehabilitation Medicine Centers of Forsyth Memorial Hospital, Winston-Salem, North Carolina.

MAINTAINING RESPIRATORY HEALTH

Six Things You Can Do to Take Care of Your Breathing System

1. **Fluid Intake.** Fluids help keep the linings of the respiratory system moist and prevent secretions from becoming thick. You should drink at least three quarts of fluid daily, but your nurse and doctor will have to coordinate the exact amount with the bladder program that is designed for you. The color of your urine is an indicator of an adequate fluid intake. Urine should be pale yellow or the color of straw.
2. **Breathing Exercises.** You should practice deep breathing three or four times each day, and you should establish a routine of doing it at the same time each day.
3. **Mobility** (movement). You should move as much as you possibly can. Activity helps to keep respiratory secretions thin and moving freely. An active lifestyle will also prevent secretions from collecting in one place in the lungs.
4. **Humidity** (moisture). Breathing in moist rather than dry air helps to prevent the drying of secretions in the respiratory system. If the air is particularly dry where you are, you may find it helpful to use a cool mist vaporizer.
5. **General Health.** If you set habits of sleep, rest, exercise, and a well-balanced diet, you will help not only the respiratory system but all of the body's systems to function as well as they can.
6. **Coughing.** Coughing assists in clearing thickened mucous secretions from the respiratory system. Be sure that you study, understand, and use the manual cough procedure if appropriate.

Notes:

Source: John C. Whitaker Rehabilitation Medicine Centers of Forsyth Memorial Hospital, Winston-Salem, North Carolina.

Chest Physical Therapy

PURPOSE

The purpose of chest physical therapy is to aid in moving secretions toward the trachea from the lungs by the aid of gravity. It is used whenever you have a chest cold, or if you cannot cough up secretions. It means placing the body in various positions to increase the drainage of all segments of the lungs.

TECHNIQUES

Percussion or vibration procedures can be used to increase postural drainage.

- *Percussion* (or clapping) is performed by cupping the hands and clapping over the rib cage. A firmly held cup is formed with each hand and will make a hollow sound when the cup hits the chest. Alternate one hand at a time. (It should sound like the sound effects of a running horse.) A towel should be placed over the area to prevent bruising. Percussion should not hurt the person.
- *Vibration* is done when the person performing the chest physical therapy tenses his or her hands, arms, and shoulders and places the hands in contact with the back for the vibratory effect. Use this method for loosening up mucous plugs. It should be done ONLY during the exhalation phase of breathing.
- *Cupping and vibration should only be done over the rib cage, NEVER on the sternum (breast bone), spinal column, stomach, or kidneys.*
- Before drainage begins, tight clothing must be removed.
- Coughing should be encouraged, particularly before each body repositioning.
- Clap (percussion) approximately 1 (one) minute—vibrate during 5 (five) exhalations—cough—repeat.
- The drainage process should last for at least 15 minutes.
- All drainage procedures must be done prior to or at least one hour after meals. Drainage may start the gag reflex and cause vomiting.
- Drainage should be done a minimum of two times daily.
- A lumberyard can make a pair of wooden blocks of specified height with saucer-like tops in which the legs at the foot of the bed can be set to prevent slipping.

Quad Coughing

Due to the paralysis of breathing muscles in people with tetraplegia and high-level paraplegia, the ability to cough may be reduced. Without an effective voluntary cough, secretions in the lungs may develop and result in further respiratory problems. To help clear these secretions, a family

continues

continued

member or friend can manually assist coughing. This is called "quad coughing" (also known as "manual" or "assistive coughing").

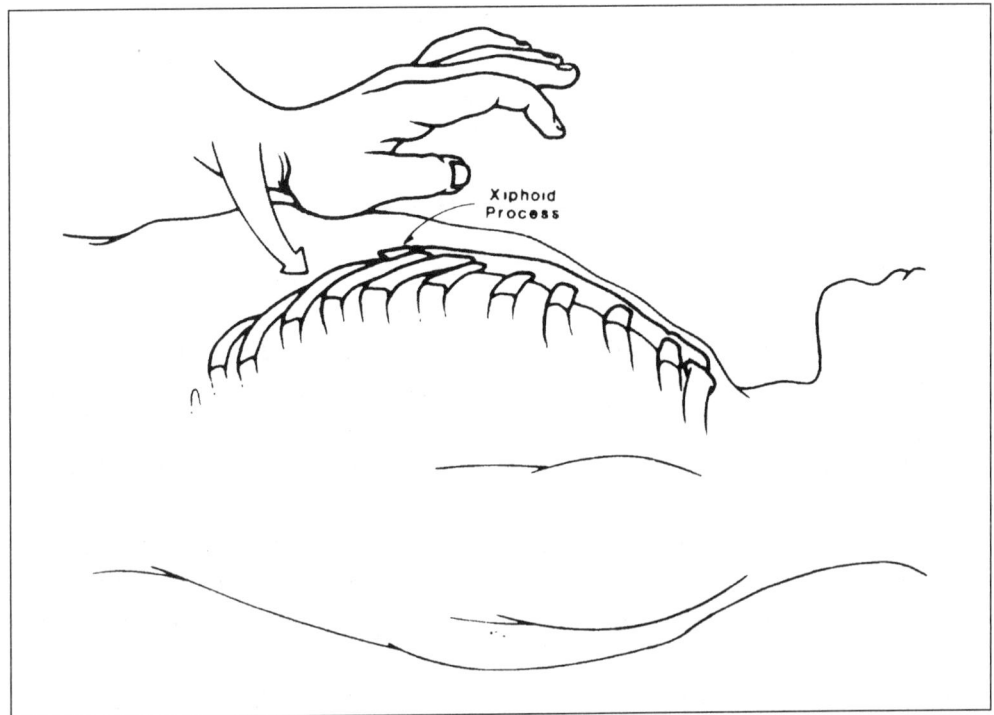

Hand Cupped over Xiphoid Process

The technique used when a person is lying on his or her back is to place the heel of one hand on the stomach at a point between the lower breastbone and the navel (known as the xiphoid process). Then place the second hand over the first. The assistant should press his or her hands into the stomach with a quick upward thrust at the same time the person tries to cough. Repeat this sequence until secretions are cleared.

Source: Virginia Spinal Cord Injury System, University of Virginia Medical Center and Virginia Department of Rehabilitative Services, *Virginia Spinal Cord Injury Care and Teaching Manual*, Fisherville, Virginia, © 1980, rev. 1985, 1988.

CLAPPING

After assuming one of the positions described, you and your assistant will need to clap your specific chest areas. This is often done along with the postural drainage to help loosen thick mucus. You cup your hand shaped as if you were drinking water from it.

Clap three to five minutes in each postural drainage position over the upper and lower

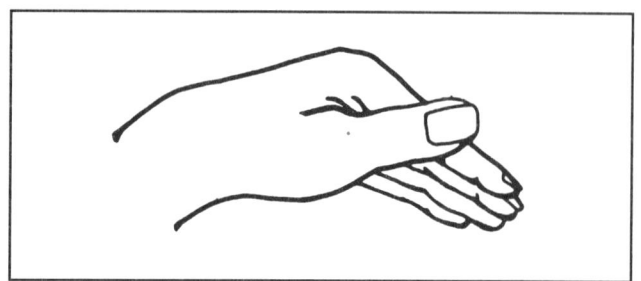

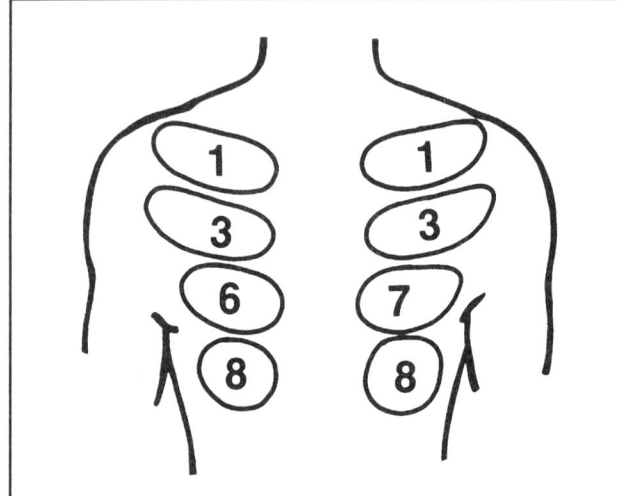

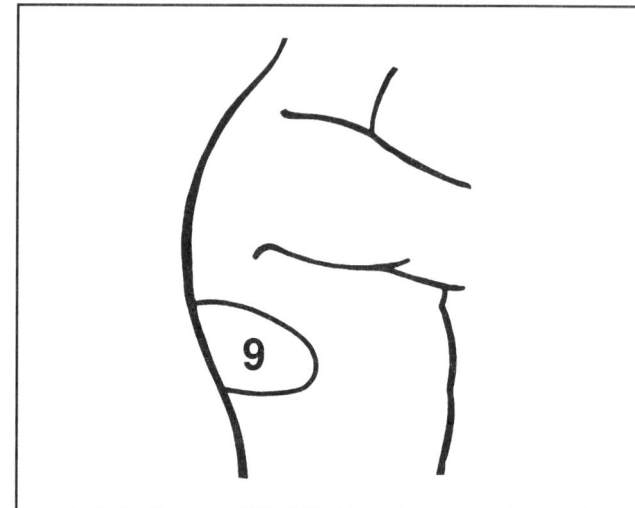

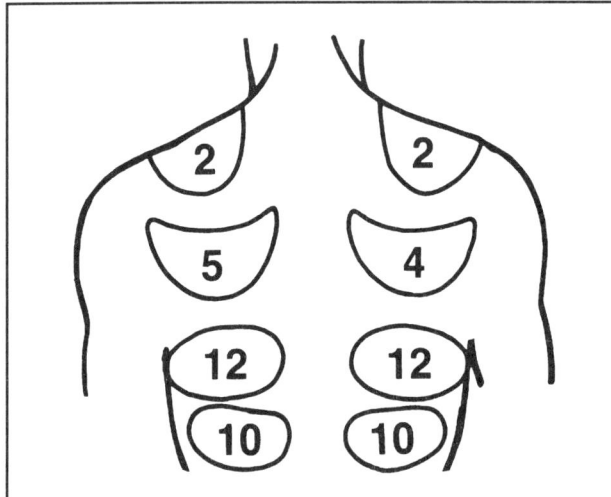

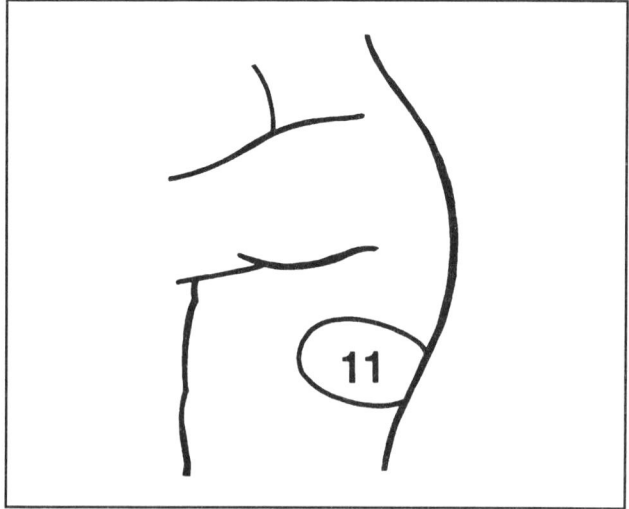

continues

continued

lobes. To prevent soreness when clapping, use a thin towel on the chest.

You should NOT clap over the following areas:

- back bone
- breast
- below the ribs

It will not be effective to clap over your shoulder blades or breast bone.

Note: Postural drainage and clapping is probably most effective if done in the morning. Do not do drainage (and clapping) right before or right after mealtime. Your stomach may be full and you do not want to get an upset stomach.

Notes:

Source: Kim Blake and Trish Fetters, Division of Nursing Services, University of Missouri-Columbia Hospital & Clinics, Howard A. Rusk Rehabilitation Center, Columbia, Missouri, © 1988. Printed with permission of the curators of the University of Missouri.

Positions for Postural Drainage

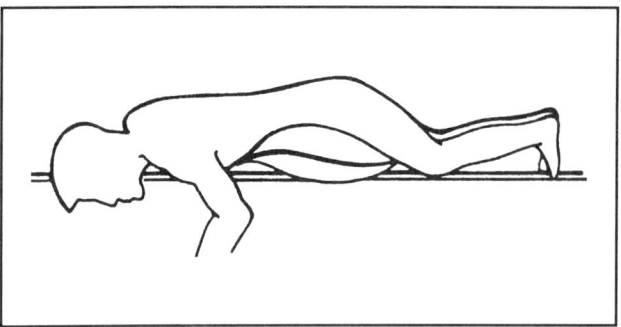

Position 1—Have someone assist you to lie on your stomach, head down. Have pillows placed under your hips, elevating them 18 to 20 inches. This position will drain the lower back portion of your lungs.

Position 2—Have someone assist you to lie on your (right/left) side, head down. Have pillows placed under your hips, elevating them 18 to 20 inches. This position will drain the lower portions of your lungs.

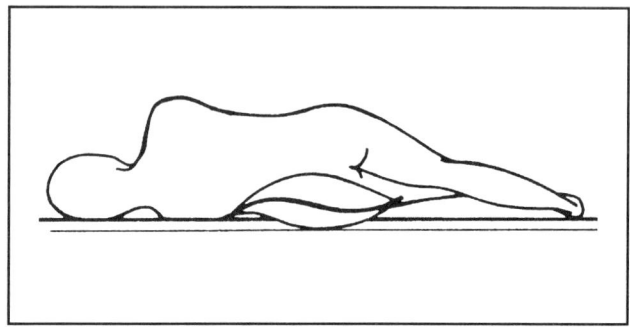

Position 3—Have someone assist you to lie on your back, face up. Have pillows placed under your hips, elevating them 18 to 20 inches. This position will drain the front lower portions of your lungs.

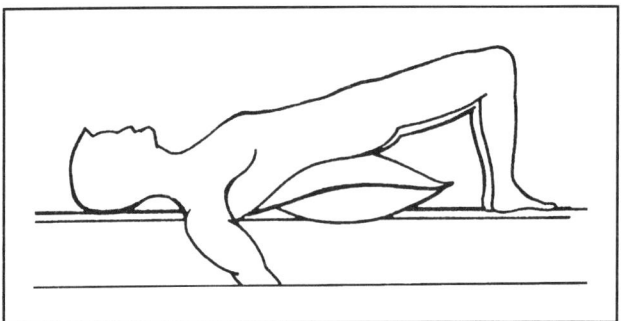

Position 4—Have someone assist you to a sitting position at a slight angle leaning back against a pillow. This position will drain the upper portions of your lungs anteriorly (in the front).

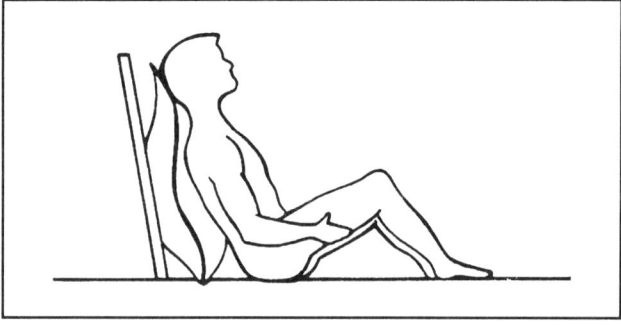

continues

continued

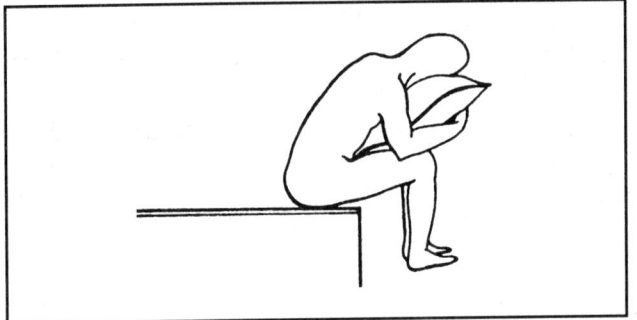

Position 5—Have someone assist you to lean forward on a pillow while sitting. This position will drain the upper portions of your lungs posteriorly (in the back).

Notes:

Source: Kim Blake and Trish Fetters, Division of Nursing Services, University of Missouri-Columbia Hospital & Clinics, Howard A. Rusk Rehabilitation Center, Columbia, Missouri, © 1988. Printed with permission of the curators of the University of Missouri.

Breathing Exercises

DEEP BREATHING

Technique: Inhale deeply through mouth, hold breath 1 to 2 seconds, exhale slowly through mouth.

Frequency: Repeat five times.

Purpose: To increase respiratory reserve.

PACED BREATHING

Technique: Inhale deeply for a count of four, hold for a count of four, exhale for a count of eight.

Frequency: Repeat five times.

Purpose: To practice a normal rhythm of the breathing cycle. Inhalation (breathing in) is a quicker process than exhalation (breathing out) and normally occurs in a ratio of 1:2.

LATERAL STRETCH

Technique: Raise right arm up, inhale deeply, lean to the left side, and stretch. Exhale and lower arm. Repeat, raising the left arm up and leaning to the right.

Frequency: Repeat five times on each side.

Purpose: To stretch the rib cage, by moving it up and out, on the side of the arm raised. This will allow the lung on that side to expand, drawing more air in. This exercise helps to draw air into the lower lobes on the side stretched.

SCAPULAR RETRACTION ("SHOULDER PINCHES")

Technique: Inhale as you round shoulder forward; exhale as you bring shoulders back.

Frequency: Repeat five times.

Purpose: To stretch chest musculature. Tight chest muscles can limit your breathing, because the lungs cannot expand fully and take in more air. This exercise also helps to improve sitting posture.

continues

continued

TRIPLE BREATH HOLDS

Technique: Take a deep breath in through your mouth, hold it and take another breath, hold it and take one more. Exhale.

Frequency: Repeat five times.

Purpose: To expand the lungs and upper airways as fully as possible. Helps to increase the vital capacity. Do not perform if there are cardiac precautions.

AIR SHIFTS

Technique: Take a deep breath, shift your stomach in and shoulders up, then stomach out and shoulders down while you hold the breath.

Frequency: Do 10 shifts on one breath. Repeat five times. Then do one for endurance, doing as many shifts as possible in one breath.

QUICK BREATHS

Technique: Inhale through your mouth as much air as you can, as quickly as you can, using two quick breaths.

Frequency: Repeat five times.

Purpose: To get air in and out as quickly as possible in order to have enough air to yell out in an emergency or to help with coughing.

NUMBER COUNTING

Technique: Inhale deeply, then count out loud until you run out of air.

Frequency: Repeat this once counting slowly with your voice at medium pitch (monotone). Then do it once shouting out loud.

ACCESSORY FOR NECK ("UGLY NECKS")

Technique: Tighten your neck muscles. The muscles and tendons should pop out. Relax.

Frequency: Repeat two sets of 15.

Purpose: To strengthen the neck accessory breathing musculature. These muscles are attached to the rib cage. When they contract they elevate the ribs and allow the lungs to expand more, increasing the vital capacity.

Source: Shirely S. Paulson, *Spinal Cord Injury Home Care Manual*, Norman B. Nelson Rehabilitation Center, Santa Clara Valley Medical Center, San Jose, California, © 1994.

SMOKING AND SPINAL CORD INJURY

Facts about Smoking and Spinal Cord Injury

WHAT EVERYONE SHOULD KNOW ABOUT SMOKING

- Lung cancer is the number one cause of cancer death among both women and men. The risk of developing lung cancer is more than 10 times greater for smokers than for nonsmokers.
- The risk of getting lung cancer if you smoke is 1 in 7. These odds are almost as bad as those in Russian Roulette.
- All forms of tobacco, including cigars, pipes, and smokeless tobacco, put the user at increased risk for cancer of any part of the oral cavity.
- Smokers have twice the risk of death from heart disease as nonsmokers.
- When parents smoke, their children have more coughs, respiratory infections, and chronic ear infections, and they are more likely to become smokers themselves.
- Smoking causes both short-term and long-term health problems:

Short Term	Long Term
—Increased heart rate and blood pressure	—Heart disease
—Decreased oxygen in body tissues	—Bronchitis, emphysema
—Decreased stamina and endurance	—Cancer

SPECIAL CONCERNS FOR PERSONS WITH SPINAL CORD INJURY

- Smoking decreases blood flow to the skin, leading to greater risk of pressure sores.
- Smoking interferes with healing of pressure sores due to decreased blood supply to skin.
- Smokers who have a Foley or suprapubic catheter are at especially high risk of getting bladder cancer.
- Smokers have 2 to 4 times the risk of hip, wrist, and spine fractures.
- Smoking can interfere with the effectiveness of medications.
- People with quadriplegia and many with paraplegia are prone to respiratory problems due to impaired cough and lowered lung capacity. Smoking can cause further deterioration of the lungs.

BENEFITS OF QUITTING SMOKING

- Smoking cessation has major and immediate health benefits for men and women of all ages. Benefits apply to persons with and without smoking-related disease.
- Former smokers live longer than continuing smokers. For example, persons who quit smoking before age 50 are half as likely to die in the next 15 years than if they had continued to smoke.

We Can Help! Talk to your doctor or nurse about programs to help you quit smoking.

Source: Julia S. Breckenridge, "Smoking Cessation and Spinal Cord Injury," *SCI Psychosocial Process*, Vol. 6, No. 4, American Association of Spinal Cord Injury Psychologists and Social Workers, Jackson Heights, New York © 1993.

VENTILATORS

Exhibit
VENTILATORY DYSFUNCTION IN SPINAL CORD INJURY

In uncomplicated spinal cord injury (SCI) the lungs are normal, and the chest wall is intact. Ventilatory failure rather than respiratory failure is more common in acute high-level SCI. Respiratory failure and impaired gas exchange, however, can occur as well with bulbar involvement, atelectasis, pulmonary embolus, or pneumonia. After any complete SCI at the cervical levels, the coordination of the ventilatory musculature is lost.

During spinal shock, when paralyzed muscles are flaccid, the paralyzed abdominal wall moves outward rather than contracting to augment chest wall expansion. Paralyzed intercostals are drawn inward with inspiration. These paradoxical movements of the intercostals and abdominal muscles result in a significant drop in the efficiency of breathing.

When the diaphragm (injuries at C4 or above) is also paralyzed and only the accessory muscles are available for inspiration, the abdominal wall is drawn inward with the negative pressure generated on inspiration, and the abdominal contents are both pushed and pulled upward. Therefore, the lungs cannot be inflated fully. Breathing in this manner is extremely inefficient and energy consuming and usually cannot maintain adequate ventilation for more than a brief period of time.

These changes in ventilatory mechanics are associated with changes in pulmonary function tests. Vital capacity, maximum static inspiratory pressure, maximum static expiratory pressure, inspiratory capacity, and expiratory reserve volume all drop significantly. Acute injuries at the midcervical levels can result in vital capacities less than 1,500 mL and not infrequently require ventilatory assistance. Injuries at the C4 level or above that result in bilateral diaphragmatic paralysis generally require long-term ventilatory assistance for survival.

Ventilator-dependent patients with SCI are sometimes classified as respiratory quadriplegics or pentaplegics. Respiratory quadriplegics have head and neck control and thus have some use of accessory muscles for breathing. Pentaplegics have no head or neck control or use of accessory muscles for breathing. Many of these individuals also have bulbar involvement because several cranial nerve nuclei extend down into the upper cervical spine. With bulbar involvement there is also loss of upper airway protection, placing these individuals at high risk for aspiration of pharyngeal and gastric secretions.

Source: Mary Elizabeth Keen, "Management of the Ventilator-Dependent Patient with Quadriplegia," in *Spinal Cord Injury: Medical Management and Rehabilitation*, Gary M. Yarkony, ed., Aspen Publishers, Inc., © 1994.

Exhibit
TYPES OF VENTILATOR SUPPORT

NEGATIVE PRESSURE VENTILATION

The iron lung was the first mechanical ventilator effectively used on a wide scale. The iron lung and a modified version called the Porta-lung are the most efficient of the negative pressure ventilators. The body below the neck is enclosed in a tank within which negative pressure is generated. Passive inspiration is induced by the pull on the chest wall. Expiration can be augmented as well if positive pressure is applied, but more commonly expiration is allowed to occur passively.

The chest cuirass and the pneumowrap (pulmowrap) are smaller and less efficient but more portable negative pressure ventilators. The tortoise shell–shaped cuirass forms a negative pressure chamber over the thorax. It can be custom made by orthotists. The plastic pneumowrap, also known as the raincoat or poncho ventilator, forms a negative pressure chamber over the chest and abdomen.

These devices are most effective in individuals with normal lungs and normal chest compliance. Achieving a comfortable fit can be difficult especially in patients who are thin or obese or who have deformities of the spine or extremities. None of these ventilators can be used in a wheelchair. They should not be used in cases of upper airway obstruction or significant bulbar weakness.

POSITIVE PRESSURE VENTILATION

Positive pressure ventilation offers several advantages over negative pressure ventilation. Ventilation volume, humidity, flow rates, and fraction of inspired oxygen can be accurately controlled. Positive pressure ventilators are less bulky and more portable. They allow improved access to the patient for medical and nursing care. They are also more effective in cases of lung pathology (e.g., pneumonia, abnormal chest wall compliance, or chest trauma). Positive pressure ventilators are most often used

continues

continued

in combination with endotracheal or tracheostomy tubes. These devices offer the advantage of airway protection, especially in cases of bulbar involvement, but they may interfere with speaking and swallowing.

There are two prototypes of positive pressure ventilators: pressure regulated and volume regulated. Pressure-regulated positive pressure ventilators deliver air for gas exchange with a stable pressure. The pressure in the system determines the tidal volume. The volume delivered changes if resistance to flow changes. For example, if there is a leak in the system, the volume delivered will be increased to maintain a stable pressure within the system. Conversely, if lung compliance decreases for some reason, the volume delivered will be decreased. Volume-regulated positive pressure ventilators deliver a specific volume of air with each cycle. These ventilators do not compensate for a leak in the system. Hence if there is a leak in the system, a lower volume of air is delivered. Variable leaks around tracheostomy tubes can be problematic and may result in hypoventilation during sleep with volume-regulated ventilators.

Portable ventilators, which are smaller and lighter than stationary ones, and console type ventilators are available for use with wheelchairs. Internal and external batteries allow freedom of movement, including community mobility.

Volume- and pressure-regulated ventilators are usually used with intubated or tracheostomized patients, but they can be used with oral or nasal interfaces as well. Researchers recently reported on 25 ventilator-dependent traumatic quadriplegic patients who were supported with noninvasive ventilatory assistance, including mouth intermittent positive pressure ventilation (IPPV). Twenty were able to have their tracheostomy sites closed. Noninvasive IPPV will not be effective in cases of severe weakness of the oropharyngeal musculature or depressed mental status. It also may interfere with the use of mouth wands. Aerophagia and abdominal distension are occasionally problematic.

DIAPHRAGMATIC ASSIST DEVICES

There are two devices in use today that assist ventilation by augmenting diaphragmatic movement: the pneumobelt, also known as the intermittent abdominal pressure ventilator (IAPV), and the rocking bed.

The pneumobelt consists of a motorized inflatable bladder secured over the abdomen. The bladder alternately expands and contracts as air is forced into and released from it. The abdomen is thus intermittently compressed, causing passive movement of the diaphragm upward and augmenting expiration (exhalation). Deflation of the bladder allows the diaphragm to descend passively and the rib cage to expand by elastic recoil. With the pneumobelt, inhalation is largely passive and dependent on gravity; hence the device is effective only when used in the sitting or standing position. The pneumobelt has been used successfully by patients with spinal cord injury who previously used tracheostomy-dependent means of ventilatory support.

The rocking bed is a motorized bed that moves continuously in the longitudinal plane. When the head is higher than the rest of the body, the diaphragm is passively pulled down by gravity, and inhalation is assisted. When the head is lower than the rest of the body, gravity pulls the abdominal contents cephalad and passively assists expiration.

PHRENIC NERVE PACING

Phrenic nerve stimulation was first used for ventilatory insufficiency in the late 1940s. A technique of radiofrequency electrophrenic respiration was first described in 1968. This system has since been successfully used in hundreds of patients with chronic respiratory failure, including many with ventilator-dependent spinal cord injury.

Phrenic pacing causes inhalation by inducing a contraction of the diaphragm through electrical stimulation of the phrenic nerve(s). A stimulating electrode is surgically placed on the phrenic nerve. Each stimulating electrode is attached to a radiofrequency receiver, which is also implanted subcutaneously. A small external transmitter supplies electrical power and stimulus through the intact skin via magnetic coupling with a loop-shaped antenna placed over the receiver. The transmitter produces a coded signal that is transmitted to the subcutaneous receiver and induces a series of electrical impulses to the phrenic nerve. Each train of impulses causes movement of the hemidiaphragm.

Diaphragmatic pacing is effective only when the lower motor neurons of the phrenic nerve are intact. Therefore, it may not be effective in cases of injury at the C3 through C5 levels. Function of the phrenic nerve can be verified via observation under fluoroscopy, measurement of phrenic nerve conduction and latency, and visualization of contraction of a hemidiaphragm at the costal insertion of the muscle when the phrenic nerve is stimulated.

High-intensity stimulation causes fatigue of the phrenic nerve and myopathic changes in the diaphragm. Low-frequency pulses and rates of stimulation with bilateral pacing produce larger minute volumes and improved air mixing at a lower intensity of stimulation.

Implantation of a pacing system is usually delayed until any spontaneous recovery is complete. Pacing is initiated gradually for the diaphragm to develop the endurance necessary for full-time stimulation. The pulse frequency can be lowered gradually as the strength and endurance of the diaphragm improve.

Advantages of electrophrenic respiration include improved cosmesis, less bulky and heavy equipment, and improved voicing. Families find phrenic pacers less intimidating than positive pressure ventilators. Problems with phrenic nerve pacing include a significant risk of system failure, risk of phrenic nerve damage during electrode implantation, and scarring and fibrosis around the electrodes. As with negative pressure devices, an adequate upper airway is necessary and should be verified by bronchoscopy.

Source: Mary Elizabeth Keen, "Management of the Ventilator-Dependent Patient with Quadriplegia," in *Spinal Cord Injury: Medical Management and Rehabilitation*, Gary M. Yarkony, ed., Aspen Publishers, Inc., © 1994.

Exhibit
VENTILATOR WEANING AND INTERVENTIONS TO IMPROVE VENTILATORY FUNCTION

A significant percentage of patients who initially present with ventilatory compromise due to high cervical spinal cord injury (SCI) do not require long-term mechanical assistance for survival. After experiencing an acute drop in vital capacity and other measures at the time of injury, many individuals with cervical SCI experience an improvement in ventilatory function over the first weeks to months after the injury. A 1986 study found that most of those who were weaned from ventilatory support developed a mean vital capacity of almost 2,000 mL. Those who remained ventilator dependent did not achieve an adequate vital capacity. Mechanisms of improvement in pulmonary function probably include neurologic recovery as swelling and posttraumatic inflammation within the injured spinal cord resolve; the development of spasticity and the recovery of stretch reflexes in the abdominal and intercostal segments, which help the diaphragm work more efficiently by stabilizing the rib cage; and recruitment of accessory muscles of the neck and upper chest to augment elevation of the rib cage and chest wall expansion.

Although ventilatory function initially may improve over time, some individuals develop progressive ventilatory failure, especially with advancing age, or experience recurrent pulmonary complications after weaning. Others develop chronic alveolar hypoventilation from nocturnal respiratory insufficiency. Therefore, patients with ventilator-dependent SCI require close follow-up and periodic reassessment of their ventilatory and respiratory status. Also, medical management of individuals with high cervical SCI requires familiarity with means to preserve, improve, or augment ventilatory function.

REST

When muscle mass is marginal for the daily work of breathing, periodic rest and ventilatory support may be necessary. Some individuals require support during times of illness, when the work of breathing is increased; others require intermittent rest during the day or may utilize nighttime ventilatory support.

POSITIONING

Although vital capacity is lower in the supine than in the upright position in normal individuals, inspiratory capacity and tidal volume are improved in the supine position in persons with quadriplegia. The abdominal contents displace the diaphragm cephalad into a mechanically more efficient position of relative stretch. The diaphragm is stretched more by the pressure of the abdominal organs, but the abdominal contents provide less resistance in the supine than in the upright position and allow more diaphragmatic excursion.

STRENGTHENING EXERCISES

Individuals with quadriplegia have reduced muscle mass available for the work of breathing. Therefore, they are susceptible to fatigue. The contractile force (strength) and resistance to fatigue (endurance) of muscles can improve with training, however. An exercise training program using inspiratory resistance has been shown to improve ventilatory function in a group of quadriplegic patients.

GLOSSOPHARYNGEAL BREATHING

Accessory muscles can be used to increase inspiratory volumes dramatically via a technique known as glossopharyngeal or frog breathing. First described in the late 1940s, it has since been used effectively by hundreds of individuals with polio, SCI, and other neurologic disorders affecting ventilation. The lips, mouth, tongue, soft palate, pharynx, and larynx are used repetitively as a pump to force air into the lungs. By closure of the larynx, air is trapped within the lungs. Frog breathing can be used to help clear secretions, to augment expiration by increasing the stretch of the chest wall and thereby increasing the elastic recoil of the chest, and to provide free time off the ventilator for minutes to hours. It has been used successfully in children as young as three years of age.

MEDICATION

Aminophylline may improve diaphragmatic contractility and fatigue resistance. Inhaled bronchodilators have also improved pulmonary function in cervical SCI, even in patients without a history of reactive airway disease. This effect may be related to unopposed parasympathetic tone causing bronchial smooth muscle constriction.

CORSETS

An abdominal corset may improve vital capacity, inspiratory capacity, and tidal volume by supporting the abdominal contents and thereby elevating the diaphragm and positioning it in a mechanically advantageous position.

ASSISTED COUGH

Among the causes of respiratory failure in high-level SCI is the inability to cough and clear secretions. Maximum expiratory pressure, a measure of expiratory function, is greatly reduced in patients with high-level SCI. Manually assisted coughing, the practice of pushing upward on the abdomen forcefully to augment expiration after a full inspiration, has been in use for decades to compensate for this difficulty. Manually assisted

continues

continued

coughing may be more effective than tracheal suctioning for removing airway secretions.

A study using functional electrical stimulation (FES) of abdominal wall muscles found that FES significantly increased the maximal expiratory pressure in a group of patients with cervical SCI. Manually assisted cough was more effective, however. Mechanical exsufflation devices have been used by polio patients for years. A study recently reviewed the use of manually assisted cough and mechanical insufflation-exsufflation (MIE) in post-polio ventilator-assisted individuals and measured the peak cough expiratory flows with these techniques. MIE was superior to manually assisted coughing in that it produced air flow and velocity more comparable with those in normal coughing with less abdominal and intrathoracic pressure.

NUTRITION

The extremes of obesity and emaciation are not uncommon among ventilator-dependent patients with quadriplegia. Either extreme can have an adverse effect on ventilatory function. Malnutrition can cause muscle weakness and increased susceptibility to infections. Hypercalcemia, a complication encountered especially among teenage patients with SCI, can cause muscle weakness and can transiently interfere with respiratory function.

Source: Mary Elizabeth Keen, "Management of the Ventilator-Dependent Patient with Quadriplegia," in *Spinal Cord Injury: Medical Management and Rehabilitation*, Gary M. Yarkony, ed., Aspen Publishers, Inc., © 1994.

4

Neuromusculoskeletal System

> Most materials in the *Spinal Cord Injury Patient Education Manual* are intended for the health care professional to share with the patient. Materials that are intended solely for the professional are labeled "Exhibit" in the table of contents.

Range of Motion

Range of Motion and Muscle
   Strengthening 67
Upper Extremity Range of Motion
   Exercises 68
Lower Extremity Range of Motion
   Exercises 73
Additional Range of Motion Exercises 75

Complications

Heterotopic Ossification 80
Heterotopic Ossification in Spinal Cord
   Injury (Exhibit) 82
Spasticity 84
Common Questions about Spasticity 85
Aging and Spasticity 87
Aging and Posture 90
Osteoporosis 93
Joint Problems 96

Questions and Answers about
   Posttraumatic Syringomyelia 97

Baclofen Injection Therapy

Facts about Baclofen Injection Therapy 99
Common Questions about the Baclofen
   Pump 100

Functional Electrical Stimulation

Functional Electrical Stimulation
   (FES): Overview 102
Overview of FES Applications 104
Guidelines for Choosing FES Products
   and Services 105

Autonomic Nervous System Disorders

Autonomic Dysreflexia 106
Autonomic Dysreflexia Reference Chart 110

Range of Motion and Muscle Strengthening

Physical and occupational therapists will work closely with you to help you keep flexibility in your joints and increase your endurance and strength in the muscles that are still functioning. As you become more active, your need for passive range of motion (ROM) will decrease.

RANGE OF MOTION

The importance of maintaining good range of motion in your joints cannot be overemphasized. Flexibility can decrease if the joints do not receive their normal amount of motion daily. The muscles and tendons then become permanently shortened, causing contractures. Contractures prevent you from being functional. For example, if your shoulders were stiff, you would be unable to get your hand to your mouth to feed yourself or to position yourself adequately for a wheelchair transfer.

Later you may develop muscle spasms. This is called "spasticity." Severe spasticity can cause contractures and make attaining full ROM difficult and painful. Daily ROM can help to decrease spasticity and prevent contractures.

The amount of ROM you need can vary and depends on your present status of joint flexibility, spasticity, and/or painful joints. Your therapist will determine how often you will need ROM and if it should be done passively to you by someone else or incorporated into your routine of performing tasks. For example, upper extremity dressing is a means of moving your shoulders through all of the normal planes of movement and thus can be used as a way to help maintain joint flexibility.

MUSCLE STRENGTHENING

Spinal cord injury prevents signals to nerves that make muscles move and can severely weaken muscles that remain. To be able to perform the necessary activities of daily living and mobility tasks, you will need to have good joint flexibility (ROM), and you will need to strengthen your remaining muscles to their absolute maximum degree of strength to compensate for lost muscle strength. Initially, this may be accomplished by working with your therapists, who will assist you in moving each specific joint until you can move that joint on your own.

When you are able to move a joint under its own power through its ROM, resistance will be added to strengthen that muscle to its fullest. Pulleys, arm skate boards, weights, and exercise "mat" classes are some of the means used by your therapists to help you achieve your muscle strengthening goals. Functional exercise such as pushing your wheelchair, dressing yourself, transfers, and other self-care tasks are very important for strengthening your muscles, maintaining that strength, and improving your overall endurance.

Source: Virginia Spinal Cord Injury System, University of Virginia Medical Center and Virginia Department of Rehabilitative Services, *Virginia Spinal Cord Injury Care and Teaching Manual*, Fisherville, Virginia, © 1980, rev. 1985, 1988.

Upper Extremity Range of Motion Exercises

It is easiest to do upper extremity range of motion (ROM) when the person is lying on his or her back. However, when this is not possible, ROM can be done while the person is sitting.

SHOULDER ROM

Shoulder motion is used for activities of daily living (ADL), positioning yourself, and moving to assist with or complete a transfer. A decrease in your ROM or the development of a contracture can severely hinder your level of independence in ADL and mobility.

1. Turn the person's palm inward and raise the arm over the head.

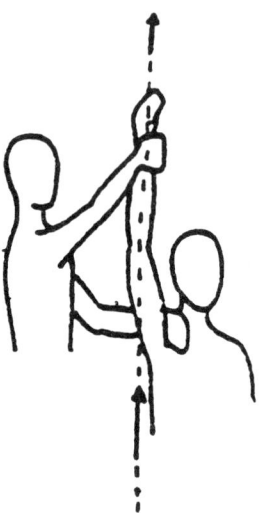

Shoulder flexion

Then return the arm to the person's side and continue the motion (if the person is sitting) as far as it will go.

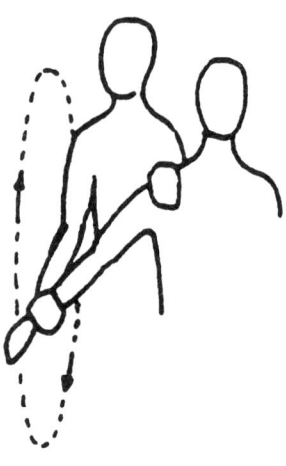

Shoulder extension

continues

continued

2. Turn the person's palm up when raising the arm out to the side. Raise the arm over the head.

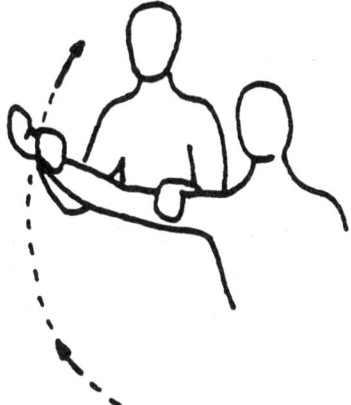

Shoulder abduction

3. Bend the person's elbow to approximately 90° and roll the hand backward as far as it will go.

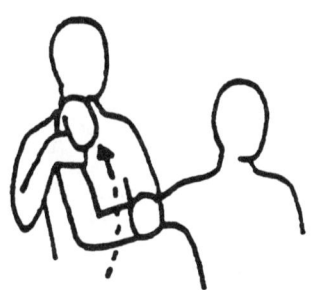

External rotation

Then roll the arm forward as far as it will go.

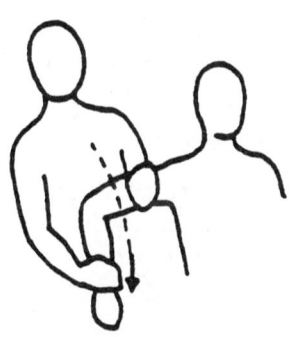

Internal rotation

continues

continued

4. Bring the arm across the body toward the opposite shoulder. Be sure to move the arm at the shoulder joint.

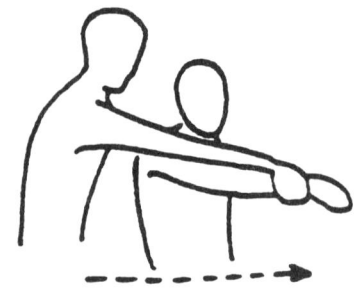

Horizontal adduction

5. Bring the straightened arm out to the side of the body at shoulder level. Alternate between this motion and horizontal adduction.

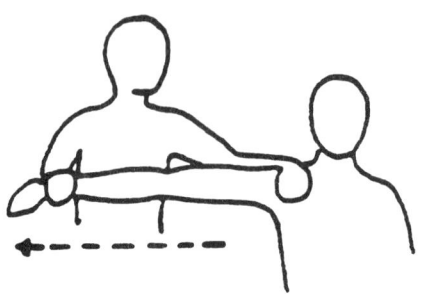

Horizontal abduction

ELBOW ROM

Flexible elbows are important for learning ADL. It is especially important that your elbows can be straightened *fully* and assume a naturally "locked" position for transfers. This can be difficult to obtain if you have very strong biceps (muscles that bend your elbow) and weak or no triceps (muscles that straighten your elbow).

1. Bring the person's hand to the shoulder.

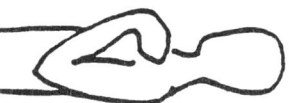

Elbow flexion

And straighten FULLY.

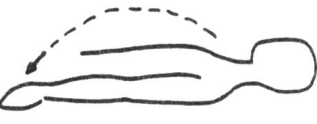

Elbow extension

continues

continued

2. With the person's elbows bent, turn the palm down.

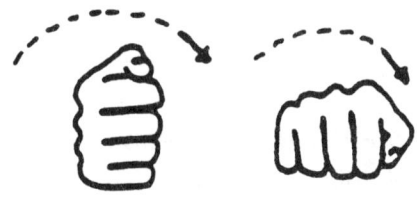

Pronation

Then roll the forearm until the palm faces up.

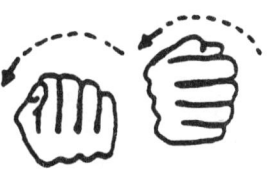

Supination

WRIST AND HAND ROM

A flexible wrist is important for ADL, positioning, and transfers. It is especially important to be able to bend your wrist backward when supporting yourself with the extended shoulders, locked elbow position necessary for transfers. Bending the wrist back also allows "tenodesis." Tenodesis is the natural bending inward (flexion) of the fingers when the wrist is extended or bent backward and can be used to pick up objects when finger movement is absent. To train the hand to assume this position, you must allow the fingers to tighten when the wrist is back. Therefore, NEVER STRAIGHTEN THE FINGERS WHEN THE WRIST IS COCKED BACK.

Wrist and hand ROM can be done at the same time. If you have some motion in your hand, you may need specific instructions from your OT.

1. Bend the wrist forward. Each finger and thumb joint should be bent and straightened. Finger joints should be spread apart and brought together.

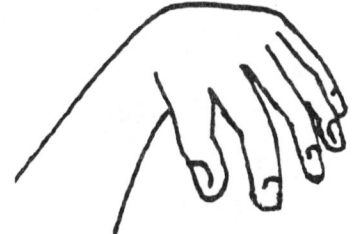

Wrist flexion and hand ROM

continues

continued

The web space between the thumb and index finger needs to be maintained. Pull the thumb away from the palm and rotate it toward the little finger and back. Hold the thumb at the base rather than the tip.

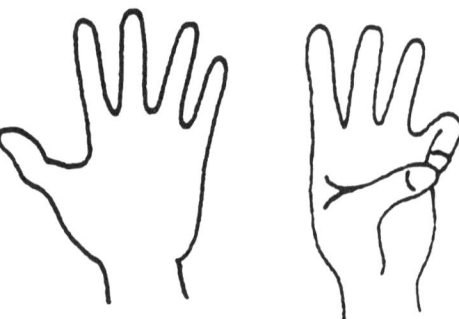

Thumb web space and rotation

2. Bend the wrist backward. Keep fingers bent.

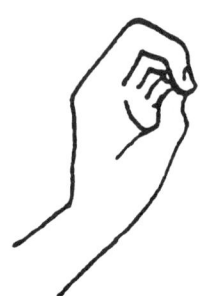

Wrist extension

Notes:

Source: Virginia Spinal Cord Injury System, University of Virginia Medical Center and Virginia Department of Rehabilitative Services, *Virginia Spinal Cord Injury Care and Teaching Manual*, Fisherville, Virginia, © 1980, rev. 1985, 1988.

Lower Extremity Range of Motion Exercises

Losing flexibility in your hips, legs, and feet can present serious problems with sitting positions, mobility for transfers, and performing activities of daily living (ADL). The following range of motion (ROM) exercises help you maintain this flexibility in your lower extremities.

HIP AND KNEE ROM

Hip and Knee Flexion and Extension: Hip Rotation

Lift leg up, bending the hip and the knee. Bring knee up toward chest as far as possible (other leg must remain flat on the bed). Keeping the knee bent and pointing toward the person's head, roll the lower leg toward you. Roll it back toward the person as far as possible. Normally, the leg will move toward the patient farther than it will toward you. Lower the leg, lift the foot upward and straighten knee. Return to starting position.

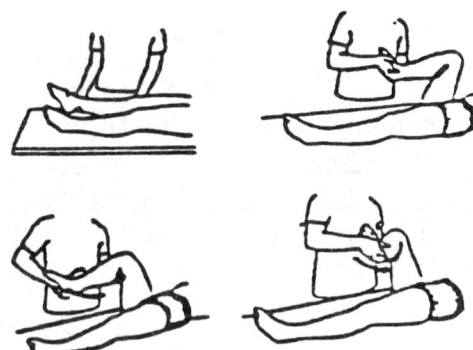

Hip Abduction

With the person lying on back, support the leg under the knee and the heel. Lift leg straight up slightly and then bring leg out to the side toward you. Keep knee and toes pointing up to the ceiling.

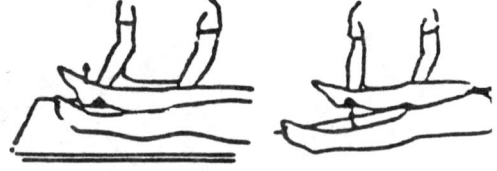

Hamstring Stretch

Stabilize the opposite leg. Hold in front of the knee joint and behind the heel. Slowly stretch the limb.

continues

continued

Most people with paraplegia and some with tetraplegia need to obtain 100° to 120° of straight leg raising. Often the heel of the person can rest on your shoulder if you have difficulty stretching the limb beyond 90°.

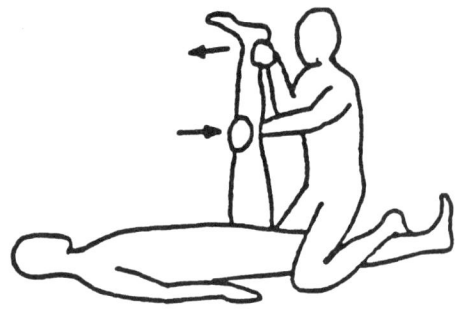

ANKLE STRETCH

Place one hand under the heel grasping the foot with the forearm against the sole. Your other hand stabilizes above the ankle joint. Gently pull down on the heel and forward with the foot.

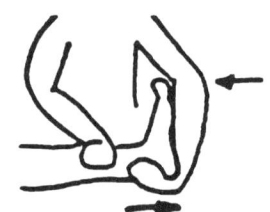

TOE STRETCH

Sometimes a person will require toe stretching with the heel cord stretching. Stretch the toes when the foot is flexed toward the body.

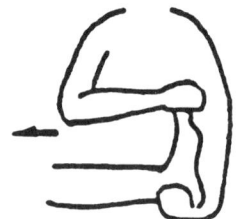

BODY STRETCH

It is a good idea to lie on your stomach every day to keep hips, knees, and shoulders stretched.

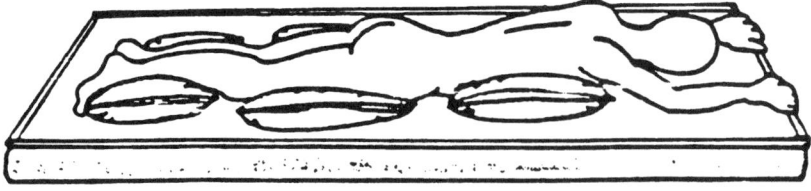

Prone

Note: Arms may be placed at sides.

Source: Virginia Spinal Cord Injury System, University of Virginia Medical Center and Virginia Department of Rehabilitative Services, *Virginia Spinal Cord Injury Care and Teaching Manual*, Fisherville, Virginia, © 1980, rev. 1985, 1988.

Additional Range of Motion Exercises

To exercise all joints to maximum capacity, you should perform the following exercises at least three times a day.

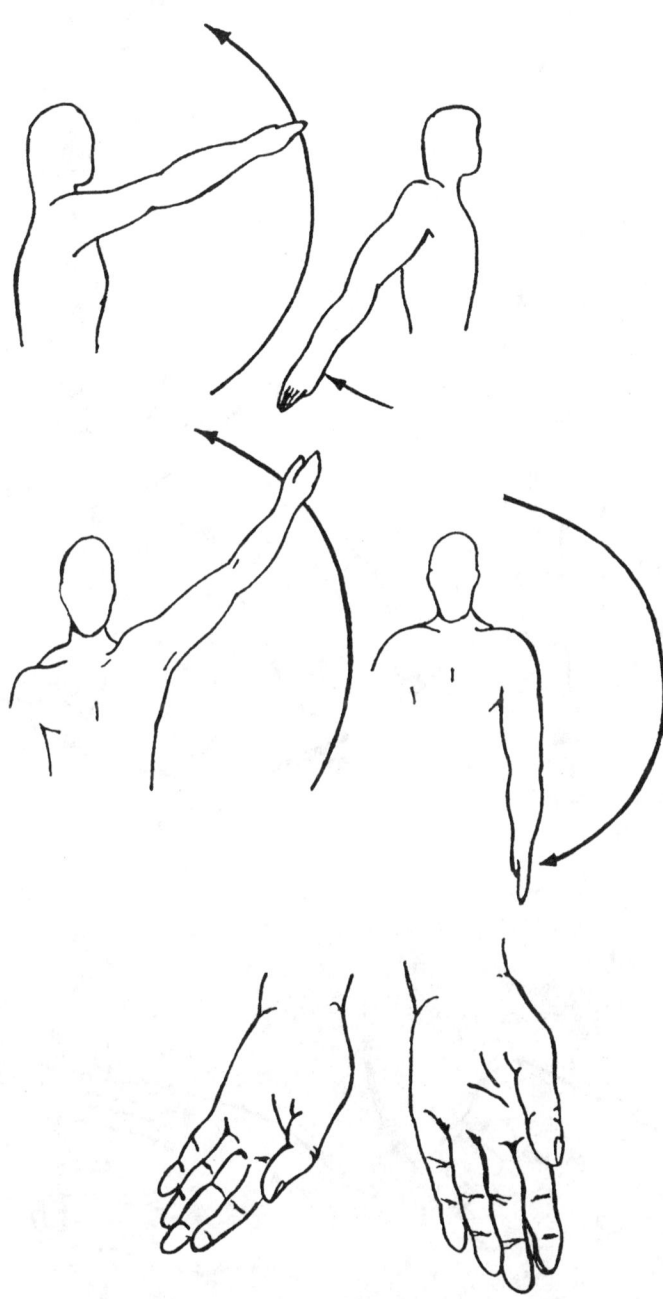

continues

continued

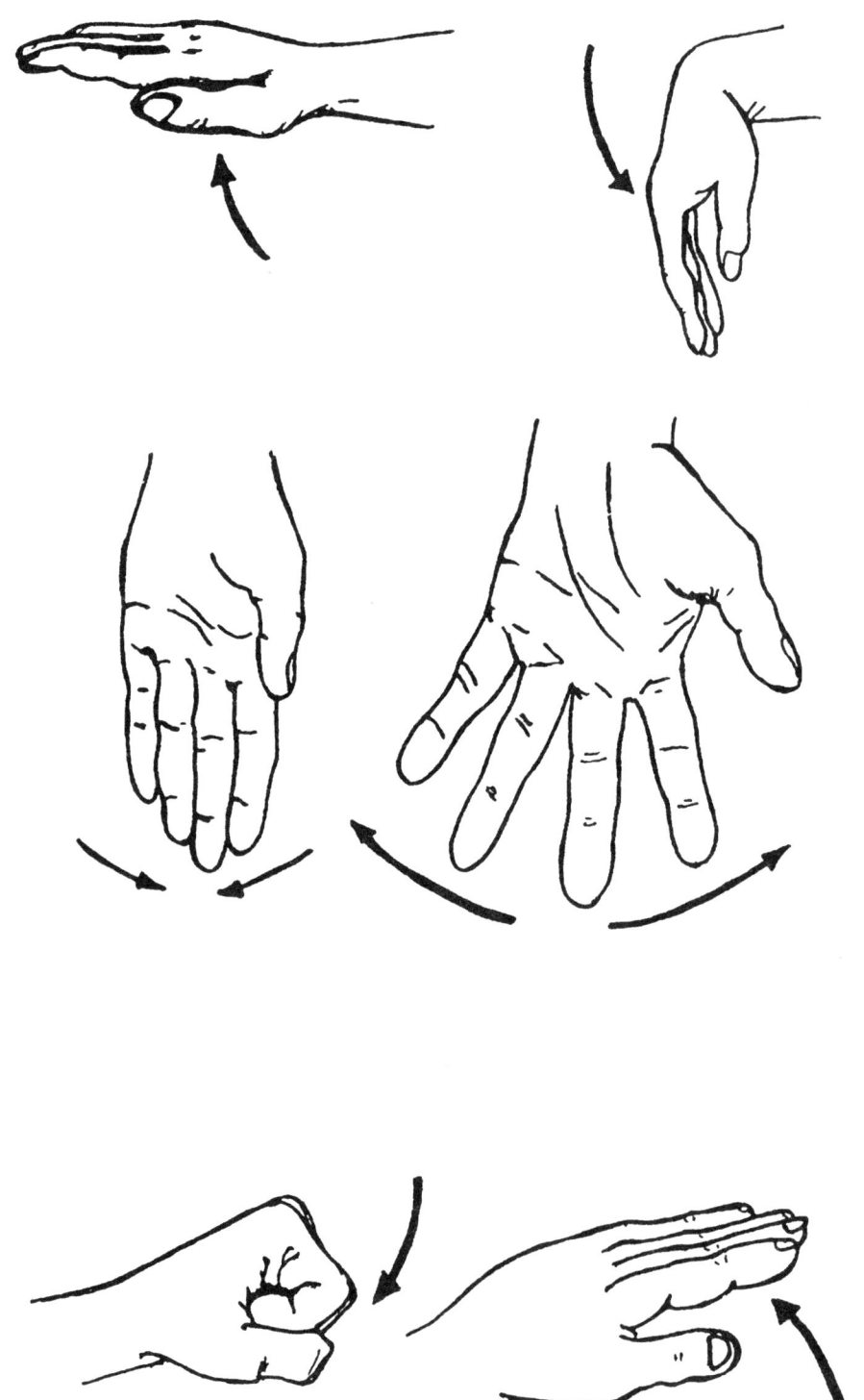

continues

continued

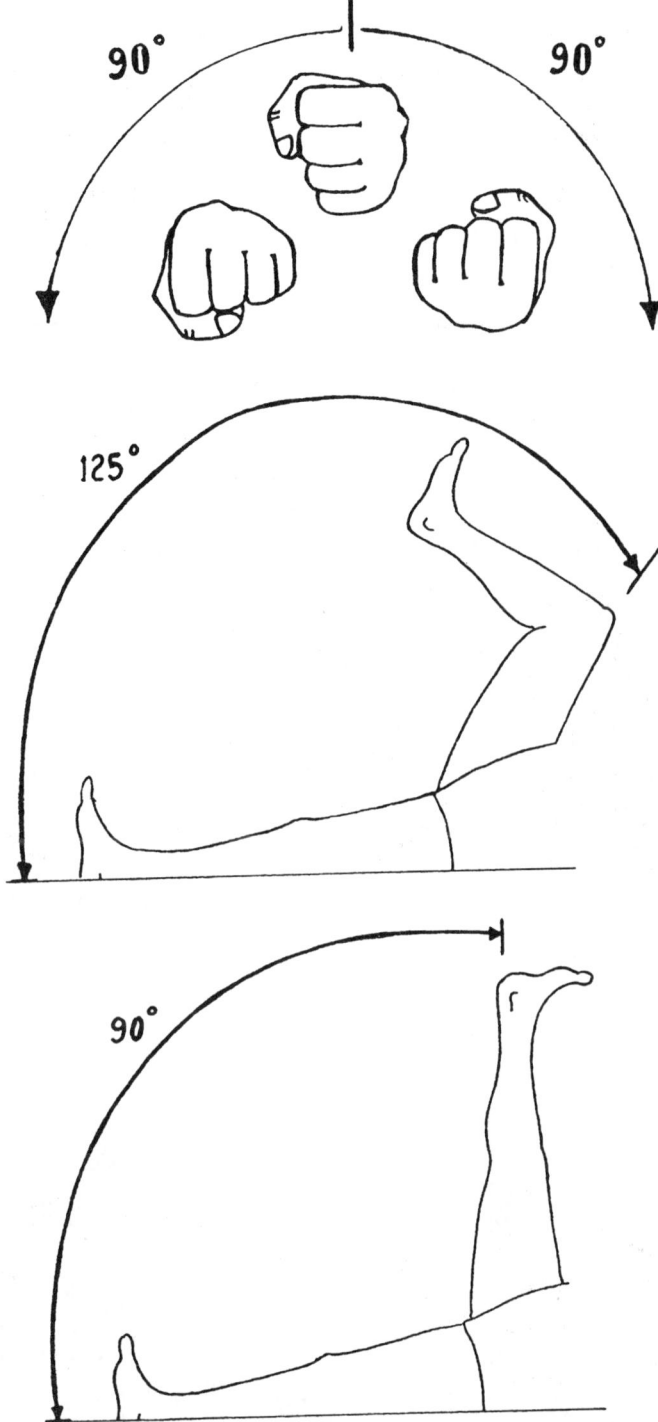

continued

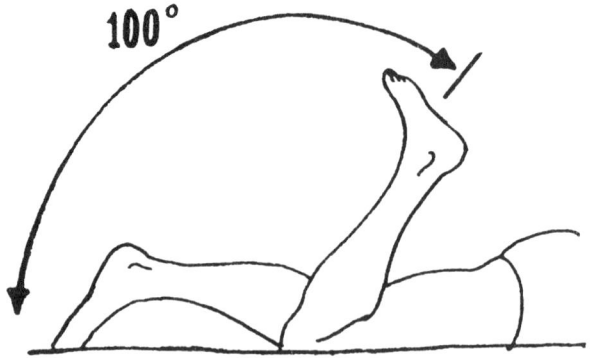

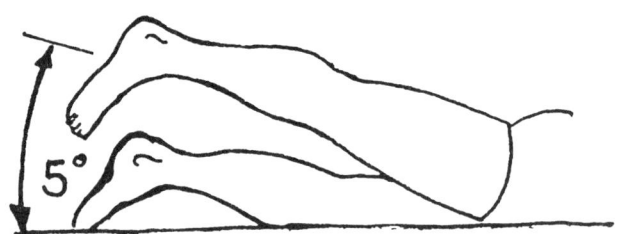

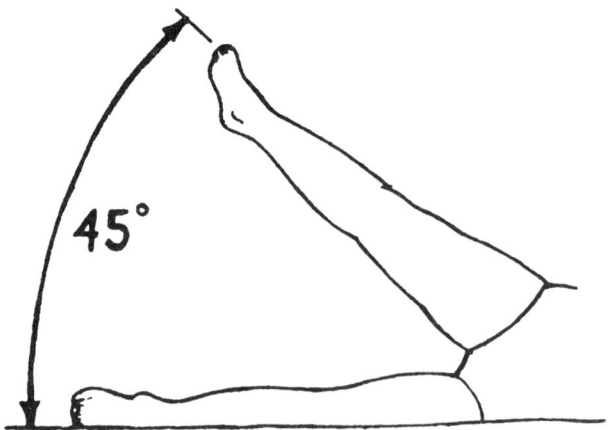

continues

continued

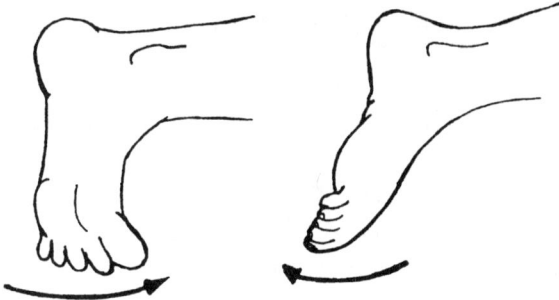

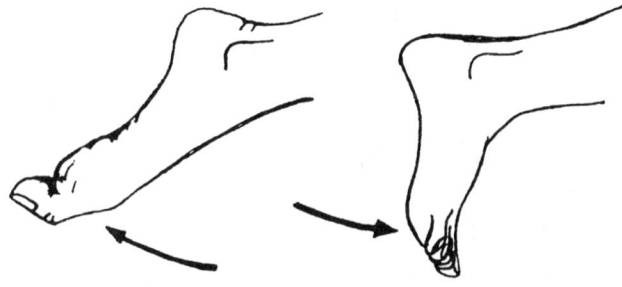

Source: Charlotte Eliopoulos, *Caring for the Nursing Home Patient: Clinical and Managerial Challenges for Nurses*, Aspen Publishers, Inc., © 1989.

COMPLICATIONS

Heterotopic Ossification

WHAT IS HETEROTOPIC OSSIFICATION?

Heterotopic ossification (HO) is the abnormal formation of bone. Pieces of bone may form around joints. This abnormal bone growth may limit movement of arms and legs; HO most often affects the hips, knees, shoulders, and elbows. HO can limit movement and independence.

Heterotopic ossification is most often seen during the first year of spinal cord illness or injury. Heterotopic ossification is also known as ectopic bone formation. If pieces of bone form between the muscles, it is known as myositis ossificans.

WHAT CAUSES HETEROTOPIC OSSIFICATION?

The cause of heterotopic ossification is unknown. It does not occur in all people who are injured. Studies have shown that HO may be caused by changes in the body due to injury. For some reason, young bone cells drift out of place. They deposit themselves outside of bones, where they mature and harden.

WHAT ARE THE SIGNS?

At the affected area, the following signs may be present:

- Swelling
- Increased temperature
- Pain
- Redness
- Stiffness
- Limited movement

These signs continue for two to four weeks, decreasing the movement of the joint. In about four to 10 weeks the new bone can be seen in a bone scan or X-rays. Over the next three to six months the new bone continues to form and grow. It may grow for years, decreasing the ability to move.

Call the doctor if:

- Changes in movement occur after discharge.
- Signs of HO occur.

continues

continued

HOW IS HETEROTOPIC OSSIFICATION TREATED?

There are many ways to treat heterotopic ossification. Doctors may treat it with medication, radiation, or, as a last choice, surgery.

Treatment includes the following measures:
- aggressive movement of joints (range of motion exercises)
  - active (person does the movement)
  - passive (assisted movement)
- joint manipulation (therapist moves the joints)
- proper positioning in bed and wheelchair

Notes:

Source: Kelly B. Wascher, ed., *Patient Education and Discharge Planning Manual for Rehabilitation*, St. Joseph Rehabilitation Hospital and Outpatient Center, Aspen Publishers, Inc., © 1995.

Exhibit
HETEROTOPIC OSSIFICATION IN SPINAL CORD INJURY

GUIDELINES FOR MANAGEMENT

Heterotopic ossification (HO) is a fairly common complication in spinal cord injury. It can range anywhere from a small amount of bone noted as an incidental finding on an X-ray to massive bone formation around a joint resulting in total ankylosis. It occurs only below the level of injury. The most common location is in the hips. Other locations in descending order of frequency are knees, shoulders, and elbows. It does not occur below the knees or below the elbows. Upper extremity involvement occurs only in tetraplegics. It can occur in either complete or incomplete injuries, with either traumatic or nontraumatic etiology. The most common time of onset is between one and four months after onset of the spinal cord injury. However, subsequent events, such as decubitus ulcers or fractures, can also stimulate the process. The etiology is unknown and there is no way to predict which patients are more likely to develop heterotopic ossification or which patients are likely to have only a mild form.

Recognition:

The onset can occur in three ways:

1. Sudden acute onset with an acute inflammatory process characterized by swelling, pain (if the patient has enough sensation to perceive the pain), and local increased temperature, which is frequently mistakenly diagnosed as thrombophlebitis.
2. Begins insidiously with no obvious inflammatory signs: The first evidence of its presence is usually discovered by an astute physical therapist who notes decreasing range of motion in a joint despite daily range of motion exercises. Any time this occurs it should be assumed to be due to heterotopic ossification until proven otherwise.
3. Knee effusion: The sudden occurrence of knee effusion with no history of trauma should always raise a suspicion of HO, which may be located in the hips or thigh quite remote from the knee.

Differential Diagnosis

1. **X-Ray:** During the early stage, an X-ray will not be helpful because there is no calcium in the matrix. (In an acute episode that is not treated, it will be three to four weeks after onset before the X-ray is positive.)
2. **Laboratory Tests:** Lab tests, also, are not very helpful. Alkaline phosphatase will be elevated at some time, but in patients who have had fractures or spine fusion recently, this is not diagnostic. The values will often be quite high, but unless weekly tests are done this peak value may not be detected. Initially the value may be only slightly elevated.
3. **Bone Scan:** The only definitive diagnostic test in the early acute stage is a bone scan. When the initial symptoms are an acute inflammatory process with swelling and increased temperature, the differential diagnosis is thrombophlebitis. It may be necessary to do a bone scan and a venogram to differentiate which is present, and it is even possible that both could be present simultaneously.
4. **Clinical Exam:** The swelling tends to be more proximal with little or no foot/ankle edema, whereas in thrombophlebitis the swelling is more uniform throughout the leg. On palpation, the swelling seems to be firmer and more localized than with thrombophlebitis. However, it must be kept in mind that it is not possible to make an absolute diagnosis on clinical examination alone—one can only have a high degree of suspicion.

Management

The most serious consequence of heterotopic ossification is permanent loss of range of motion in the affected joint. The potential for this depends on location of the ossification—whether it occurs around a joint or along the shaft of a long bone—and on the amount of bone deposited. Therefore, treatment is directed toward prevention of this loss of motion. There are two suggested factors in treatment of heterotopic ossification:

1. Vigorous physical therapy to maintain as much range of motion in the joint as possible, keeping in mind the risk of fracture due to osteoporosis
2. Didronel, at a dosage of 20 mg/kg body weight for 14 days then reduced to 10 mg/kg body weight for a minimum of 3 to 6 months in a confirmed case of heterotopic ossification

To get effective drug absorption, it is very important for the tablets to be given all at one time (once daily) on an empty stomach and for no food to be taken for at least two hours afterward. Therefore, the usual administration time is two hours before breakfast. Juice may be used to help swallow the tablets.

The effect of the Didronel is to prevent calcium from being deposited in the bony matrix that has already been formed. Therefore, it is essential to make the diagnosis as soon as possible (preferably before any calcium shows up on X-ray) and start the Didronel immediately. Didronel will do nothing to remove calcium that has already been deposited. It is a preventive drug and has no effect on existing ossification. It also has no effect on the underlying process that produces the bony matrix. There are no known side effects that would prohibit usage. Many physicians

continues

continued

recommend prophylactic use of Didronel in all acute spinal cord injuries, but because of the cost this may not be practical. Some patients complain of nausea the first week, but this is rarely severe enough to stop treatment and usually subsides in a few days.

Duration of Treatment

There is no uniform agreement on how long the Didronel should be continued. In most cases, there will be a brief flare-up of the heterotopic ossification following discontinuing of the Didronel and some increase in the amount of calcium deposited. There are no completely reliable tests to indicate that the heterotopic ossification is inactive and treatment can be safely stopped. However, if the treatment was continued long enough, this calcium deposition will be of minimal clinical significance. The patient needs to be observed closely for signs of recurrence whenever treatment is discontinued.

Courtesy of Shirley McCluer, MD, Medical Director, Arkansas Spinal Cord Commission, Little Rock, Arkansas, December 1990.

Notes:

Spasticity

WHAT IS SPASTICITY?

Spasticity is an abnormal increase in muscle tension. Tone is the normal state of tension in a muscle.

- *Normal* muscle tone is needed for sitting up and standing straight.
- *High* muscle tone is an abnormal increase in muscle tension. Muscles are so tight (spastic) that movement is hard.
- *Abnormal high* muscle tension makes the muscle so tight that the body part is hard to move.

If not managed, spasticity may lead to:

- joint tightness
- skin breakdown
- trouble moving

Spasticity often happens after damage to the brain or spinal cord. The amount of spasticity ranges from mild (with little effect on ability to move) to severe (preventing easy movement).

HOW IS SPASTICITY MANAGED?

Many treatments can be used. Some treatments include:

- exercises to move the joints (range of motion exercises)
- positioning programs
- casts or splints
- using the body weight through exercise (weight bearing)
- medication

Source: Kelley B. Wascher, ed., *Patient Education and Discharge Planning Manual for Rehabilitation*, St. Joseph Rehabilitation Hospital and Outpatient Center, Aspen Publishers, Inc., © 1995.

Common Questions about Spasticity

Q. What causes spasticity?

A. In common terms, spasticity is an exaggeration in muscular tension and reflexes that occurs in certain types of paralysis. In spinal cord injury this typically results from injury to the spinal cord in the thoracic or cervical region of the spine. Although we commonly think of the function of spinal cord neurons in the control of movement as being a simple direct pathway from the brain down the spinal cord and, via peripheral nerves, out to muscle, there are more subtle neurologic influences on muscular contraction that control muscular tone and reflexes. After a spinal cord injury, the interruption of neurologic impulses coming down the spinal cord not only affects the direct voluntary ability to contract muscles but also interrupts these more subtle descending influences on tone and reflexes. Withdrawal of this influence leads to an exaggeration of these phenomenon, which is manifest as spasticity.

Q. Does all spasticity require treatment?

A. The complete lack of spasticity is termed flaccidity. This can occur in paralysis that results from injury to the nerve roots below the spinal cord in the lumbar spine or even in spinal cord injury during the early phase, termed "spinal shock." In the case of cauda equina or nerve root injury, this flaccid paralysis does not evolve into spasticity over time. In the case of true spinal cord injury of the thoracic and cervical levels, however, the initial flaccid state of spinal shock usually evolves into a state of spasticity, over several weeks or months. Especially in higher levels of injury, it is typically felt that some degree of muscular tone in the form of spasticity may be helpful to create postural integrity. Without some muscle tone, in other words, there would be no muscular component to trunk postular support, leaving one with a "rag doll" like system of postural support. For this reason, most physicians do not prescribe antispasticity medications for moderate degrees of spasticity, waiting until the exaggeration of tone and reflexes begins to interfere with the safety of transfers, awakens the individual during sleep, and so forth, prior to recommending medications.

Q. Are medications the only form of conservative treatment for spasticity?

A. While medications such as baclofen (Lioresal), dantrolene (Dantrium), and diazepam (Valium) are commonly prescribed to treat spasticity, we should not overlook the possibility that other conservative treatments may be effective in reducing the severity of this phenomenon. Specifically, positioning and range of motion may be simple considerations for use in the home that may be effective. It is known that certain postures promote or inhibit specific reflex patterns. The prone position, for example, tends to inhibit flexor spasms and promote those in extension. In the supine and side lying positions, reflex patterns tend to be more extensor in nature. In the standing position, extensor patterns are facilitated. For this reason,

continues

continued

the standing posture may be beneficial as a treatment of spasticity counteracting the flexor tendency promoted by the sitting position. Many patients who routinely use standing devices report that it may have a beneficial effect on their spasticity. Passive range of motion may be beneficial not only to promote relaxation of spastic musculature but also for the prevention of contractures. In addition to these simple treatments, there are anecdotal reports from patients that other treatments such as acupuncture or chiropractic have helped to relieve spasticity.

Q. If medications and conservative treatments prove inadequate, what are the surgical options for treatment?

A. In the past, surgical treatment options have been largely limited to destructive procedures wherein the surgeon interrupted reflex arcs or sensory inputs to the spinal cord by cutting, burning, or chemically injuring peripheral nerves, nerve roots, or the spinal cord itself. While these procedures can be effective in the hands of an experienced clinician, many persons with spinal cord injury experiencing spasticity have been reluctant to agree to such procedures, not wanting to accept further damage to their nervous system for philosophical and other reasons. More recently, the availability of intrathecal baclofen pumps has opened a new avenue for treatment that, while requiring a surgical procedure, is in essence a pharmacologic treatment that is not destructive to nervous tissue. In this form of treatment, a totally implanted pump and catheter system infuses liquid baclofen into the spinal canal at the lower end of the spinal cord. This treatment can be much more effective than oral medications but comes at the cost of requiring a surgical procedure for implantation of the pump, monthly or bimonthly pump refills by trained individuals, replacement of the pump every four to five years, the cost of the pump, and related maintenance expenses.

Source: "Common Question about Spasticity," *Spinal Cord Injury Life,* National Spinal Cord Injury Association, Cambridge, Massachusetts, © 1994. *SCI Life* printing courtesy of Eastern Paralyzed Veterans Association. For more information, contact NSCIA at 545 Concord Avenue, Suite 29, Cambridge, MA 02138.

Aging and Spasticity

Thirty and 40 years ago, no one "in the know" believed that aging with a spinal cord injury (SCI) would be something we'd care about. Back then, no one believed any of the survivors would survive long enough for it to matter. Now that assumption has been disproved and the tune has changed. We're identifying and learning about the issues and concerns facing survivors—problems like fatigue, upper extremity pain, urinary system problems, and caregiver issues. But spasticity doesn't seem to have a place on that list. There hasn't been much research into spasticity and aging, and what SCI survivors tell us varies. Some say their spasticity has gotten worse over time, some say it has lessened, and most don't say much of anything.

It seems that as people age with SCI, they *focus* less on their spasticity. When none of the treatments that are acceptable to them work, many begin to think that spasticity is like the weather: You can complain all you want, but there isn't a whole lot you can do about it. So, even though spasticity doesn't necessarily stop being a problem, it's not mentioned when survivors visit their physicians, it's not documented if it is mentioned, and the researchers don't have any real information to sink their teeth into. Instead we rely on clinicians' observations and some good sound logic and intuition based on what we know about spinal cord physiology.

WHAT WE DO KNOW

At least in theory, there's reason to suspect that just getting older may lead to an overall *decrease* in spasticity. Nerve conduction slows down over time, anterior horn cells may degenerate, muscle mass and fiber size may decrease, and blood circulation within the cord itself can diminish. All of these should lessen spasticity.

Even more important, many people, over time, learn to deal more effectively, or become more "comfortable" with their spasticity. As they get stronger, they learn to overpower their spasms, they learn what triggers their spasms, and they avoid those things.

Some people even use their spasticity—to empty their bladders, to transfer, to dress, even to stand and walk. Others say it keeps their muscles toned and improves circulation. Some suspect it helps keep bones stronger and better mineralized. True or not, spasticity may not be entirely bad.

WARNING SIGNS

Changing spasticity—regardless of your age—is often a symptom as much as a problem. Sensations that you may not even be able to perceive, but which your nervous system senses when something is wrong, make spasticity increase.

Within the nervous system itself, perhaps the most serious complication is a cyst or cavity in the spinal cord (sometimes called posttraumatic syringomyelia). Increased spasticity is a common symptom of this complication. However, *decreasing* or disappearing spasticity can also sometimes be a sign of a cyst.

continues

continued

Other diseases that may develop in the spinal cord—tumors, Guillain-Barre syndrome, transverse myelitis, a spinal cord stroke—also may cause spasticity to change.

Other types of problems *outside* your nervous system also can make spasticity increase, for example, a urinary tract infection, an over-full bladder, or a skin sore.

Finally, *you* may change in ways that make spasticity become *more of a problem*, even though the spasticity itself doesn't get any worse. Things like shoulder joint pain, fatigue, or general weakness may make it harder to deal with what once was a reasonable amount of spasticity. The result is the same as if the spasticity actually had increased.

The bottom line is: don't ignore a significant change in your spasticity.

TWO PERCEPTIONS

So how much spasticity is *too* much? Unless you're one of those people who "walk on their spasticity," uncontrollable spasms can make life pretty miserable.

Ask John, who has an incomplete C6 spinal cord injury. He thought long and hard about the function and quality of life issues and finally got to the point where no spasticity treatment would have been too drastic. After too many years of incredible spasms and megadoses of antispasmodics, he was ready to take a look at dramatic, nerve-destroying surgical procedures, even if it meant potentially sacrificing sensation and sexual function that he had below his injury site.

"Life was nearly impossible," he says, "I feared staying in bed; my legs would launch me out of it." His hip was dislocating because of the spasticity and he was taking so many antispasmodics that his memory was failing. He tried rhizotomies with only short-term success, and now he's waiting to have a pump implanted.

Phil has pretty bad spasticity too; he blames it, at least in part, for his worsening scoliosis. Though he's independent in his wheelchair, he describes his spasticity as "very interfering." Still, unlike John, he thinks most any intervention is too drastic. In the more than 20 years since he broke his neck, he has tried various oral medications; some worked a while, some didn't, and overall he didn't like the side effects. He won't consider a rhizotomy because of its permanence. Besides, he says his spasticity helps him with his transfers. He has given a bit of thought to the baclofen pump, but he's still very hesitant, taking a "wait and see" approach.

Two different survivors; two different approaches to dealing with their spasticity. Both seem to have ended up at least thinking about the baclofen pump, but that's probably coincidental. The pump is generally effective, but countless people have had excellent results with rhizotomies too. Regardless, the purpose here is not to promote one type of spasticity management over another or to tell you *what* you should do about spasticity. Instead we'd like to help you learn to recognize *when* it's time to do something.

continues

continued

QUESTIONS

You might want to ask yourself some of the following questions.

Is spasticity limiting your function? Are there things that the spasticity keeps you from doing for yourself? Is the job of your attendants or helpers made harder because of spasticity? Are you using more personal assistance—to keep you positioned in your chair, to pick you up when a spasm throws you on the floor? Are there other safety risks—losing control while driving your power wheelchair, car, or van?

Is the treatment you're currently using as bad as the problem itself? Are antispasmodic drugs affecting your memory, concentration, or energy level? Are your sleeping and waking cycles out of kilter? Has the amount of money you spend—on medications, on attendant care, on treating related skin problems—gotten out of control?

Are your spasms becoming harder and harder for you to cope with? Does shoulder pain make it harder for you to fight them? Are they frustrating your personal assistant also? Are they becoming more than your aging caregiver can handle? Can you no longer stay alone because of your spasms? Does someone always have to be around to reposition you in your chair? Have the oral medications stopped working, or do other medications make them ineffective?

PARTING THOUGHTS

Think about it. Having a satisfying life is what it's all supposed to be about. Only you know what it takes to give you the quality of life you want. If you decide it's time for a change, educate yourself about the pros and cons of each option. Then, find a health care provider who understands both spinal cord injury and spasticity and who will look with you at the big picture.

You may be getting older and your spasticity may be keeping you company all the way. But if you're knowledgeable about your alternatives and their implications, that long-term companion of yours need not be such bad company.

Source: The Rehabilitation Research and Training Center on Aging with SCI, a joint project of Craig Hospital and the Department of Rehabilitation Medicine at the University of Colorado Health Sciences Center. Funded by the National Institute on Disability and Rehabilitation Research. For more information about the "SCI & Aging" publications, contact the RRTC at 800-5-REHAB-8.

Aging and Posture

You may find it harder to sit up straight at the table. You may notice a certain crookedness when glancing in a mirror or store window. The lower back pain or forward lean seems to have gotten worse over the past year. Or your back just seems constantly tired. These symptoms all point to posture problems, which are common with both aging and spinal cord injury. Getting older with a spinal cord injury? Pay attention.

THE PROBLEMS

Many posture problems are associated with spinal cord injury, ranging from chronic pain and fatigue to scoliosis and kyphosis, as well as skin and respiratory problems. Just like the problems, the causes are numerous.

- Lack of trunk muscles puts your body in a constant slump.
- Muscle imbalance or spasticity pulls your body to one side or the other.
- Inactivity or lack of exercising drastically decreases physical fitness, leaving you fatigued or in chronic pain.
- Habitual functional activities done the same way every day, such as hooking the same arm on the chair back for support, can cause contractures and severe muscle imbalances.
- Poorly fitted equipment—wheelchair, cushion, or back—places your body in a poor position.

When left unaddressed, the problems magnify, possibly causing worse problems. Sitting crooked means uneven weight distribution and possible skin sores. Slumping or slouching makes the lungs work harder, compromising respiratory function. Poor posture while sitting or wheeling puts extra strain on the neck and spine, causing pain and discomfort. The more slumping or leaning or slouching in *response* to pain, the more pain or fatigue that is *produced*.

EVALUATION

Determining whether you've got a problem may be as easy as asking, and honestly answering, a few questions.

- Do you have a chronic pain in the neck, lower back, or trunk?
- Is your fatigue more in the trunk and back, rather than in your arms or shoulders?
- Do you sit crooked? Are you leaning to one side or the other? Is one hip higher than the other? Is one hip or knee more forward than the other?
- Are you always leaning a bit forward or is balance a problem?
- Do you have breathing problems or trouble getting full breaths?

continues

continued

Thinking about these questions is a good first step. Answering yes to any of the questions means you may need to go further.

Looking at how you're sitting is a good second step. Get someone to help. When facing a mirror, is more of the chair back visible on one side or the other? When viewing a profile, do your ear lobe, shoulder joint, and hip joint form a straight vertical line above the chair axle? Remember: living in your body day to day makes it difficult to always recognize or feel the small changes that can result in big problems. You may need to make a conscious effort to observe and evaluate how you sit.

The third step is seeking the opinion and evaluation of a physical or occupational therapist or a physician trained in spinal cord injury.

GETTING STRAIGHT

Changes in the body often require new or different equipment. "Gravity is not your friend," says Craig Hospital physical therapist Cindy Smith. Lack of trunk muscles, or just minor trunk muscle imbalances can, over the course of years, cause major problems with posture. Smith compares the spine to building blocks. Stack them slightly off kilter and they'll probably be okay. Put some weight on them and problems develop incrementally, over time.

Eventually, gravity takes its toll and the price is poor posture, chronic pain, decreased energy, and skin problems. We can address the problems in a number of ways—what we sit *in*, what we sit *on*, and possibly even the types of weight shifts we do.

Starting at the bottom and working up, many solutions exist to address posture problems. New or modified cushions can ensure proper weight distribution and begin to solve hip unevenness. Solid chair backs can provide the support necessary to compensate for weakness in the trunk. Lateral supports or "wings," will serve to support the trunk and keep it straight. Chest belts can ensure stability and help with balance. Corsets can counteract muscle imbalances, straighten out the trunk, reduce fatigue, and assist with balance. One, several, or all of these solutions can be used to deal with poor posture.

THE PAYOFFS

There are rewards for making these changes: reduced fatigue and thus more energy, decreased pain, fewer skin problems, reduction of spinal curvature or hip obliquity, and in general, an overall better and more "normal" appearance.

Wearing a corset may provide the trunk stability necessary to make sports or other activities fun rather than work. Lateral supports and a chest belt may reduce pain and fatigue enough to make sitting at a desk for hours feasible and thus make employment possible. Proper posture leads to even weight distribution, fewer potential skin problems, and safer driving. Proper posture affects body physics and places you in a more efficient wheeling position.

continues

continued

And not all the effects are physical. Posture is often a reflection of how people feel about themselves. Sitting up straight, just like walking tall, speaks forcefully to others about your confidence, competence, and self-image in general. Height, whether sitting or standing, is related to self-esteem.

Everyone ages, and as they do, their bodies change. Responding to these changes with appropriate equipment can allow you to avoid future problems and enjoy yourself as you age.

Notes:

Source: The Rehabilitation Research and Training Center on Aging with SCI, a joint project of Craig Hospital and the Department of Rehabilitation Medicine at the University of Colorado Health Sciences Center. Funded by the National Institute on Disability and Rehabilitation Research. For more information about the "SCI & Aging" publications, contact the RRTC at 800-5-REHAB-8.

Osteoporosis

Rick was getting dressed one morning—just sliding on his pants and pulling up a sock. He heard a loud snap. He had a broken hip, just like that. He was under 40, very active for his C6 injury, and hadn't had a lot of other injuries. He did have osteoporosis.

WHAT IS OSTEOPOROSIS?

Throughout our lives our bones continually break themselves down and rebuild themselves. In the process, several vital minerals, especially calcium, are lost and then replaced. For Rick and others with osteoporosis, the breaking down process happens faster than the rebuilding, and the net loss of minerals causes bones to become brittle. Fractures can happen for almost no reason—during range of motion, after a minor fall, even after a bad spasm. Hip bones (femurs) are often affected, but so are the back bones (vertebrae) and wrist bones. Osteoporosis can limit your function, and if your sitting posture is affected, it can increase your risk for skin and respiratory problems.

SPINAL CORD INJURY AND OSTEOPOROSIS

Osteoporosis occurs in almost everyone who ages. However, in the nondisabled population, older women who have gone through menopause have many more problems with osteoporosis than men. With spinal cord injury, it's an entirely different story.

Soon after the injury—regardless of your age or your sex—bones begin to lose minerals and become less dense. Researchers don't know for sure why this happens, but they have some theories. First, all the things that are risks for osteoporosis in nondisabled people are risks for spinal cord injury survivors too: diabetes; long-term use of steroid medications; being thin, light-skinned, or fair-haired; vitamin D deficiency; smoking; having had scoliosis; excessive alcohol or caffeine use; and following a diet extremely high in fiber or protein or low in calcium.

Second, spinal cord injury itself seems to pose additional risks. New spinal cord injuries tend to keep people in bed, and osteoporosis and inactivity go hand in hand. We also know that bearing weight on bones helps keep them strong, but many survivors who use wheelchairs go years without putting much weight on their legs. Finally, researchers believe that there is something about spinal cord injury itself—something in addition to not being active and not bearing weight. That something is probably a change in the autonomic nervous and circulatory systems. One reason they suspect this is the speed with which osteoporosis appears. Within days of the spinal cord injury, the body starts dumping out minerals, primarily in the urine, which means that bone is being broken down. And these chemicals are dumped in a different order and at a different pace than in persons on bedrest who do not have spinal cord injury.

continues

continued

The Good News

The rapid bone loss that starts after your injury usually stops at about 2 years; people injured 30 to 40 years really don't have any more osteoporosis than those hurt less than a decade. And just because you have osteoporosis, it doesn't mean you'll have a fracture. Only about 1 percent to 6 percent of persons with spinal cord injury have brittle bone—related fractures. That may seem to be a lot, but statistically the odds still are in your favor.

DIAGNOSING OSTEOPOROSIS

Osteoporosis can be diagnosed through blood work and urinalysis, X-rays, and high-tech procedures called photon absorptiometry and quantitative computerized tomography. But doctors don't agree on which test is best, or on how aggressively to pursue diagnostics. This is because these tests often cost a lot of money and only tell doctors what they already know: if you have a spinal cord injury, you have osteoporosis. Frequently the tests fail to tell you and your doctor what you *need* to know: will *you* be one of the survivors who actually has a fracture. If it turns out that you actually do have a fracture, then your doctor may choose to do tests to get a sense of your risk for future fractures and to rule out other possible causes for your fracture.

TREATING OSTEOPOROSIS

Unfortunately, osteoporosis probably can't be cured. The general consensus is that lost minerals can't be brought back into bones. But there probably *are* things you can do to help keep your bones from getting *more* demineralized.

- Increase your physical activity, especially with weight-bearing or resistance exercises.
- If you're a woman who has been through menopause, estrogen supplements might help. If your doctor does prescribe these, be faithful in your checkups, for estrogen has side effects. For men and women alike, there are other drugs that might be available. Talk to your doctor.
- You can probably eat more calcium: milk, ice cream, shellfish, etc. Doctors don't worry as much about the possibility of these foods causing kidney and bladder stones as they used to, but you still will need close follow-up.
- Get more vitamin D from the sun and from eating food like fish and green leafy vegetables.
- Quit smoking. It speeds up bone loss.
- Limit alcohol. It also speeds up bone loss.

Standing: In theory, standing helps. Bones respond to weight bearing, and one researcher's findings suggest that this is true; however, others believe that it's not possible to stand enough on a daily basis to make a difference.

continues

continued

Spasticity: Spasms exert force on bones. Like weight bearing, this should maintain bone strength. People without spasticity often have more problems with leg fractures than do people with spasticity, a fact that seems to verify this. However, at the same time, spasms themselves have caused bones to break. The message here is that some spasticity probably is good; too much is bad.

Be Careful: Sometimes osteoporotic fractures just happen, even without serious trauma. Don't worry too much; just be a little more careful. Remember to take your feet out of the heel loops or toe straps on your footrests before transferring. When you're in bed, move slowly as you turn or come to sitting if your legs are already bent, crossed, or twisted.

WHAT TO DO IF YOU THINK A BONE HAS BROKEN

Stay calm. Usually a broken bone is not an emergency; you probably do not need an ambulance. It might be an emergency:

- if you're prone to autonomic hyperreflexia and you're having symptoms
- if you're in incredible pain
- if the bone has poked through the skin, or if it hasn't poked through the skin, but it looks like there's a lot of bleeding happening under the skin
- if there has been a lot of swelling rapidly
- if you feel lightheaded, nauseated, or otherwise really "crummy"

Even if you decide it's not an emergency, call your doctor. You'll need an X-ray as soon as possible. Treat the bone gingerly; don't try to line it back up the way it was before. If it's your leg, avoid twisting it more. Elevate it if you can. If it's an arm, keep it positioned in close to your body. Don't struggle into socks, pants, or sweaters that will be hard to get off later, but do get enough clothing or blankets on to stay warm. If you live alone, this would be a good time to call a friend to help you to the doctor's office!

PARTING THOUGHTS

Osteoporosis and spinal cord injury is a fact of life. Although the risk is very real, most survivors are not breaking bones. Thousands have made it to ripe old ages without fracturing anything. The odds are in your favor.

Source: The Rehabilitation Research and Training Center on Aging with SCI, a joint project of Craig Hospital and the Department of Rehabilitation Medicine at the University of Colorado Health Sciences Center. Funded by the National Institute on Disability and Rehabilitation Research. For more information about the "SCI & Aging" publications, contact the RRTC at 800-5-REHAB-8.

Joint Problems

People with spinal cord injuries often begin to have joint problems about 15 years after their injuries. Those in wheelchairs or on crutches use their wrists, shoulders, and elbows a great deal. Because these joints are repeatedly performing tasks, they can wear out. Frequent rests and gentle stretching can alleviate the overuse and misuse of joints. It's also wise to seek out the help of a health care professional if joint problems are suspected.

Often changes in one's living space can relieve some stress on the joints. Countertops, desks, and work surfaces at home and on the job should be low enough for a person sitting in a wheelchair. Reaching up to kitchen counters and bathroom sinks stresses the shoulder, neck, and elbow joints.

To find out what financial help is available for the purchase of equipment to redesign living or work spaces, contact any Independent Living Center. ILCs often have access to grants from the U.S. Office of Housing and Urban Development. There are also publications on designing accessible environments, available from the Center for Accessible Housing (North Carolina State University, Box 8613, Raleigh, NC 27695-8613). In addition, many states have an Assistive Technology Center that can offer other ideas and solutions.

Meanwhile, here are some joint-preserving tips:

- Pay attention to pain. Rest joints that hurt or look red or swollen. Avoid stressing them again until signs of fatigue have gone. If pain persists or returns, contact your doctor.
- Warm up with stretching. Bend and flex the wrist, elbow, and shoulder joint, especially if you anticipate wheeling a long distance.
- Stay fit and be sure you work all muscle groups evenly. Exercise to keep the muscles along the back of the shoulder as strong as those at the front, for example.
- Ease into new sports or activities. Muscles need a chance to familiarize themselves gradually with new demands.
- Pay attention to posture. If you're doing something that has you holding your arms at chest level or higher, be sure your back is straight and your shoulders are level.
- Install grab bars in bathrooms, dressing areas, and other places where transfers are likely to be made.
- Ask a physical therapist about strengthening and stretching exercises for keeping joints flexible.

Source: "Joint Problems," *Spinal Cord Injury Life*, National Spinal Cord Injury Association, Silver Spring, Maryland, © Winter 1995. *SCI Life* printing courtesy of Eastern Paralyzed Veterans Association.

Questions and Answers about Posttraumatic Syringomyelia

Q: I have heard of a medical complication called syringomyelia that individuals with spinal cord injury can get. What is syringomyelia?

A: In individuals without spinal cord injury (SCI), syringomyelia is a chronic and progressive disorder that mainly involves the spinal cord. A cavity develops in the spinal cord. As cerebrospinal fluid leaks into the cavity, pressure builds up inside the cavity and it expands. As the cavity expands, adjacent nerve fibers are damaged. This may cause a loss of strength, function, and sensation in the body systems affected by these nerves.

In individuals with SCI, the condition is called posttraumatic syringomyelia (PTS). PTS develops at the site of the initial SCI. This may occur because the fluid does not move freely around the spinal cord at the site of injury. Pressure may increase, forcing the fluid into the cord and the syrinx (cavity).

Q: What are my chances of getting PTS?

A: Current figures show that only about 3 percent of individuals with SCI have PTS. It is more likely to occur in individuals with cervical or upper thoracic injuries.

PTS can develop any time after SCI. It may be months or years before it occurs. A spinal cyst can remain stable for years, develop slowly over many years, or grow rapidly. Individuals with SCI may have a spinal cyst but may never develop any symptoms. This is why it is important to report any symptoms to your doctor so the symptoms can be closely monitored.

As life expectancy of individuals with SCI increases, more cases of PTS are being diagnosed. This may be attributed to the use of magnetic resonance imaging (MRI), which improves the ability to diagnose PTS.

Q: What are the symptoms that I may have if I am developing PTS?

A: You should watch for signs that include a loss of feeling in the extremities, muscle weakness and spasticity, continued pain that is new or different, and changes in patterns of sweating. Some people with syringomyelia suffer from chronic pain and headaches.

Early detection is very important. Further loss of function can be very harmful to an individual with SCI.

Q: How is PTS treated?

A: The main treatment has been surgery. The surgery involves inserting a shunt tube into the spinal cavity to drain the fluid or relieve the pressure. Over time the surgery is not always successful. New cavities may form in the spinal cord, the drainage tube may plug up, and other complications may develop. There is not a standard operative treatment for this condition. More

continues

continued

research is needed in this area. There has been little success in regaining lost function or stopping the progression of the symptoms.

Q: Where can I go for information and/or treatment if I think I may have symptoms of PTS?

A: You should first see a physician who specializes in the care of individuals with SCI. Ask your physician to be tested for PTS. The tests normally done are an MRI, an electromyography (EMG), and nerve conduction.

For further information on syringomyelia you can contact:

American Syringomyelia Alliance Project (ASAP)
P.O. Box 1586, Longview, TX 75606-1586
903-236-7079

This nonprofit organization provides a clearinghouse for information about syringomyelia. ASAP has a hotline where you can call and leave a message requesting information: 1-800-272-7282.

Notes:

Source: *Pushin' On Newsletter*, Vol. 12, No. 2, Summer 1994, published by the Medical RRTC in Secondary Complications in SCI, housed at the Department of Rehabilitation Medicine, University of Alabama at Birmingham-Spain Rehabilitation Center, Birmingham Alabama, © 1994, Board of Trustees of the University of Alabama. Supported in part by a grant (#HI33B80012) from the National Institute on Disability and Rehabilitation Research, U.S. Department of Education. Opinions expressed in this document are not necessarily those of the granting agency.

BACLOFEN INJECTION THERAPY

Facts about Baclofen Injection Therapy

WHAT IS BACLOFEN INJECTION?

Oral baclofen is usually taken as a tablet for managing spasticity. However, some patients experience intolerable side effects such as drowsiness, dizziness, weakness, and nausea or do not receive adequate control of their spasticity. Baclofen injection is a liquid form of baclofen that can be delivered to the area surrounding your spinal cord (the intrathecal space). The pump is a device that pumps the drug directly to this area. Baclofen injection is for the management of severe spasticity of spinal cord origin in people who are unresponsive to oral baclofen therapy or who experience intolerable central nervous system side effects at effective doses.

HOW DO I KNOW IF BACLOFEN INJECTION WILL WORK FOR ME?

Your physician will give you a "test dose" of baclofen injection to see how you respond. The test dose is given in the hospital so you can be closely watched for changes in spasms, rigidity, and any side effects you may have from the drug. The test dose is given with a small needle into the intrathecal space in your lower back. The needle is taken out as soon as the drug is injected, or a small tube (catheter) may be placed for a short time. If baclofen injection decreases your spasms or rigidity, you and your physician will then decide if receiving the drug on a long-term basis by the pump is right for you.

Notes:

Source: *Lioresal® (Baclofen) Intrathecal (Injection) Synchromed® Infusion: Questions and Answers for Prospective Patients,* Medtronic, Inc., Minneapolis, Minnesota, © 1992.

Common Questions about the Baclofen Pump

Q. Will people be able to see that I have a pump?

A. Your pump is placed near the surface of your skin, usually in the abdomen, so it will be visible if not covered with clothes. On occasion someone might notice it because it may bulge under fitted clothes. Depending on your size and shape and where your pump is located, it may not show at all under regular clothes.

Q. How will the pump affect my spasticity?

A. The pump is just a tool for automatic delivery of the drug. Let your physician know if you have not received adequate control of your spasticity. It may take a few adjustments to find the best dose for you.

Q. Can I stop taking other medications once I have the device?

A. Your physician will determine what medications you need. It is **very** important that you follow his or her directions.

Q. How will alcohol or other drugs affect me?

A. The depressant effects of baclofen injection may be additive to those of alcohol and other central nervous system depressants.

Q. Will I have to change my daily routine because of the pump?

A. Control of spasticity may give you more independence in your daily routine. There are no special procedures for taking care of your pump other than returning to your physician for follow-up visits. Drowsiness and weakness have been reported in patients on baclofen injection. Caution should be used in the operation of automobiles or other dangerous machinery, and in activities made hazardous by decreased alertness.

Q. Can this therapy be used during pregnancy?

A. There are no adequate and well-controlled studies in pregnant women. Baclofen injection should be used during pregnancy only if the potential benefit justifies the potential risk to the fetus. If you are considering becoming pregnant, be sure to discuss your plans with your physician.

continues

continued

Q. Will I be able to take hot baths or showers?

A. Yes. A hot bath or shower will not interfere with the pump's operation.

Q. Will having the pump prevent me from traveling?

A. Your physician will tell you how often you must return to the clinic. If you plan to travel, notify your physician. It may be necessary to schedule a refill before you travel.

Q. Will my pump set off the metal detector at the airport?

A. It might, so present your implanted device identification card to airport security personnel for clearance.

Q. Will my pump need to be replaced?

A. The battery that powers the pump will last three to five years, depending on the amount of medication the pump must deliver. When the pump needs to be replaced, your physician will arrange for replacement.

Notes:

Source: *Lioresal® (Baclofen) Intrathecal (Injection) Synchromed® Infusion: Questions and Answers for Prospective Patients,* Medtronic, Inc., Minneapolis, Minnesota, © 1992.

FUNCTIONAL ELECTRICAL STIMULATION

Functional Electrical Stimulation (FES): Overview

BACKGROUND

Functional electrical stimulation (FES) is a general term that refers to more than two dozen different clinical applications in which electricity is applied to the body to produce a specific outcome. The term "functional" is often used in conjunction with "electrical stimulation" because the goal of the stimulation is to restore or improve an individual's ability to function in activities of daily living. FES applications have a broad range of use. Some of these applications are highly experimental. Others are used regularly in the clinic or in the home.

Certain FES applications may be more familiar to you than others. Cardiac pacing is an example of FES in which electrical stimulation is used to initiate and control heart muscle contractions. TENS (transcutaneous electrical nerve stimulation) is another application that is used by many physicians and therapists to provide relief of chronic pain.

FES is not for everybody. In the United States, most FES is prescribed by a physician and requires a medical evaluation to determine if it is a suitable treatment option. Some people cannot tolerate certain types of electrical stimulation because it causes discomfort. In some cases, FES is experimental and will not be reimbursed by health insurance. Some FES treatments, even though they are available, are controversial because their success is not well documented.

TECHNOLOGY

Although FES applications differ considerably from one another, they have several things in common. First, all FES systems either mimic or adjust the tiny electrical currents that are naturally generated in the body. These currents are carried throughout the body by certain tissues and by nerve fibers that provide motor (muscle) and sensory (sight, hearing, touch, etc.) function.

Second, FES systems use devices called stimulators to generate electrical current that is transmitted to the body through electrodes. The electrodes are attached to a particular part of the body, depending on the specific application. The electrodes may be placed on the skin, inserted through the skin, or implanted in the body. For a cardiac pacemaker, the stimulator is implanted under the skin in the chest and one or more electrodes are attached directly to the heart. In TENS systems, the stimulator is a box about the size of a hand-held calculator. The electrodes are connected to the stimulator by thin cables and are placed directly on the skin over the nerves to be stimulated.

Finally, all FES systems require some method of controlling the amount of electrical current that is passed through the electrodes and into the body. For example, a TENS system usually comes with a box that has an on/off switch and knobs for adjusting the level of current. More complex stimulators may be automatically controlled by a microprocessor, a miniaturized computer. Certain stimulators use information from sensors to control the level of stimulation. Some

continues

continued

stimulators implanted in the body, like the pacemaker, can communicate through radio frequency with computers in the operating room, doctor's office, or laboratory.

STATUS

Most FES applications are not nearly as widely available as TENS systems and pacemakers. There are many factors contributing to limited availability. Some FES systems are much more complicated than others and designing systems that are safe and effective takes longer. For example, a single electrical pulse can cause the heart to beat, yet an FES system to provide hand grasp in people with paralysis requires coordinated movement of many muscles.

Before medical device manufacturers can sell a stimulator in the United States, they must prove to the Food and Drug Administration that their product is safe and effective. This is often a lengthy process that delays product availability. Even if the FES system is available commercially, considerations such as candidate selection, ease of use, appearance, cost-effectiveness, and training determine how widely it is used. There may be a shortage of clinicians with expertise in evaluating candidates and applying the system, which limits its availability. In other cases, there may be a sufficient number of clinicians to meet the demand, but they may be located at one or more specialized medical centers scattered across the country.

There are other reasons why obtaining FES systems may be difficult. In some cases, the limiting factor may be the lack of appropriate technology. For example, the sensors that are needed to use electrical stimulation to restore sensation for people who have lost feeling due to central nervous system damage do not exist. In other cases, scientists are still trying to understand what causes a body system to malfunction or how the "normal" body system works. For example, scientists have spent decades conducting experiments to learn how cells in the visual cortex of the brain can be electrically activated to recreate a visual image for individuals who are blind. In some cases, such as the use of FES to restore walking in people with paraplegia, a combination of the above factors results in problems of access and availability.

IMPLICATIONS

FES is an exciting rehabilitation technology that has helped thousands of individuals live more independently, but FES is not for everyone. Its appropriateness must be evaluated on a case-by-case basis. For some people, a practical FES solution to their problem does not exist yet. Some individuals have medical conditions that prevent FES from working the way it was designed to work. Other people may not have physical access to clinicians providing FES. In some cases, the cost of the FES system is prohibitive.

Individuals who think that FES may help them, now or in the future, should try to get as much information as possible about the particular application that interests them. That information should be shared with a knowledgeable clinician. Remember, as with any medical innovation, the media usually provides dramatized rather than factual coverage. Try to get the facts. In the process of investigating FES, it is possible that other more appropriate options may be found.

Courtesy of the FES Information Center, Cleveland, Ohio.

Overview of FES Applications

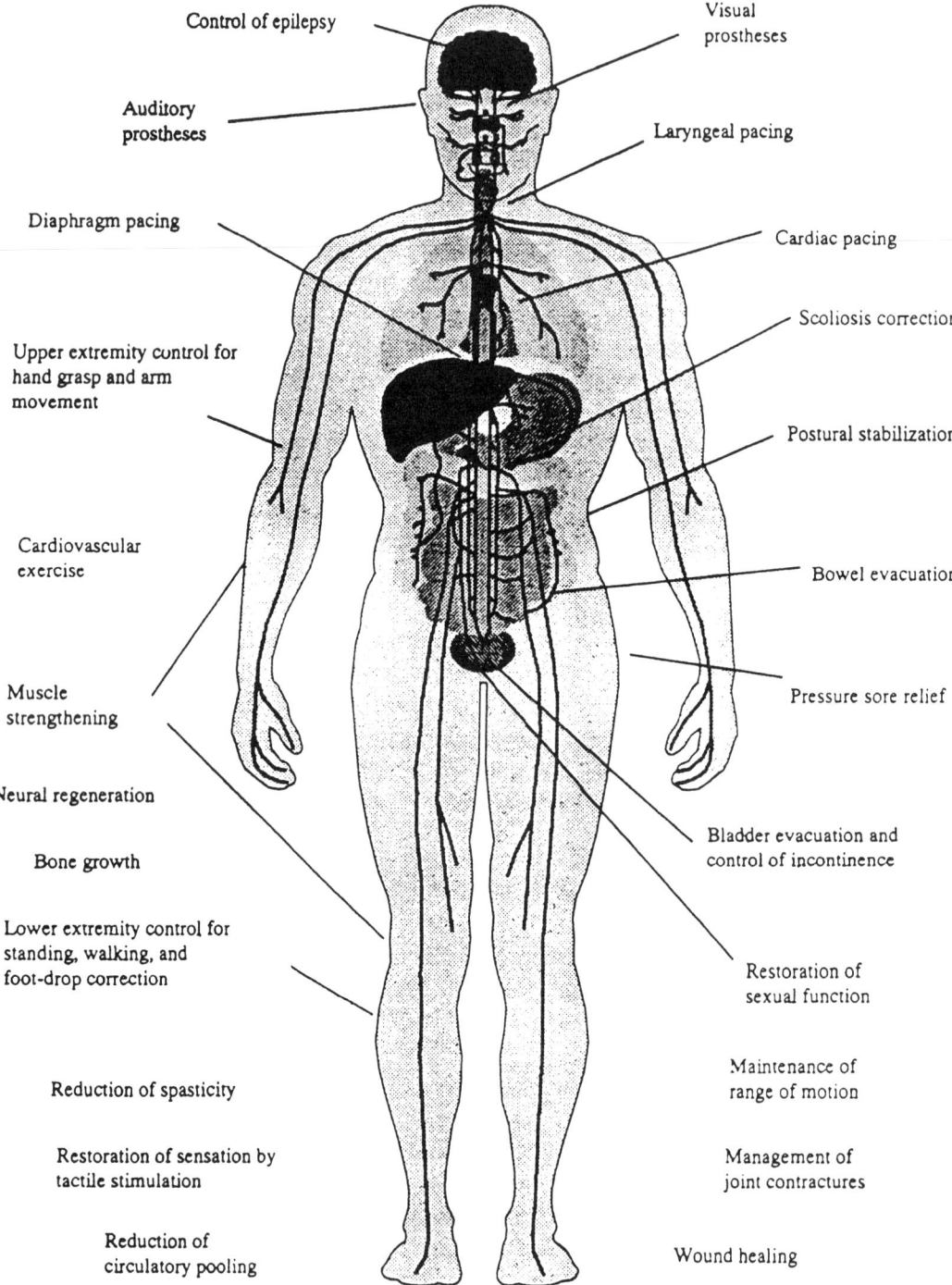

Courtesy of the FES Information Center, Cleveland, Ohio.

Guidelines for Choosing FES Products and Services

"Caveat emptor!" "Let the buyer beware!" We're all familiar with the need to be informed consumers, whether we're purchasing a VCR or buying a used car. We must be educated consumers as well when selecting FES products and services.

Be aware that evaluating FES options can be a complicated process. FES is generally a specialized treatment, offered by few providers. Third-party payers are often reluctant to cover innovative treatments like FES because it can be difficult to prove that the benefits of the treatment outweigh the costs. Add in the emotional involvement, and you can see how complicated the decision becomes.

To assist you with responsibly identifying appropriate functional electrical stimulation options, we offer the following guidelines based on interviews with FES consumers. Remember, you are your own best advocate!

- DO check out the credentials of FES service providers or product manufacturers. How long have they been in business, how many customers have they had, are they accredited with a professional organization or review board, has the Better Business Bureau received any complaints?
- DON'T rely on a provider's or manufacturer's claims. Interview customers, tour the facility, arrange for demonstrations; look for clear evidence that the product/service is safe and effective.
- DO obtain, in advance, a written good-faith estimate of all costs that you may incur. Check out your insurance coverage immediately. Beware of hidden costs such as equipment that you must purchase for home use and transportation and accommodation expenses.
- DON'T get carried away by your emotions. Be as realistic as possible about the benefits you can expect to receive from your purchase, as well as the risks.
- DO obtain written documentation describing your treatment plan. A typical plan should describe the initial evaluation, treatment goals, frequency and duration of treatment, how progress will be measured, and when the treatment will be terminated, for example, upon failure to show gain.
- DO find out if your use of FES will require permanent or irreversible surgery. Discuss the proposed treatment plan with clinicians whose opinion you respect.
- DO explore all the alternatives to FES. More traditional treatment plans may well be just as effective, and less expensive.

In addition, if you volunteer to participate in an experimental FES project, make sure that you completely understand your commitment to the project and the risks and benefits of the treatment. This should be documented in an informed consent form, which you will be asked to sign. Find out in advance what expenses will be incurred and who will cover them, how your daily activities might be affected, and what FES, if any, will be available to you on termination of the research project.

In closing, FES is an exciting technology that demonstrates much potential for enhancing the health, well-being, and quality of life for many of us. In the words of one FES user, "Become well informed, and if everything looks good, go for it!"

Courtesy of the FES Information Center, Cleveland, Ohio.

AUTONOMIC NERVOUS SYSTEM DISORDERS

Autonomic Dysreflexia

WHAT IS AUTONOMIC DYSREFLEXIA?

Autonomic dysreflexia is an overreaction of the nervous system. This happens below the level of spinal cord injury. It is due to an irritation or stimulus. This may also be called "Hyperreflexia."

WHAT CAUSES AUTONOMIC DYSREFLEXIA?

The most common cause of autonomic dysreflexia is a full bladder. Other common causes include:

- Bladder:
  - Infection
  - Foley catheter plugged, kinked, or overfilled
- Bowel:
  - Constipation
  - Impaction
- Skin:
  - Pressure sores
  - Burns
  - Open wounds
  - Tight or wrinkled clothing
  - Painful stimulation (cuts, bruises, pressure on body)
  - Temperature changes
- Other:
  - Sexual activity
  - Menstruation (periods)
  - Ingrown toenail

People with spinal cord injuries above the 6th thoracic level (T6) may have this problem. Some people with spinal cord injuries will never have dysreflexia.

WHAT HAPPENS?

Signals from the irritated area try to send messages to the brain. Because of the spinal cord injury, the message does not reach the brain. A reflex begins. The body continues to try and send the message to the brain. This reflex becomes "hyper."

The reflex makes blood vessels squeeze or tighten, making blood pressure rise. Normally, the blood vessels widen to lower high blood pressure. Because of the spinal cord injury, the blood

continues

continued

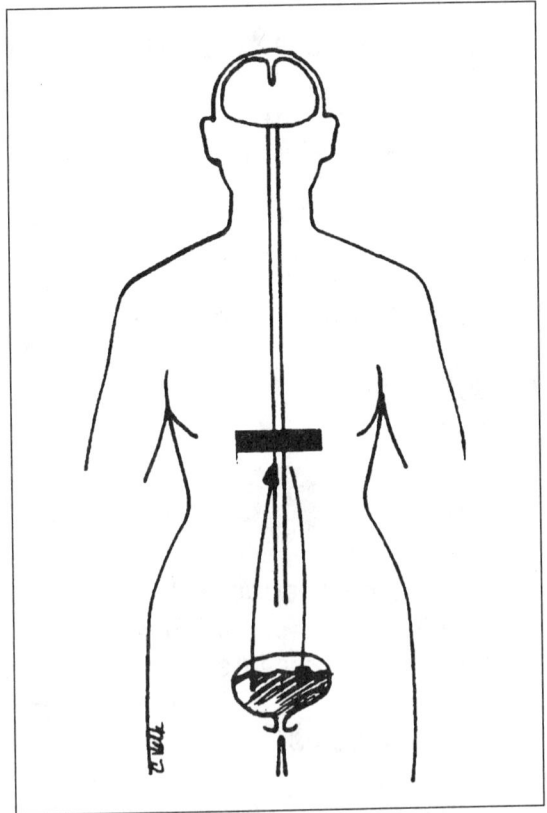

vessels below the level of injury cannot widen. The blood pressure keeps rising. This uncontrolled high blood pressure may cause a stroke, seizures, or death.

WHAT ARE THE SIGNS OF AUTONOMIC DYSREFLEXIA?

- High blood pressure (*hypertension*)
- Pounding headache (caused by high blood pressure)
- Flushed face
- Red blotching of the chest
- Sweating above the level of the injury
- Goose bumps
- Cool, clammy skin
- Nasal stuffiness
- Nausea
- Slow pulse
- Anxiety

continues

continued

WHAT HAPPENS BELOW THE LEVEL OF INJURY

Stimulus

(Full bladder or bowel, or skin irritation.)

Body Reacts to Stimulus
1. Sensory nerves send message to spinal cord.
2. Message cannot get to brain.
3. Reflex happens.

What Happens?
- Blood vessels tighten (constrict), which causes:
  —VERY high blood pressure
  —Cool, clammy skin
- May have goose bumps.

If blood pressure stays high, call doctor.

WHAT HAPPENS ABOVE THE LEVEL OF INJURY

Body Tries to Lower Blood Pressure

What Happens?
- Blood vessels widen, causing red, blotchy skin
- Sweating
- Pounding headache
- Slow heart (again, to try to lower blood pressure)
- Nausea
- Nasal stuffiness
- Anxiety

continues

continued

HOW IS AUTONOMIC DYSREFLEXIA TREATED?

1. **SIT UP** or raise the head of the bed RIGHT AWAY.
2. **LOOK FOR THE CAUSE:**
   - **Bladder**
     - Is intermittent catheterization needed?
     - Does Foley tubing need kinks or plugs removed? irrigation? to be changed (if unable to drain bladder)?
     - Is leg bag full and should it be emptied?
   - **Bowel**
     - Is constipation a problem?
     - Has it been more than three days since last bowel movement, or is there stool in the rectum?

     If so
     - Use xylocaine jelly.
     - Remove stool gently.
   - **Skin**
     - Check for pressure sores, painful stimulus (cut, bruise, pressure on body), or ingrown toenails.
     - Make sure to relieve pressure and loosen clothing.
   - **Sexual Activity:** Talk with your doctor about use of medication:
     — Xylocaine jelly
     — Nitropaste patches

Prevention Is the Best Way to Avoid Dysreflexia

- Empty the bowel and bladder regularly.
- Take care of the skin.

Medication may be used to lower the blood pressure if needed.

Be prepared to explain autonomic dysreflexia to hospital staff who may not know about dysreflexia.

Source: Kelley B. Wascher, ed., *Patient Education and Discharge Planning Manual for Rehabilitation*, St. Joseph Rehabilitation Hospital and Outpatient Center, Aspen Publishers, Inc. © 1995.

Autonomic Dysreflexia Reference Chart

EMERGENCY SITUATION. Life-threatening high blood pressure due to overactive nervous system (hyperreflexia), usually caused by a full bladder. Seen in spinal cord injuries at T6 and above.

Signs	Cause	Treatment	Prevention

• Increase in blood pressure
• Pounding headache (due to an increase in blood pressure)
• Flushed face
• Red blotching of the chest
• Sweating above the level of injury
• Goose bumps
• Cool, clammy skin
• Nasal stuffiness
• Nausea
• Slow pulse
• Anxiety
	Bladder
	• Stretching of the bladder due to:
	  1)—Plugged or kinked catheter
	  2)—urine retention
	  3)—overfilled leg bag
	• Bladder infection
	Bowel
	• Stretching of the bowel due to constipation or impaction
	Skin
	• Burns or skin sores
	• Ingrown toenails
	• Tight clothes or irritating pressure
	Sexual Activity
	• Overstimulation during sexual activity
	• Contractions of uterus before and during menses (female)
	• Labor and delivery (female)
		1. SIT UP!
		2. Identify and remove source of irritation.
		3. **Bladder:**
		  • Check catheter.
		  • Remove kink in catheter.
		  • Empty catheter.
		  • Irrigate catheter if not draining.
		  • Change catheter.
		  • Drain no more than 500 cc at a time.
		4. **Bowel:**
		  • Digital check (using hemorrhoidal cream).
		  • Remove stool.
		5. **Skin:**
		  • Loosen clothing.
		  • Check for pain and pressure.
		6. Call the doctor right away if signs continue!
			• Keep catheter equipment clean.
			• Follow a regular bladder program.
			• Follow a regular bowel program (never go longer than three days between bowel programs).
			• Check skin daily:
			  —Look for pressure areas.
			  —Wear loose-fitting clothing.
			• Check for painful stimulus.

Source: Kelly B. Wascher, ed., *Patient Education and Discharge Planning Manual for Rehabilitation,* St. Joseph Rehabilitation Hospital and Outpatient Center, Aspen Publishers, Inc., © 1995.

5

Bladder and Bowel Management

> Most materials in the *Spinal Cord Injury Patient Education Resource Manual* are intended for the health care professional to share with the patient. Materials that are intended solely for the professional are labeled "Exhibit" in the table of contents.

Bladder Management

Bladder Program: Overview	113
Bladder Program Checklist	118
Common Bladder Problems	119
Common Urinary Tests	122
Intermittent Catheterization	124
How to Do a Clean IC—Male	125
How to Do a Clean IC—Female	130
Indwelling Catheters	134
How to Put in an Indwelling Catheter (Foley)—Male	135
How to Put in an Indwelling Catheter (Foley)—Female	137
How to Do a Suprapubic Catheterization—Male or Female	139
How to Apply a Condom	141
How to Apply a Self-Adhesive Condom	144
How to Apply a Two-Piece Self-Adhesive Condom	146
Helpful Hints about Condoms	149

Common Urological Problems: Leakage Around a Catheter	150
Common Urological Problems: Frequent Catheter Changes	151
Leg/Bedside Drainage Bag Care	154
Selecting Proper Urological Supplies	155

Bowel Management

Bowel Program: Overview	157
Ensuring Success of Your Bowel Program	160
Digital Stimulation	163
Constipation	165
How to Give a Suppository	168

Hygiene

General Hygiene	170
Male Hygiene	171
Female Hygiene	172

BLADDER MANAGEMENT

Bladder Program: Overview

HOW YOUR BODY MAKES, STORES, AND RELEASES URINE[*]

When you eat and drink, your body absorbs the liquid. The kidneys filter out waste products from the body fluids and make urine.

Urine travels down tubes called ureters into a muscular sac called the urinary bladder, which stores the urine.

When you are ready to go to the bathroom, your brain tells your system to relax.

Urine travels out of your bladder through a tube called the urethra. You release urine by relaxing the urethral sphincter and contracting the bladder muscles. The urethral sphincter is a group of muscles that tightens to hold urine in and loosens to let it out.

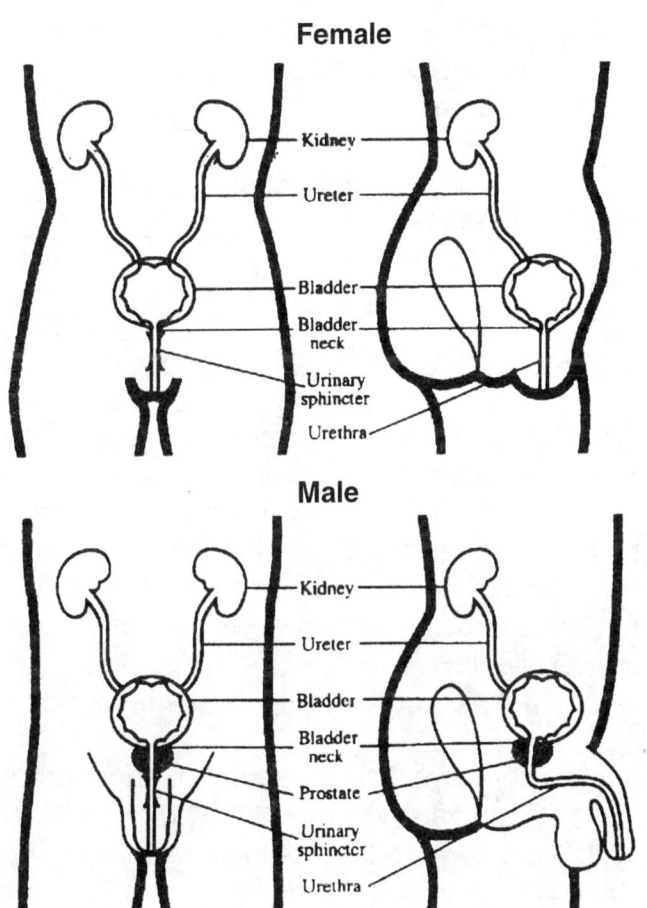

continues

continued

WHEN SOMETHING GOES WRONG**

Any illness or injury that affects the nervous system in your body also can affect the way your bowel and bladder work, resulting in a "neurogenic" condition.

The reflexes dealing with sexual activity as well as with the bowel and bladder are supplied from the reflex arc in the spinal cord near the bottom of your spine. When a signal goes to the reflex arc announcing that it is time for the bowel or bladder to empty, the signal is also sent up the spinal cord to the brain, the body's "big computer." When the signal has reached the arc, a message *can* be sent back to the sphincter muscles telling them to relax and let the waste out of the body. This happens *unless* the brain *overrides* the release signal with a different message.

When you have an injury to the spinal cord, the path of communication between the brain and any part of the body *below* the injury has been interrupted. Therefore, where the spinal injury is located will determine how your bowel and bladder will function.

If the communication break is *above* the reflex arc, then you will have a "reflex" or "spastic" bladder. That means that messages can still get through from the bladder to the arc, and some messages are sent back to the bladder telling it to empty. However, the link to the brain is gone, and those *overriding* messages cannot get through. You cannot control when or where the bladder will empty.

If your injury is low enough in the spine to have damaged the reflex arc itself, you have a "nonreflex" or "flaccid" bladder. That means messages cannot get through from the bladder to the spine and back *or* to the brain. Your body will not even know when the bladder is full and needs to be emptied.

WHY HAVE A BLADDER PROGRAM?**

A normal bladder empties itself of all urine. After a spinal cord injury, however, or after an illness or disease resulting in neurological damage, you may not be able to feel fullness. You may not be able to tighten or relax the sphincter muscle at the base of the bladder that controls the exit of urine from your body. If some urine does come out, the bladder may not get it all out, leaving "residual." In some cases, the bladder may not empty of any urine at all.

When the bladder does not work properly, there is the danger of urine stagnating in the bladder, getting infected, and backing up into the kidneys. If this happens, the kidneys will not be able to do their job of getting waste out of the blood. Leaving waste in your body can make you very ill (sepsis and uremia).

Based on your specific injury and your particular needs, a bladder program will be designed for you at the rehabilitation center. The primary purpose of the program will be to get the urine out of your body and then to help you regulate yourself, with the eventual goal of restoring "continence," which simply means putting you in control of elimination. Your bladder training program will be successful when you are able to use specific methods to empty the bladder without "incontinence," or loss of control.

continues

continued

DIFFERENT NEEDS AT DIFFERENT TIMES[**]

Just as no two patients are the same, individual patients' needs will vary at different times during the rehabilitation process. This is certainly true of your bladder program.

Immediately after your injury or illness, an internal catheter was probably put into your bladder. This catheter had a small balloon on the end that was blown up with a small amount of water to act as an anchor and keep it in the bladder. During that time you depended on the internal or "indwelling" catheter to drain the urine out of the body.

Later, you may have been taught intermittent catheterization so that you had some control over when the urine was removed from your bladder.

As you progress with your bladder program, you will be taught other methods of attempting to eliminate urine. Be aware that you may require not just one but a combination of methods, including catheterization, at different times during and following rehabilitation. The methods prescribed for you will depend on your condition and needs at a particular time. To help you understand, let's look in more detail at the phases the paralyzed bladder goes through.

Flaccid Bladder Phase

The word "flaccid" means "soft or flabby," and "limp or asleep." That is an accurate description of the bladder in the phase that occurs immediately following spinal injury or illness. You may also hear the bladder in this phase called "nonreflex," "autonomous," or "atonia." While the flaccid phase may vary in length of time for different individuals, if the spinal injury has occurred in the lower thoracic or lumbosacral area (at L2 or below), the motor branch of the reflex arc may be injured and the bladder will remain flaccid.

In the bladder that is flaccid, the reflex may be sluggish or absent, and there may be no sensation of bladder fullness. The flaccid bladder cannot develop enough pressure to overcome the resistance of the sphincter muscle that keeps urine from flowing out of the body through the urethra. The bladder becomes stretched too far beyond its normal capacity (overdistention), and the stagnant and infected urine may back up through the ureters to the kidneys. When the flaccid bladder is overstretched, or overdistended, the muscle tone of the organ is damaged and may change a partially functioning bladder to one that will not work at all. It is very important not to let the bladder stay distended and to relieve it by catheterization.

A person with a flaccid bladder sometimes may be able to empty it satisfactorily by applying pressure over the bladder area with his or her fist. This is a method called Crede, and it may be taught to you while you are in the rehabilitation center. Be aware, however, that this does not always result in *complete* emptying. Depending on "true residuals" (the amount of urine left in the bladder immediately after Credeing or voiding), you may be advised to catheterize yourself. If your bladder is flaccid, you should never allow more than 400 cc of urine to accumulate in the bladder.

continues

continued

During the flaccid bladder phase, keep in mind this brief checklist:

- Be sure to drink a minimum of three quarts of fluids every 24 hours.
- Keep an accurate fluid intake and output record. This should include:
  - spontaneous voiding (the urine that comes out without any stimulation)
  - triggered or Crede voiding (the urine that comes out from using the Crede method or any other form of stimulation you are taught to provoke a reflex action) Only use the Crede method if recommended by your physician.
  - residual (the amount of urine left in the bladder immediately after spontaneous or triggered voiding has occurred)
- Check urine daily for odor, eggshell-like particles, and color. Urine should be clear and light in color.
- Promptly report any sign of infection to your doctor.

Spastic Bladder Phase

If your reflex arc is still intact (or your spinal injury is above T12), you may have a spastic bladder. You may also hear this phase referred to as "automatic" or "reflex." When the spastic bladder is full, the sphincter muscle automatically relaxes and the bladder empties itself, but this type of bladder is unreliable. When it will empty is uncertain, and urination often may be in small amounts.

Just as the muscles of the legs may have spasms, the muscle of the spastic bladder may respond to any mild stimulation. In fact, spasms of the leg muscles may stimulate spasms of the bladder, or vice versa. The spastic bladder may contract once a certain degree of filling is reached and empty again spontaneously. The presence of a small amount of urine in the bladder, a small stone, or a mild infection may cause it to tighten or spasm.

If it can be established for sure that spasms are *not* forcing urine back up through the ureters to the kidneys, a male patient may be able to wear a condom catheter attached to a leg bag to keep himself dry when he is out of bed. He may use a bedside drainage bag when he is in bed. For female patients, a catheter may be necessary to stay dry, since there is no satisfactory external apparatus for the female. Sometimes, the use of absorbent pads and waterproofed pants is satisfactory. Fortunately, the prolonged use of a catheter is less troublesome for women than for men, because the female urethra is shorter and straighter. Some female patients may be able to manage their bladder with a combination of intermittent catheterization and medications that help them retain urine.

One of the goals for a patient in the spastic bladder phase is to experiment and find ways to trigger the reflex arc by stimulation. Some of the ways that have been found to be effective are:

- massaging or tapping the abdomen
- leaning forward to change position
- doing push-ups from the chair

continues

continued

- pulling the pubic hair
- pinching or stroking the inner thigh
- inserting a gloved finger into the rectum

It is important to remember that when you have found a successful method of stimulation, the spastic bladder will contract and maintain a fairly adequate contraction. Once the contraction has started, there is no way to stop the reflex emptying of the bladder, so be sure you are on a toilet or have a receptacle ready before starting stimulation.

Notes:

[*]Source: "Urinary Incontinence in Adults: A Patient's Guide," Clinical Practice Guidelines, U.S. Department of Health and Human Services, Public Health Service, Agency for Health Care Policy and Research, Rockville, Maryland, 1992.
[**]Source: John C. Whitaker Rehabilitation Medicine Centers of Forsyth Memorial Hospital, Winston-Salem, North Carolina.

Bladder Program Checklist

The following tips will be helpful in your bladder program:

- You must drink the prescribed volume of liquid daily to ensure a good output of urine. This will help to prevent kidney infection and the formation of stones. A good beginning is to drink a glass of liquid every hour.
- Attempt voiding, beginning with every hour. Apply gentle pressure over the bladder area or any of the other methods of stimulation you have been taught and have found to be effective.
- Observe if your bladder capacity is small. If it is, you will need to void more often to prevent urinary incontinence.
- Be aware of any sensations that may occur before the act of voiding. Make note of any of these and tell your doctor:
  —chilliness
  —sweating
  —a vague full feeling
  —muscular twitching
  —flushing or feeling warm
- The sitting position is helpful when trying to void. After you are seated, bend forward in a slow, rhythmic fashion. This creates pressure on the bladder.
- Try to get relaxed. You may find that reading or listening to water running will help you.
- If you have a flaccid bladder, begin to limit your liquid intake in the early evening (around 6:00 P.M.) This will help to eliminate having to catheterize during the night. Make a routine of emptying your bladder as the last thing you do before bed.

Notes:

Source: John C. Whitaker Rehabilitation Medicine Centers of Forsyth Memorial Hospital, Winston-Salem, North Carolina.

Common Bladder Problems

URINARY TRACT INFECTION*

A urinary tract infection, or UTI, is an infection in the bladder or other part of the urinary tract.

Signs of a UTI

- Cloudy urine
- Foul-smelling urine
- Fever
- Sweating and chills
- Voiding more often or incontinence (different than usual)
- More spasms
- Bloody urine (urine will be pink, red, or rusty in color)
- Leaking around Foley catheter (due to bladder spasms)
- Burning feeling when you void.

A bladder infection can spread into your kidneys, causing an infection called pyelonephritis. Signs of a kidney infection are chills, fever, back pain, pain in your scrotum or inner thighs, nausea, and vomiting.

What to Do

- Call your doctor so you can get a prescription for an antibiotic. You will need to give your doctor a urine sample.
- Drink at least two to three glasses **more** of fluid a day.
- Take all the medication your doctor orders even if you feel better. This is important so that all of the infection will be gone.
- The doctor may want another urine sample to make sure the infection is gone.

Prevention

- Drink enough fluids, at least six to eight glasses per day (if you have a Foley, at least eight glasses per day). Fluids flush your kidneys and bladder. This helps to prevent bacteria from collecting and growing.
- Use a clean catheter every time you cath.
- Be sure to wash your hands and the opening of your urethra, along with the area around it, before and after you cath.
- Give a urine sample to your doctor when he or she orders one or when you think you have an infection.

It is very important to prevent infections and to treat them early. Severe infections can damage the kidneys and cause kidney failure, which can cause death.

OVERFULL BLADDER**

The bladder is a muscular organ that is like a balloon. When the bladder gets over-

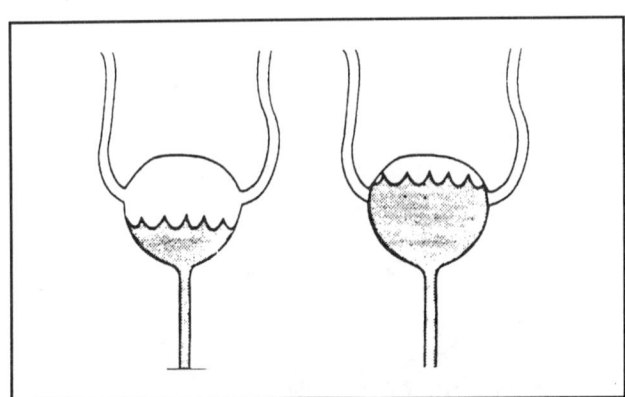

Full Bladder

continues

continued

full, it will become overstretched. A continuously stretched bladder will lose its ability to contract well. The bladder will become thickened and flabby. This also means that blood flow to the muscle wall is decreased, which makes the bladder more likely to become infected. Urine that stays in the bladder too long causes germs to grow, and this leads to infections. Infections can travel up to the kidneys and can also cause stones to form in the bladder and kidneys. Stones can block the flow of urine out of the bladder and can interfere with the filtering system in the kidneys.

Causes

- Not doing intermittent catheterizations (ICs) on time
- Not emptying bladder when doing IC

Signs

- Increased amount of urine when you do your IC (over 500 cc)

What to Do

- Do ICs on time.
- Be sure to totally empty the bladder when doing an IC.
- Limit fluid intake after last IC of the day or before bedtime.

Prevention

- Empty the bladder on a regular schedule and empty completely.
- Call your doctor or the rehabilitation center if you reflex more often with small amounts of urine.

BLADDER OR KIDNEY STONES**

Bladder or kidney stones can cause serious problems. Stones that form in the bladder can block the flow of urine. Stones in the kidneys can interfere with the filtering of the blood and with drainage of urine to the bladder.

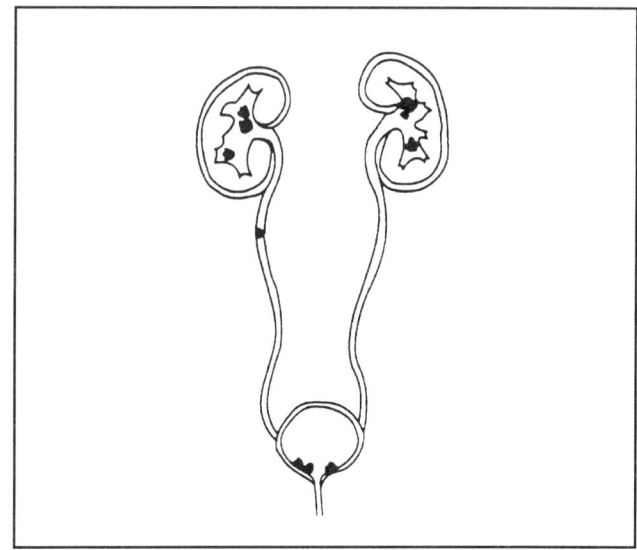

Bladder and Kidney Stones

Causes

- Not doing ICs on time
- Not doing ICs correctly
- Urine sitting in the bladder too long
- Many urinary tract infections
- Not enough exercise
- Backup of urine into the kidneys
- Not drinking enough water or other liquids

Signs

- Blood in the urine
- Increased spasms
- Increased sweating
- Seeing stones passed in the urine
- Many urinary tract infections

continues

continued

- Pain in the lower back or abdomen (may be present if spinal cord injury is incomplete)

What to Do

- Call the doctor right away if you think you might have a bladder or kidney stone.

Prevention

- Do ICs correctly and on time.
- Drink six to eight glasses of water every day.
- Exercise as much as possible every day.
- Have an intravenous pyelogram done every two years until the doctor decides otherwise.

REFLUX**

Reflux is the back flow of urine into the ureters and the kidneys.

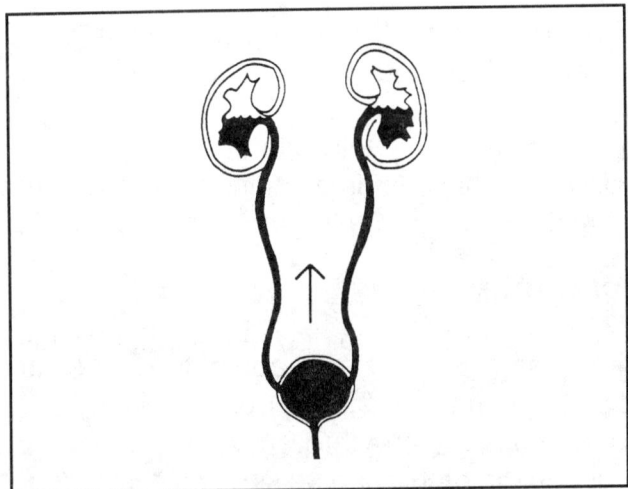

Urine Backing up into the Kidneys

Causes

- An overfull bladder (from not emptying completely and on time)
- Sphincter dyssynergia, which increases pressure in the bladder

Signs

- Many urinary tract infections with fever

What to Do

- Call the doctor right away.

Prevention

- Do ICs on time and correctly.
- Have annual checkups.

Remember, prevention is the key.

HYDRONEPHROSIS**

Chronic reflux of urine into the kidneys causes a condition called hydronephrosis. Hydronephrosis means water (urine) on the kidneys. This may lead to severe infections of the urinary system and kidney failure. The damage may be permanent. Taking good care of the urinary system and preventing infections is the key to healthy kidneys.

SPHINCTER DYSSYNERGIA

When there is bladder-sphincter dyssynergia, the sphincter does not relax when the bladder is squeezing. This blocks the flow of urine and may cause the urine to back up through the ureters into the kidneys (reflux).

---

*Source: *Spinal Cord Injury Manual*, University of Rochester, Strong Memorial Hospital Rehabilitation Unit, Rochester, New York, © 1986, rev. 1994.
**Source: Donna Schachtel, et al., *Key to Independence Personal Care Manual*, Shepherd Spinal Center, Atlanta, Georgia, © 1989. To order a complete version of the manual, contact the Shepherd Center at 404-350-7361.

Common Urinary Tests

CULTURE AND SENSITIVITY*

The culture and sensitivity (C&S) test shows the number and type of germs growing in the urine. It will also show which antibiotic will kill the germs.

URODYNAMICS*

A urodynamics test shows how much urine the bladder holds and how much urine will cause the bladder to reflex. It shows if the sphincter is working with the bladder as it should.

RENAL SCAN AND ULTRASOUND**

The scan and ultrasound help your doctor check for any problems or changes in your urinary tract. Some examples of these are kidney or bladder stones and damage in the kidneys, ureters, or bladder.

The scan is done by first putting a dye into a vein. Your body gets rid of the dye through your kidneys. As the dye goes through your kidneys, it can be seen on X-ray. The scan lets your doctor know what your kidneys look like, how well they are working, and their blood supply.

The ultrasound is done by using sound waves. The sound waves bounce off your kidneys and bladder. This lets your doctor know what your urinary tract looks like.

The renal scan and ultrasound are usually done before you are discharged home, to check your urinary tract. After discharge, these tests are done when you are having problems or if your doctor feels your urinary tract should be checked again. The doctor will be able to tell if what these tests show is new or if it was shown on the test done before discharge. This can help your doctor find the cause of your urinary tract problem.

A renal scan and ultrasound are more likely than an intravenous pyelogram (IVP) to be done to check your urinary tract. This is because you usually do not have to do anything special before the scan and ultrasound and because some people have problems with the IVP dye (see "IVP").

INTRAVENOUS PYELOGRAM**

An IVP is a test that helps your doctor check for any changes in size or shape of the kidney or for problems, such as kidney or bladder stones and damage in the kidneys or ureters.

To do the test, a dye is put into a vein. Your body gets rid of the dye through your kidneys. As the dye goes through your kidneys and the rest of your urinary tract, it can be seen on X-ray. Your bowels must be empty for the test.

Your doctor will tell you what you need to do before having the test. Your doctor may choose to check your urinary tract by doing an IVP instead of a renal scan and ultrasound. If so, the IVP

continues

continued

will be done before you are discharged home. After discharge, an IVP is done when you are having problems or if your doctor feels your urinary tract should be checked again. The doctor will be able to tell if what the X-ray shows is new or if it was there before. This can help your doctor find the cause of your urinary tract problem.

Some people have problems with the IVP dye (these problems do not last long). The dye may cause you to feel hot all over, nauseated, nervous, and headachy.

CYSTOSCOPY[**]

Cystoscopy lets your doctor look inside your bladder. To do this, the doctor uses a cystoscope. The cystoscope is about the size of a catheter (but longer) and has a light on the end of it. It is put into the bladder through the urethra.

CYSTOMETRICS[**]

Cystometrics is done to see if the muscles of your bladder and urethra are working, and how well they are working.

To do the test, a catheter is put into your bladder. After your bladder is empty, a gas is slowly put into your bladder.

Any muscle action in the bladder or urethra will show up on the special machine that is used. Signals of muscle action are picked up by a very thin needle that is put into a muscle near your rectum. This needle is hooked to the machine by a wire. This machine lets the doctor see when there is a muscle action and it can be recorded on paper.

[*]Source: Donna Schachtel, et al., *Key to Independence Personal Care Manual*, Shepherd Spinal Center, Atlanta, Georgia, © 1989. To order a complete version of the manual, contact the Shepherd Center at 404-350-7361.

[**]Source: *Spinal Cord Injury Manual*, University of Rochester, Strong Memorial Hospital Rehabilitation Unit, Rochester, New York, © 1986, rev. 1994.

Intermittent Catheterization

WHAT IS INTERMITTENT CATHETERIZATION?

Intermittent catheterization (IC) is draining the bladder at set times. It almost always is used to empty a nonreflex or flaccid bladder but may be used to help drain a reflex or spastic bladder. Intermittent catheterization is putting a rubber tube through the urethra to drain urine from the bladder. Once the bladder is drained, the tube is taken out.

An intermittent catheter looks like this:

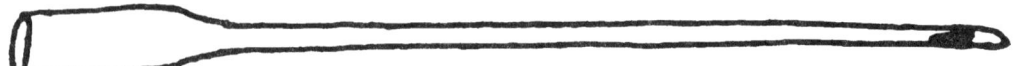

WHY USE INTERMITTENT CATHETERIZATION?

Intermittent catheterization can be used for treating urinary retention. Intermittent catheterization is used because:

- It allows the bladder to fill and empty as before.
- It maintains the muscle tone in the bladder.

IMPORTANT

- Catheterize regularly (usually every four to six hours).
- Drink the amount of fluid prescribed by your doctor.

HOW IS INTERMITTENT CATHETERIZATION DONE?

There are two ways to do intermittent catheterization:

1. Sterile
2. Clean

Source: Kelly B. Wascher, ed., *Patient Education and Discharge Planning Manual for Rehabilitation,* St. Joseph Rehabilitation Hospital and Outpatient Center, Aspen Publishers, Inc., © 1995.

How to Do a Clean IC—Male

SUPPLIES NEEDED

- Catheter
- K-Y jelly
- Soapy washcloth and wet cloth
- Handiwipes or Babywipes (use only when soap, water, and washcloths are not available)
- IC bag or container
- Clean paper towel or hand towel (See Figure 1.)

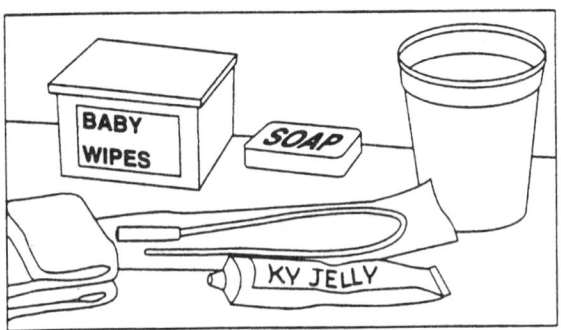

Figure 1. Urinary Supplies

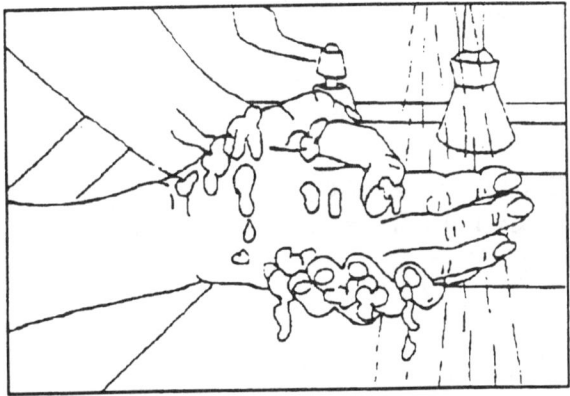

Figure 2. Washing Your Hands

WHAT TO DO

1. Wash your hands with soap and water. Handwashing is one of most important steps in the prevention of bladder infections. (See Figure 2.)
2. Prepare all needed supplies.
3. Place catheter, K-Y jelly, IC bag or container, Handiwipes, the soapy cloth, and the wet cloth on a clean paper towel or hand towel. Always have your supplies ready before beginning an IC (See Figure 3.)

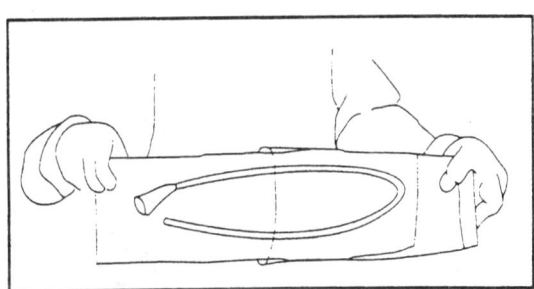

Figure 3. Opening a New Catheter

4. Open the K-Y jelly and squeeze 1 inch onto the tip of the catheter. Do not let the tube touch the catheter. (See Figure 4.)

continues

continued

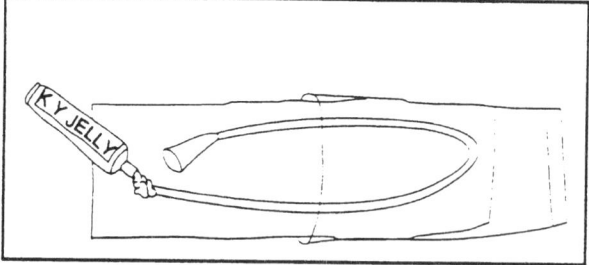

Figure 4. Lubricating the Catheter

5. Connect the IC bag to the catheter or place the container within reach.
6. Wash penis with soapy cloth and then rinse penis with the wet cloth. Pull the foreskin back and clean the head of the penis well. (See Figure 5.)

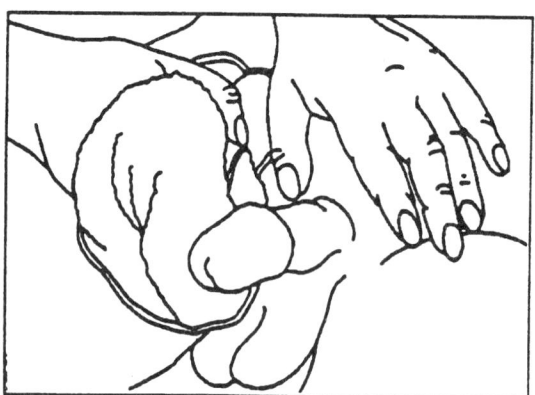

Figure 5. Washing the Penis

7. Wash your hands with a clean, soapy washcloth or a Handiwipe. (See Figure 6.)

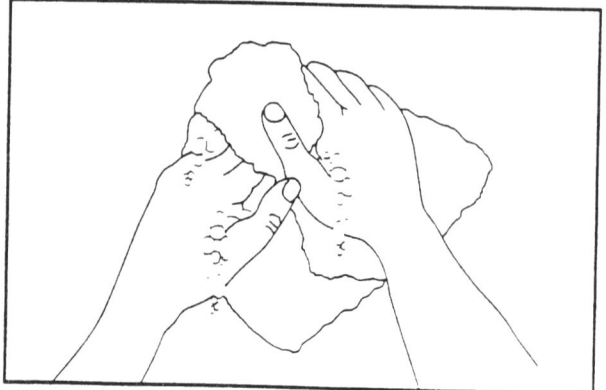

Figure 6. Washing Your Hands

8. Pick up the catheter directly behind the jelly about 2 to 3 inches from the tip. When using a container, make sure the other end of the catheter is in the container. (See Figure 7.)

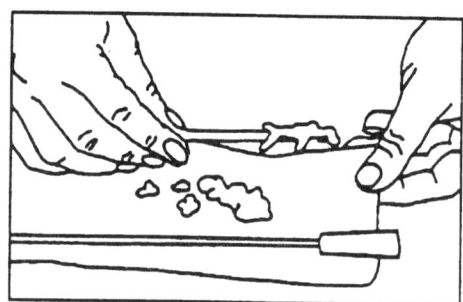

Figure 7. Picking Up the Catheter

9. Hold penis straight up with the other hand and insert the catheter. (See Figure 8.)

continues

continued

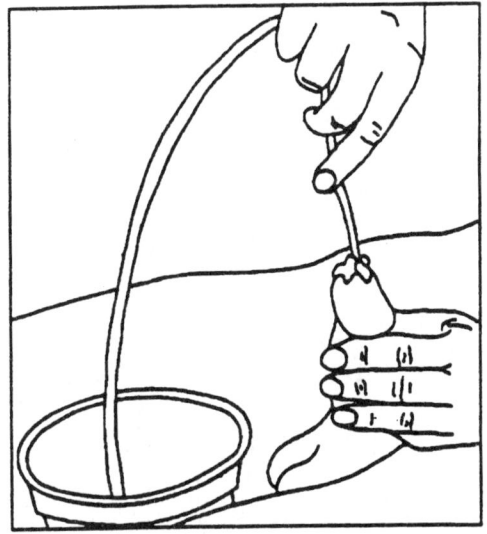

Figure 8. Inserting the Catheter

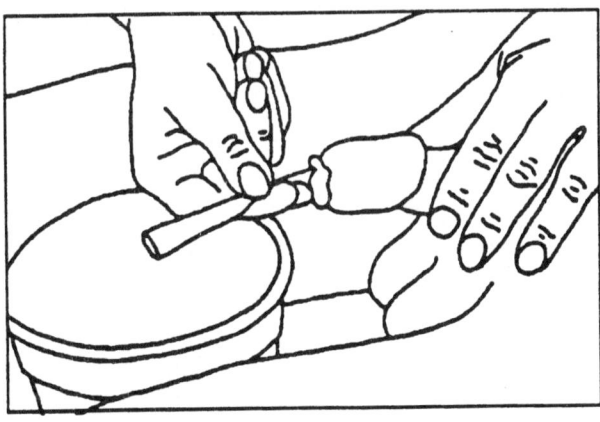

Figure 9. Insert the Catheter until Urine Flows

10. As the catheter is pushed down, pull up on the penis with the other hand. This straightens out the passageway to the bladder, allowing the catheter to pass more easily. It will also help prevent damage to the urethra and sphincter.
11. Keep pushing the catheter in until urine flows through the catheter. Then insert the catheter 2 to 3 inches more and allow urine to drain. The bladder will empty better by letting the penis come down and by holding the catheter in place. (See Figure 9.)
12. When the urine flow stops, gently push down on the bladder area. Pushing down on the bladder may be necessary to completely empty the bladder. Withdraw the catheter slowly. Removing the catheter slowly helps to empty the bladder completely. This will prevent urine from remaining in the bladder. Urine left in the bladder can cause an infection. Remove the catheter when the urine flow has stopped. (See Figure 10.)

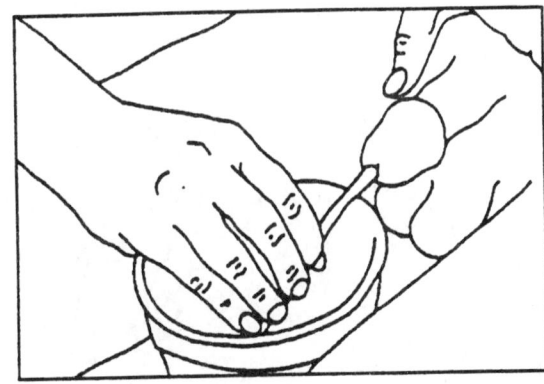

Figure 10. Press Gently on the Bladder

continues

13. While you are at the rehabilitation facility, a new catheter is used for each IC. After discharge, a catheter can be used for seven days. After each use, clean the catheter with soap and water. Rinse with clean water, air dry, and store the catheter in an envelope or paper bag (not a plastic bag). (See Figure 11.)

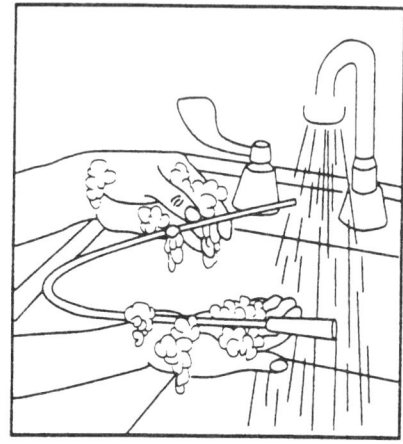

Figure 11. Washing the Catheter

14. Wash the penis with a soapy cloth and rinse with a wet cloth. Dry penis well. Remember to pull the foreskin back down over the head of the penis. (See Figure 12.)

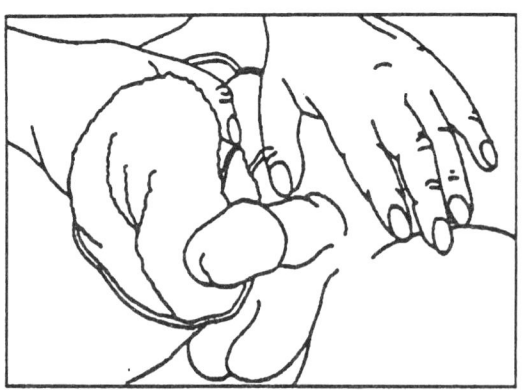

Figure 12. Washing the Penis

15. Empty the IC bag or container. Rinse it out and clean with bleach water (1 tablespoon of bleach to 1 quart of water). (See Figure 13.)

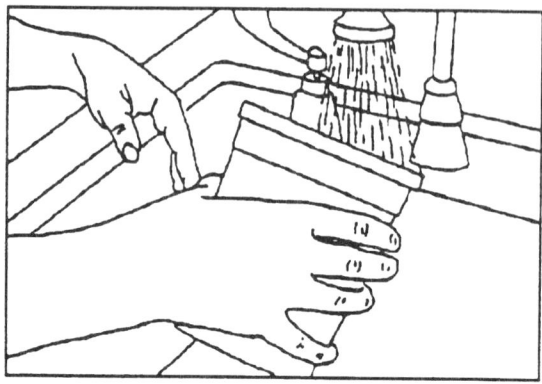

Figure 13. Washing the Urine Container

16. Wash your hands. (See Figure 14.)

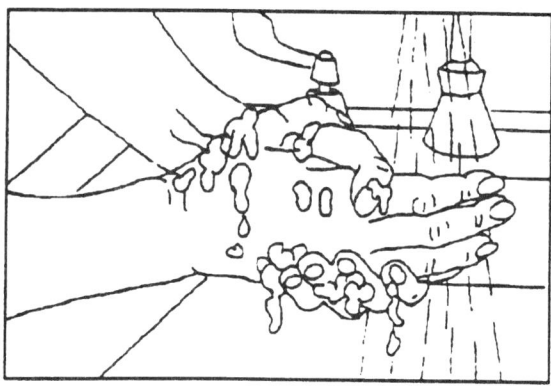

Figure 14. Washing Your Hands

continues

continued

> **KEY POINTS**
>
> 1. If you drop your catheter, clean it with soap and water before using again.
> 2. If a spasm occurs while doing the IC, stop and wait for the spasm to pass before pushing the catheter any farther.
> 3. If the catheter will not go in easily, call your doctor or rehabilitation facility. Do not force the catheter into the bladder.

Notes:

Source: Donna Schachtel, et al., *Key to Independence Personal Care Manual*, Shepherd Spinal Center, Atlanta, Georgia, © 1989. To order a complete version of the manual, contact the Shepherd Center at 404-350-7361.

How to Do a Clean IC—Female

SUPPLIES NEEDED

- Catheter
- Mirror (if needed)
- K-Y jelly
- Handiwipes or Babywipes (use only when soap, water, and washcloths are not available)
- Soapy washcloth and wet cloth
- IC bag or container
- Clean paper towel or hand towel (See Figure 1.)

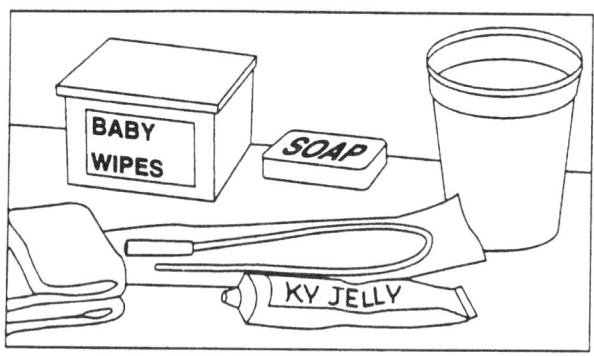

Figure 1. Urinary Supplies

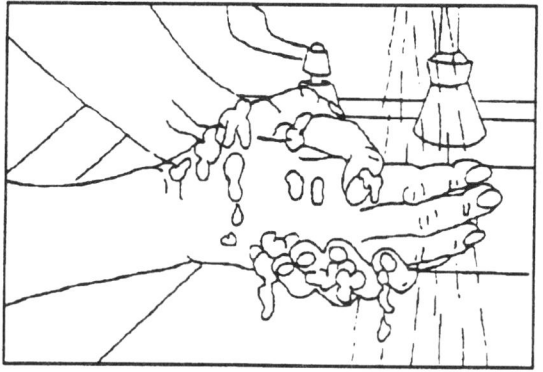

Figure 2. Wash Your Hands

What to do

1. Wash your hands with soap and water. Handwashing is one of the most important steps in the prevention of bladder infections. (See Figure 2.)
2. Prepare all needed supplies.
3. Place catheter, K-Y jelly, IC bag or container, Handiwipes, the soapy cloth, and the wet cloth on a clean paper towel or hand towel.

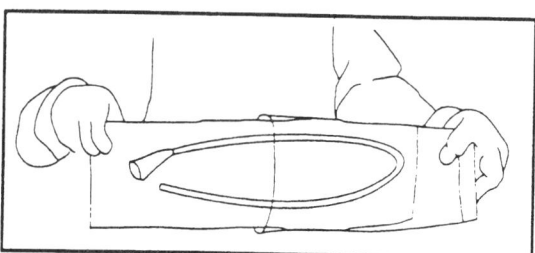

Figure 3. Opening a New Catheter

4. Open the K-Y jelly and squeeze 1 inch onto the tip of the catheter. (See Figure 4.)

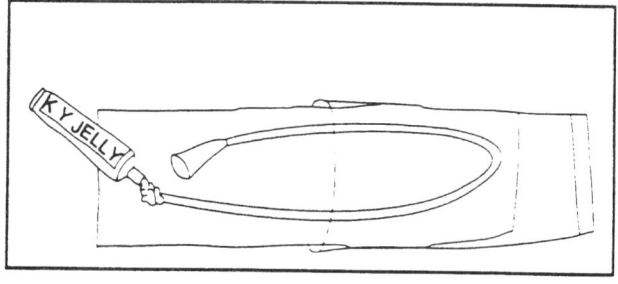

Figure 4. Lubricating the Catheter

5. Place IC container within reach of catheter or connect catheter to IC bag.
6. Wash around the urinary opening with the soapy washcloth and rinse off the soap

continues

continued

with the wet cloth. Wash from above the urinary opening to the area above the anus. Always wash from the front to the back. This prevents any germs from the rectal area from entering the urethra. (See Figure 5.)

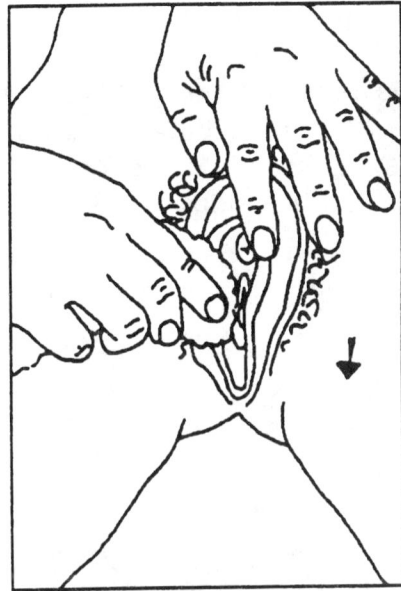

Figure 5. Cleaning the Urethra

7. With one hand, spread the labia apart with your ring finger and pointer finger. Locate the urethral opening with the finger located between the ring finger and the pointer finger. The third finger serves as a landmark for inserting the catheter. (See Figures 6 and 7.)

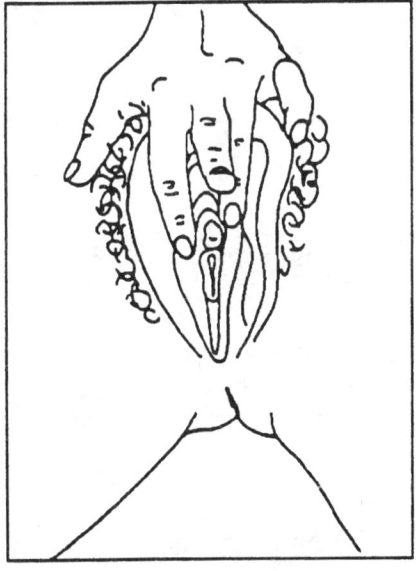

Figure 6. Spreading the Labia

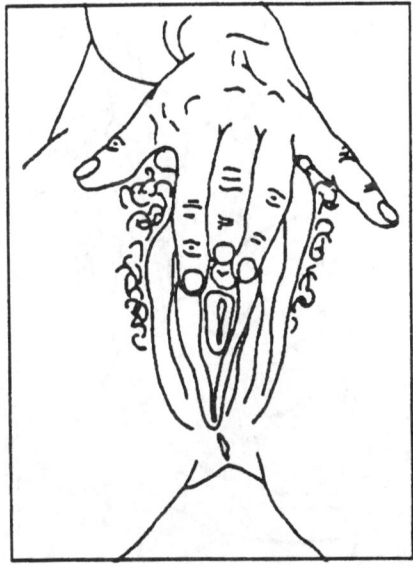

Figure 7. Finding the Urethra

8. With your other hand, pick up the catheter by the clear tip directly behind the K-Y jelly. If using a container, make sure the

continues

continued

other end of the catheter is in the container. (See Figure 8.)

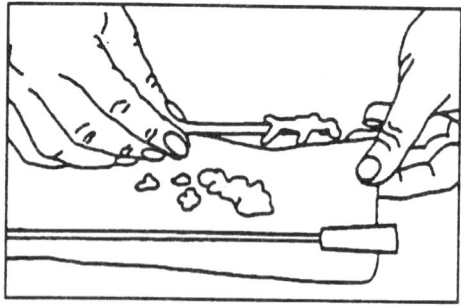

Figure 8. Picking Up the Catheter

9. Insert the catheter into the urethral opening until urine begins to flow. (See Figure 9.)

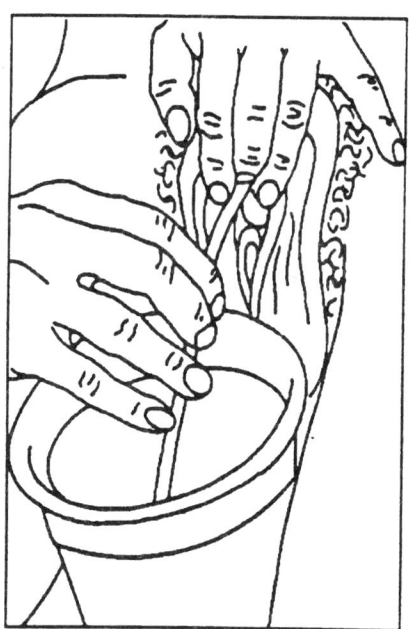

Figure 9. Inserting the Catheter

10. Insert the catheter another 2 to 3 inches and allow urine to drain. Hold the catheter in place. This will help the bladder empty better.

11. When urine flow stops, gently push down on the bladder area with your free hand. Pushing down on the bladder may be necessary to completely empty the bladder. Withdraw the catheter slowly. Removing the catheter slowly helps to empty the bladder completely. This prevents urine from being left in the bladder. Urine left in the bladder can cause an infection. Remove the catheter when urine flow has stopped. (See Figure 10.)

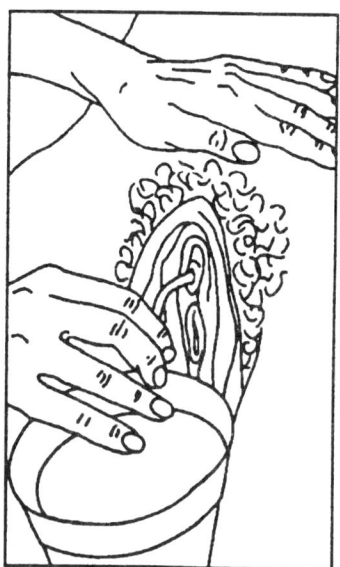

Figure 10. Press Gently on the Bladder

12. While you are at the rehabilitation facility a new catheter will be used for each IC. After discharge, a catheter can be used for seven days. After each use, clean the catheter with soap and water. Rinse with clean water, air dry, and store the cathe-

continues

continued

ter in an envelope or paper bag (not a plastic bag). (See Figure 11.)

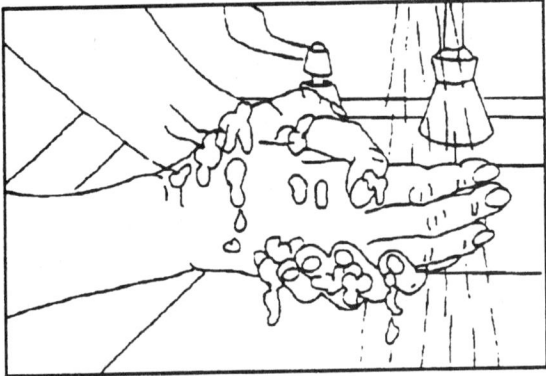

Figure 11. Washing the Catheter

13. Wash around uretheral opening with a soapy cloth and rinse with a wet cloth. (See Figure 12.)

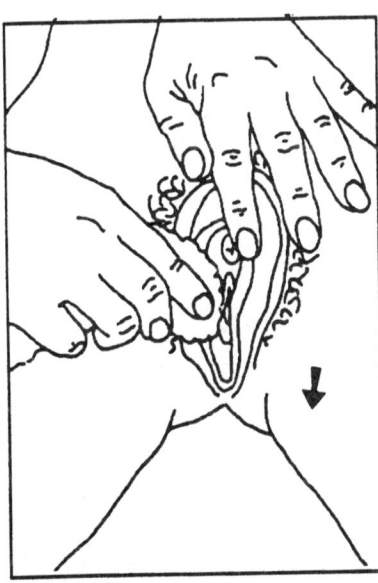

Figure 12. Cleaning the Urethra

14. Empty IC bag or container. Rinse it out and clean it with bleach water (1 tablespoon of bleach to 1 quart of water).
15. Wash your hands. (Figure 13.)

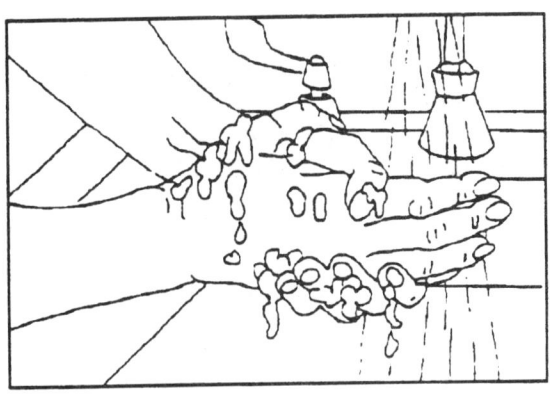

Figure 13. Washing Your Hands

KEY POINTS

1. If you drop your catheter or insert it into the vagina by mistake, start over and use a clean catheter. You may want to leave the first catheter in the vagina to avoid inserting the new catheter there.
2. If a spasm occurs while doing an IC, stop and wait for the spasm to pass before pushing the catheter any farther.
3. If the catheter will not go in easily, call your doctor or the rehabilitation facility. Do not force the catheter into the bladder.

Source: Donna Schachtel, et al., *Key to Independence Personal Care Manual*, Shepherd Spinal Center, Atlanta, Georgia, © 1989. To order a complete version of the manual, contact the Shepherd Center at 404-350-7361.

Indwelling Catheters

CHARACTERISTICS

- Indwelling catheters are used for males and females.
- The catheter is left in the bladder and drains the bladder continuously.
- Balloon sizes are:
  - 5 cc (filled with 10 cc sterile water)
  - 30 cc (filled with 30 cc sterile water)
- Types of material include:
  - latex catheters with coating
  - all-silicone catheters

TYPES OF INDWELLING CATHETERS

Foley

The catheter goes into the bladder through the urethra. A Foley catheter is used early after a spinal cord injury. It can also be used for females who have a reflex bladder or who are unable to do ICs. If a Foley is worn long term, then a leg strap is necessary to keep the catheter in place.

Suprapubic

The catheter goes in through the abdomen into the bladder. A suprapubic catheter is used when some problem makes it impossible to enter the bladder through the urethra.

Notes:

Source: Donna Schachtel, et al., *Key to Independence Personal Care Manual,* Shepherd Spinal Center, Atlanta, Georgia, © 1989. To order a complete version of the manual, contact the Shepherd Center at 404-350-7361.

How to Put in an Indwelling Catheter (Foley)—Male

SUPPLIES NEEDED

- Indwelling catheter tray with a 10 cc balloon (The most common size adult catheter is a 16 fr.)
- A syringe to deflate the old balloon
- Soapy washcloth and wet cloth

WHAT TO DO

1. Wash your hands with soap and water.
2. Prepare all needed supplies.
3. Lie flat on back with legs flat.
4. If there is already a catheter in place, remove it by deflating the balloon. Attach syringe to end of catheter not attached to drainage bag. Remove water from the balloon using the syringe. Gently remove the old catheter.
5. Wash penis with the soapy washcloth and rinse with the wet cloth.
6. Wash your hands again.
7. Open the indwelling catheter tray and set up supplies.
   a. Place pad between legs and under hips.
   b. Put on gloves if not a self-catheterization.
   c. Wet cotton balls with Betadine.
   d. Remove the plastic cover from the catheter and squeeze 1 inch of K-Y jelly onto the catheter tip.
   e. Remove the rubber cap from the syringe with water in it.
   f. Connect the catheter to the drainage bag in the kit.
8. Hold the penis with the other hand. This hand is now considered "dirty." Do not touch catheter with this hand.
9. Squeeze cotton balls to get rid of excess Betadine. Clean the urinary opening with the cotton balls soaked with Betadine. Use one cotton ball per wipe. Wipe from the tip of the penis to the shaft of the penis. Never reuse the cotton ball.
10. Insert the catheter slowly and gently into the urethral opening until you see urine flow into the catheter. Insert the catheter to the "Y" section of the catheter.
11. Blow up the balloon with the full 10 cc of sterile water from the syringe found in the tray.

KEY POINT

Do not blow up the balloon of the catheter until you have urine flowing from the catheter. Flowing urine means the catheter is in the bladder.

---

continues

continued

12. Clean off any Betadine left on the skin. Betadine can irritate the skin.

CATHETER CHANGING SCHEDULE

The changing schedule should be designed to meet individual patient needs. Catheters may stay in for an indefinite period of time as long as encrustations or leaking do not occur. Patients need to discuss this with their doctor.

KEY POINTS

1. **Change the catheter following the schedule given by your doctor.**
2. **Use a size 16 fr. catheter unless the doctor has ordered a different size.**
3. Save the syringe from the tray. Clean it with soap and water. Use this syringe to deflate the balloon of the catheter the next time the catheter is changed.
4. If a spasm occurs while putting in the catheter, stop and wait for the spasm to pass before pushing the catheter any farther.
5. If the catheter will not go in easily, call your doctor or rehabilitation facility. Do not force the catheter in.

Notes:

Source: Donna Schachtel, et al., *Key to Independence Personal Care Manual*, Shepherd Spinal Center, Atlanta, Georgia, © 1989. To order a complete version of the manual, contact the Shepherd Center at 404-350-7361.

How to Put in an Indwelling Catheter (Foley)—Female

SUPPLIES NEEDED

- Indwelling catheter tray with a 10 cc balloon (The most common size adult catheter is a 16 fr.)
- A syringe to deflate the old balloon
- Soapy washcloth and wet cloth

WHAT TO DO

1. Wash your hands with soap and water.
2. Gather supplies.
3. Lie flat on back with legs flat but apart.
4. If there is already a catheter in place, remove it by deflating the balloon. Attach the syringe to the end of the catheter not attached to the drainage bag. Remove water from the balloon using the syringe. Gently remove the old catheter.
5. Wash the urinary opening with the soapy washcloth and rinse with the wet cloth.
6. Wash your hands again.
7. Open the indwelling catheter tray and set up supplies.
   a. Place pad between legs and under hips.
   b. Put on gloves if not a self-catheterization.
   c. Wet cotton balls with Betadine.
   d. Remove plastic cover from syringe and squeeze 1 inch of K-Y jelly on the catheter tip.
   e. Remove rubber cap from syringe with water in it.
   f. Make sure the catheter is connected to drainage bag in the kit.
8. Using the other hand, spread the labia apart so you can find the urinary opening.
9. Clean around the urinary opening with cotton balls soaked in Betadine. Squeeze cotton balls to get rid of excess Betadine. Use each cotton ball only once. Wipe with cotton ball from front (above the opening) to back (below the opening).
10. Insert catheter slowly and gently into the urethral opening. When urine flows into the catheter, insert the catheter two more inches. If you insert the catheter into the vagina by mistake, start over and use a new catheter kit.
11. Blow up the balloon with the full 10 cc of sterile water. **Do not** blow up the balloon until you see urine flowing from the catheter tube. Flowing urine means the catheter is in the bladder.
12. Clean off any Betadine left on the skin. Betadine can irritate the skin.
13. Daily care around the urethra and catheter should be done using plain (unscented) antibacterial soap and water. The area should be dried thoroughly. Avoid using powders. The area will need to be washed after bowel movements.

continues

continued

CATHETER CHANGING SCHEDULE

The changing schedule should be designed to meet individual patient needs. Catheters may stay in for an indefinite period of time as long as encrustations or leaking do not occur. Patients need to discuss this with their doctor.

> **KEY POINTS**
>
> 1. Change the indwelling catheter following the schedule given by your doctor.
> 2. Use a size 16 fr. catheter unless the doctor has ordered a different size.
> 3. Save the syringe from the tray. Clean it with soap and water. Use this syringe to deflate the balloon on the catheter the next time the catheter is changed.
> 4. If a spasm occurs while putting in the catheter, stop and wait for the spasm to pass before pushing the catheter any farther.
> 5. If the catheter will not go in easily, call your doctor or rehabilitation facility. Do not force the catheter in.

Notes:

Source: Donna Schachtel, et al., *Key to Independence Personal Care Manual,* Shepherd Spinal Center, Atlanta, Georgia, © 1989. To order a complete version of the manual, contact the Shepherd Center at 404-350-7361.

How to Do a Suprapubic Catheterization—Male or Female

SUPPLIES NEEDED

- 16 fr. catheter tray or other size catheter and add-a-Foley tray (The doctor may order a different size based on your needs.)
- A syringe to deflate the old balloon
- Soapy washcloth and wet cloth

WHAT TO DO

1. Wash your hands with soap and water.
2. Gather supplies.
3. Lie flat on back with legs flat. This position lines up the opening in the abdomen with the opening in the bladder.
4. Remove the old catheter tube by deflating the balloon with the syringe. Gently remove the old catheter.
5. Remember how much of the old tube was in the bladder. This will help you know how far to insert the new one.
6. Wash around the opening with the soapy washcloth and rinse with the wet cloth.
7. Wash your hands again.
8. Open tray and set up supplies.
   a. Place pad around opening.
   b. Put on gloves if not a self-suprapubic catheterization.
   c. Wet cotton balls with Betadine. Squeeze out excess Betadine.
   d. Remove plastic cover from the catheter and squeeze 1 inch of K-Y jelly on the catheter tip.
   e. Connect catheter tubing to leg bag.
   f. Remove the rubber cap from the syringe that has water in it.
9. Cleanse around the opening site with cotton balls soaked in Betadine. Use each cotton ball only once.
10. Wash your hands.
11. Insert catheter into the opening, push straight. Go in about 4 inches. You should be able to feel the catheter hit the bottom of the bladder.
12. While holding the catheter in place, blow up the balloon with the full 10 cc of sterile water.
13. Gently pull back on the catheter until it stops.
14. Clean off any Betadine left on the skin. Betadine can irritate the skin.
15. Wash your hands.

continues

continued

> **KEY POINTS**
>
> 1. Change the suprapubic catheter once a month, or more often if needed.
> 2. If the catheter tube is not draining well, flush the catheter with tap water. If it still does not drain well, change the catheter. Call your rehabilitation facility if the problem continues.
> 3. At first there may not be any urine in the catheter because the bladder has not had time to collect any more urine since you removed the old one.
> 4. Cover the opening with a piece of gauze.
> 5. Save the syringe from the Foley tray. Clean it with soap and water. Use this syringe to deflate the balloon of the catheter the next time it is changed.

Notes:

Source: Donna Schachtel, et al., *Key to Independence Personal Care Manual,* Shepherd Spinal Center, Atlanta, Georgia, © 1989. To order a complete version of the manual, contact the Shepherd Center at 404-350-7361.

Bladder and Bowel Management 141

How to Apply a Condom

SUPPLIES NEEDED

- Condom (The correct size—small, intermediate, medium, large—is very important. See Figure 1.)
- Condom holder
- Soapy washcloth and wet cloth.

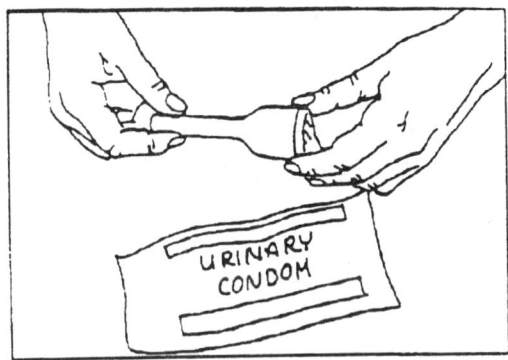

Figure 1. Urinary Condom

WHAT TO DO

1. Gather supplies.
2. Wash hands with soap and water. (See Figure 2.)

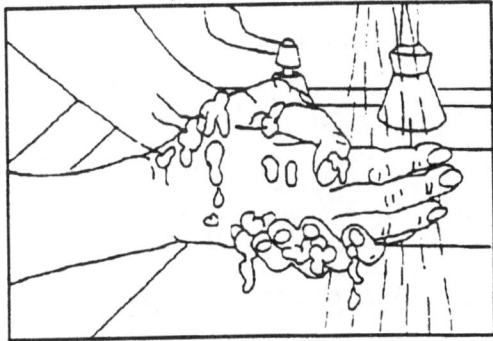

Figure 2. Washing Your Hands

3. Take off old condom. Roll it down the penis. Do not pull the condom off because it may hurt the skin.
4. Wash penis with the soapy washcloth and rinse with the wet cloth. Pull the foreskin back and clean the head of the penis well. (See Figure 3.)

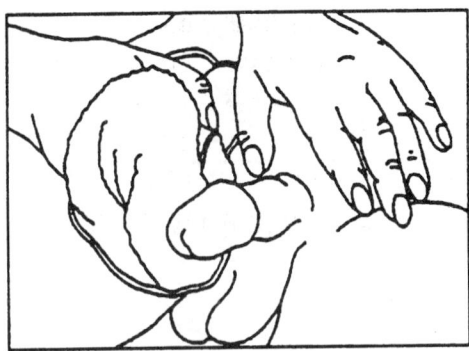

Figure 3. Washing the Penis

5. Dry penis well. Remember to pull the foreskin back down over the head of the penis to prevent swelling of the foreskin.
6. Roll the condom up close to the funnel-shaped end of the condom. (See Figure 4.)

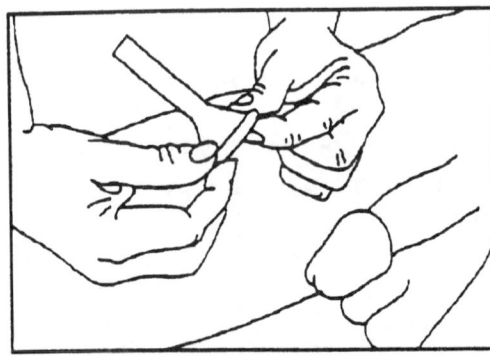

Figure 4. Rolling Up the Condom

continues

continued

7. Place the funnel end of condom on penis. Be sure the head of the penis is close to the funnel tip. (See Figure 5.)

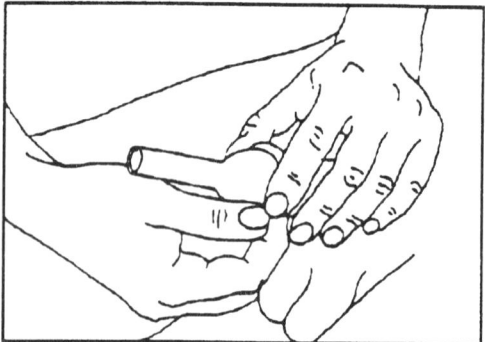

Figure 5. Applying the Condom

8. Roll the condom over the penis to the base of the penis. (See Figure 6.)

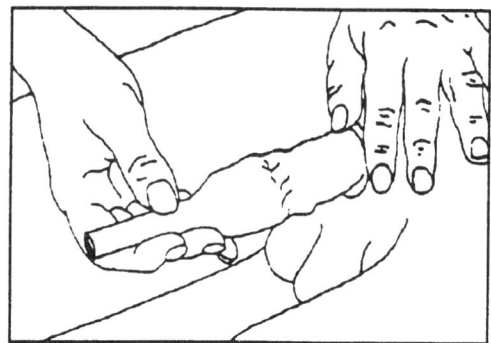

Figure 6. Rolling the Condom

9. Wrap the condom holder about one inch above the base of the penis. (See Figure 7.)

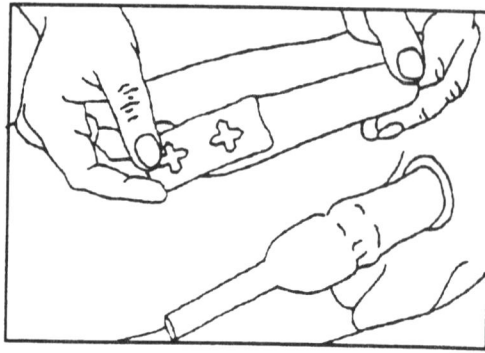

Figure 7. Condom Holder

10. Pull the white strap over one finger to make sure the strap is not too tight. Fasten the white elastic strap to the Velcro (See Figures 8 and 9.)

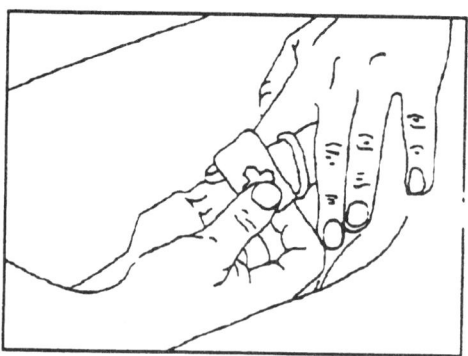

Figure 8. Applying Condom Strap

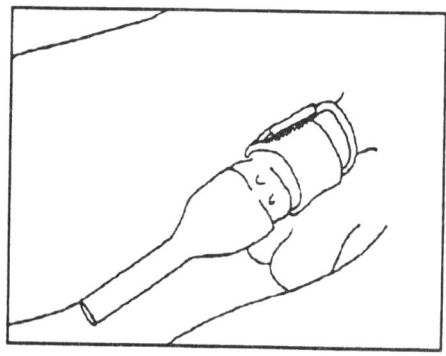

Figure 9. Condom and Condom Holder

continues

continued

11. Connect the condom to a leg bag or a bedside bag. (See Figures 10 and 11.)

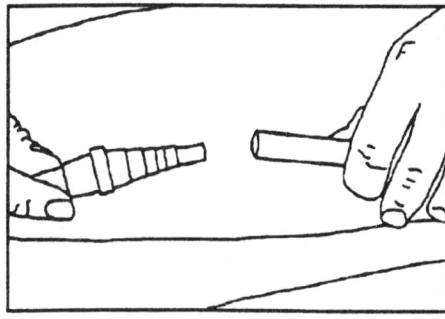

Figure 10. Connect Leg Bag

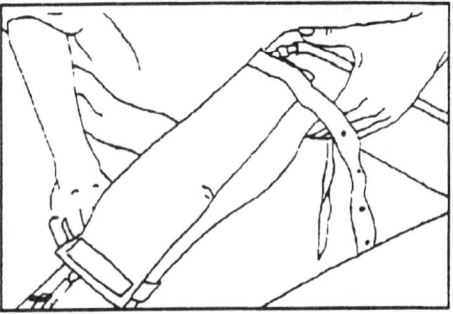

Figure 11. Apply Leg Bag

HELPFUL HINTS

- Handwash the condom holder with soap and water, air dry, and use again.
- To reuse a condom, wash by hand with soap and water. Make sure there are no tears in the condom before using it again.
- Always be sure to check the condom holder to make sure it is not too tight or too loose.
- Change the condom at least once a day to check the penis for skin problems and for cleaning.
- After each IC, use a clean, dry condom.
- If you become sensitive to the condom, try a skin prep or change to a different brand condom.
- Always apply the leg bag with the arrow pointing up to the top. This keeps urine from backing up from the leg bag. It is best that the leg bag be worn below the knee. This helps the urine to drain better.

Source: Donna Schachtel, et al., *Key to Independence Personal Care Manual*, Shepherd Spinal Center, Atlanta, Georgia, © 1989. To order a complete version of the manual, contact the Shepherd Center at 404-350-7361.

How to Apply a Self-Adhesive Condom

SUPPLIES NEEDED

- Self-adhesive condom—small, intermediate, medium, large (See Figure 1.)
- Soapy washcloth and wet cloth

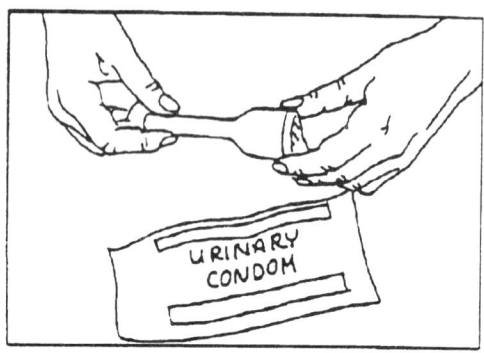

Figure 1. Urinary Condom

WHAT TO DO

1. Gather supplies.
2. Wash hands with soap and water. (See Figure 2.)

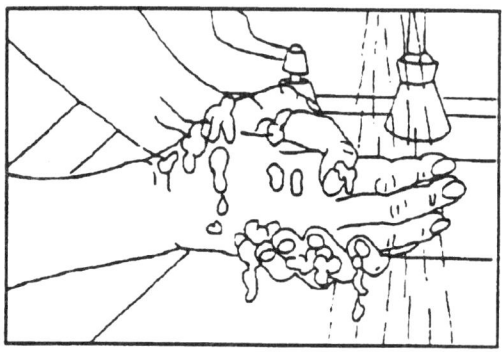

Figure 2. Washing Your Hands

3. Take off old condom. Roll it down the penis. Do not pull the condom off because it may hurt the skin.
4. Wash penis with the soapy washcloth and rinse with the wet cloth. Pull the foreskin back and clean the head of the penis well. (See Figure 3.)

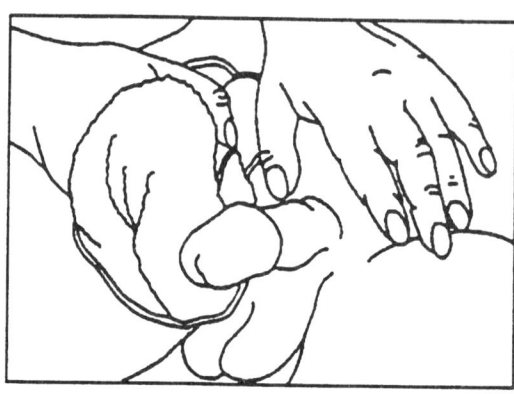

Figure 3. Washing the Penis

5. Dry penis well. Remember to pull the foreskin back down over the head of the penis to prevent swelling of the foreskin.
6. Roll the condom up close to the funnel-shaped end of the condom. (See Figure 4.)

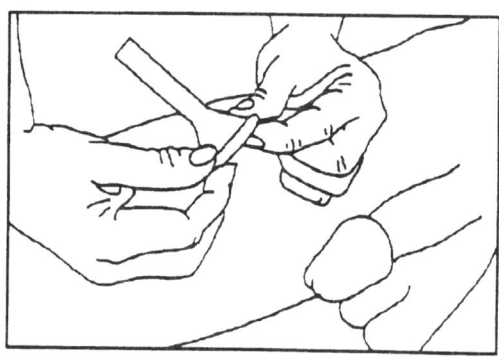

Figure 4. Rolling Up the Condom

continues

continued

7. Place funnel end of condom on penis. Be sure the head of the penis is close to the funnel tip. (See Figure 5.)

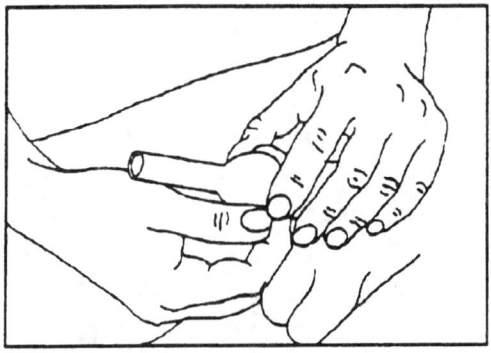

Figure 5. Applying the Condom

8. Roll the condom over the penis to the base of the penis. (See Figure 6.)

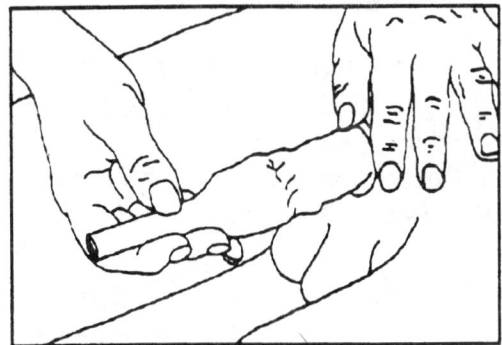

Figure 6. Rolling the Condom

9. Hold your hand around the condom for 10 seconds. (See Figure 7.)

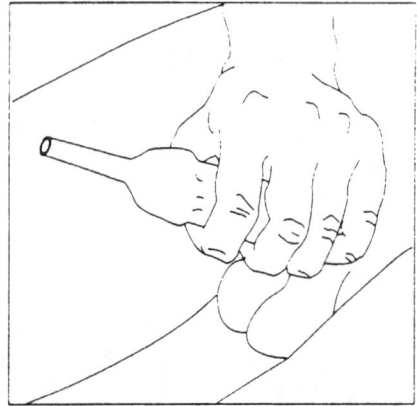

Figure 7. Bond Adhesive for 10 Seconds

10. Connect the condom to a leg bag or bedside bag. (See Figures 8 and 9.)

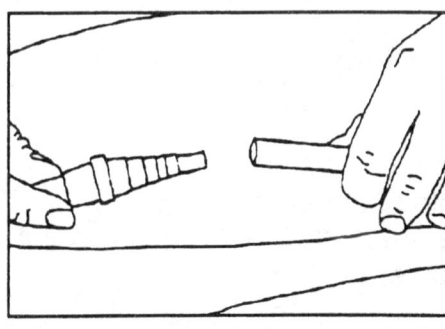

Figure 8. Connect Leg Bag

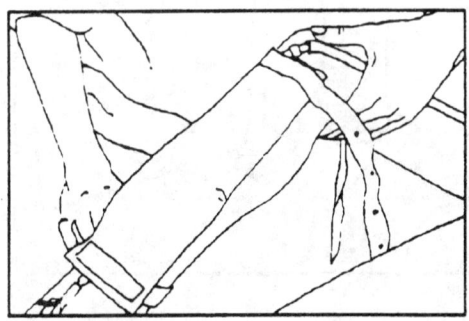

Figure 9. Apply Leg Bag

Source: Donna Schachtel, et al., *Key to Independence Personal Care Manual*, Shepherd Spinal Center, Atlanta, Georgia, © 1989. To order a complete version of the manual, contact the Shepherd Center at 404-350-7361.

How to Apply a Two-Piece Self-Adhesive Condom

SUPPLIES NEEDED

- Two-piece self-adhesive condom—small, medium, large (See Figure 1.)
- Soapy washcloth and wet cloth.

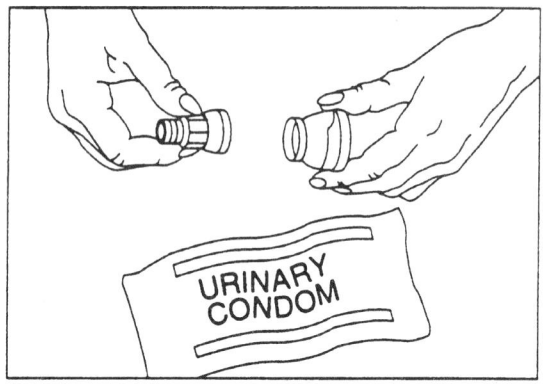

Figure 1. Urinary Condom

WHAT TO DO

1. Gather supplies.
2. Wash hands with soap and water. (See Figure 2.)

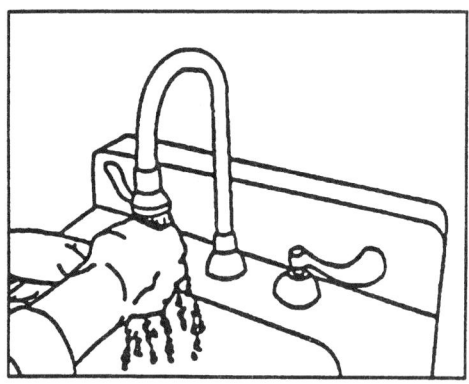

Figure 2. Washing Your Hands

3. Take off old condom. Roll it down the penis. Do not pull the condom off because it may hurt the skin.
4. Wash penis with the soapy washcloth and rinse with the wet cloth. Pull the foreskin back and clean the head of the penis well. (See Figure 3.)

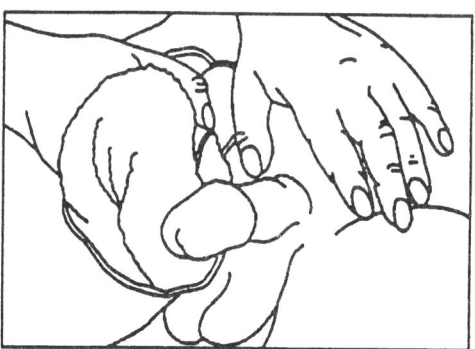

Figure 3. Washing the Penis

5. Dry penis well. Remember to pull the foreskin back down over the head of the penis to prevent swelling of the foreskin.
6. Roll the condom up close to the open end. (See Figure 4.)

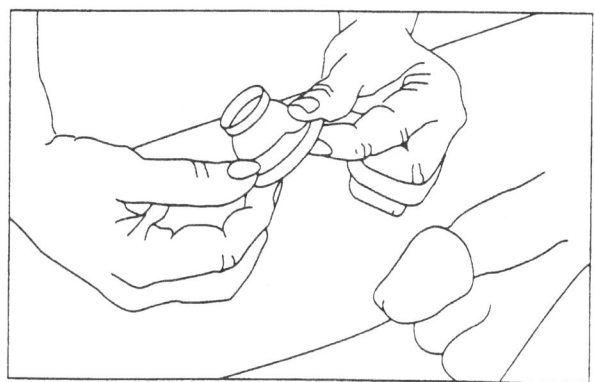

Figure 4. Rolling up the Condom

continues

continued

7. Place end of condom on penis. (See Figure 5.)

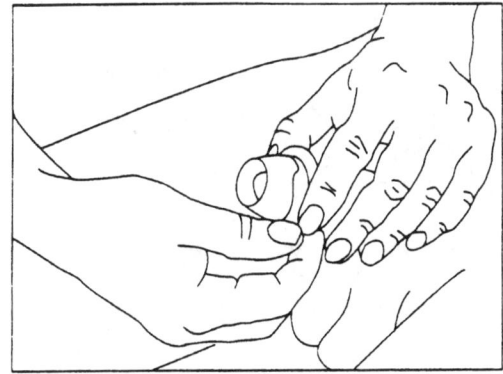

Figure 5. Applying the Condom

8. Roll the condom over the penis to the base of the penis. (See Figure 6.)

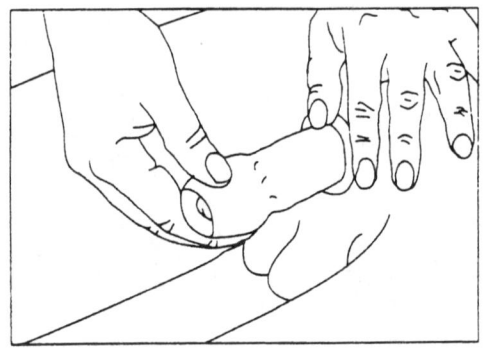

Figure 6. Rolling the Condom

9. Hold your hand around the condom for 10 seconds. (See Figure 7.)

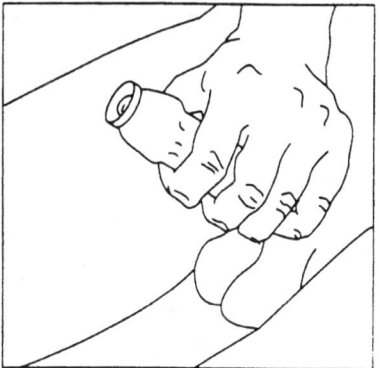

Figure 7. Bond Adhesive for 10 Seconds

10. Screw adapter onto condom. (See Figure 8.)

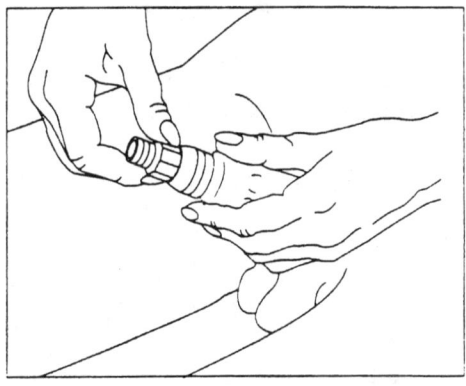

Figure 8. Screw Adapter onto Condom

11. Connect the condom to a leg bag or bedside bag. (See Figures 9 and 10.)

continues

continued

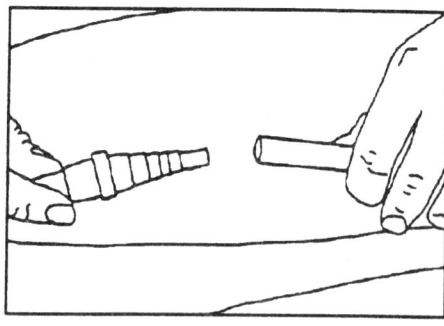

Figure 9. Connect Leg Bag

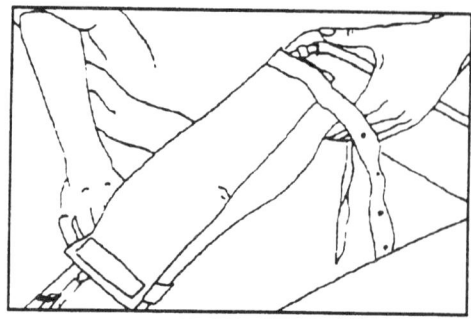

Figure 10. Apply Leg Bag

Notes:

Source: Donna Schachtel, et al., *Key to Independence Personal Care Manual*, Shepherd Spinal Center, Atlanta, Georgia, © 1989. To order a complete version of the manual, contact the Shepherd Center at 404-350-7361.

Helpful Hints about Condoms

- Condoms, also called Texas catheters, should be taken off every day to check and clean your skin.
- A stretchy tape is used to hold a condom on so that if there is an erection, blood supply to the penis is not stopped. Coban is one kind of stretchy tape used. There are many kinds of tape and condoms. You need to find what works best for you.
- The tape should not be so tight that there is swelling or redness when the condom is taken off.
- When putting on the condom, leave a space between the tip of the penis and the end of the condom. This is because there is some suction on the condom when you void. If the tip of the penis is too close to the end of the condom, you can get a sore.
- If you have any sores or a lot of red areas, it is best to prop a urinal at night instead of wearing a condom. This lets the skin dry out and heal. It also keeps pressure off the sore and red areas. Also, use thin Duoderm. This helps protect the penis.
- If the sores do not go away, it is best to keep a condom off as much as you can. If you have to wear a condom, wear it only as long as needed. Also keep the tape off the sore as much as you can.

Notes:

Source: *Spinal Cord Injury Manual*, University of Rochester, Strong Memorial Hospital Rehabilitation Unit, Rochester, New York, © 1986, rev. 1994.

Common Urological Problems: Leakage Around a Catheter

Leakage around a catheter is much more common in women than men, but it can occur with anyone using a catheter. It is a fairly simple problem to solve if one understands the reason, which is nearly always one of the following things.

Blocked Catheter

A blocked catheter may be due to a kink in the tubing or pressure on the tubing causing obstruction, which is easily relieved by repositioning, or the catheter may be blocked from the inside and need to be changed. If there is any question about whether the catheter is blocked, it is usually best to go ahead and change it.

Bladder Spasms

If an individual has a spastic bladder that contracts suddenly, the urine may not be able to flow fast enough through the tubing and some of it flows around the catheter instead. This happens in women more often than in men because the urethra is so short. If the spasms are severe enough, they may even force the catheter out with the balloon still inflated.

The treatment for this is medication for the bladder spasms. The most commonly used medications are Probanthine (up to 15 mg four times a day) or Ditropan (5 mg four times a day).

Do not treat this by putting in a larger catheter or a larger balloon, because this usually makes the problem worse rather than better. Some bladders are even strong enough to force a 30 cc balloon out while it is still inflated. This just results in stretching the opening of the bladder and can be harmful. Also, the larger balloon causes the spasms to be even worse.

Do not use a balloon larger than 5 cc (although it is all right to put 5 to 8 cc in the balloon as most people do).

Small Bladder Capacity

Individuals who have used a catheter for many years will often develop a small, contracted bladder that no longer has the ability to relax and expand. In such situations medication will not be effective and a surgical procedure such as bladder enhancement may be indicated. This should be discussed with your urologist.

Courtesy of Shirley McCluer, MD, Medical Director, Arkansas Spinal Cord Commission, Little Rock, Arkansas, December 1990.

Common Urological Problems: Frequent Catheter Changes

There is no uniform agreement on how frequently catheters should be changed, but once a month is most commonly recommended. If you are having to change your catheter regularly more often than once a month, you should try to find out why. The following are some of the possibilities.

1. **Not enough fluids.** This is nearly always the cause. Any person with a catheter should put out at least three quarts of urine in 24 hours. Drink more water! Remember that in summer when you are sweating you will need to drink even more than during cool weather.
2. **Wrong kind of fluids.** You should try to avoid all "fizzy" drinks like Coke, 7-Up, etc. If you absolutely must drink them, have no more than one a day. Water is always the best, but other acceptable liquids are tea, coffee, lemonade, fruit juice, cranberry juice, etc. (See number 7, below.)
3. **Cause of the obstruction.** Each time you have to take your catheter out because it stopped up, you should cut the catheter open lengthwise and look inside to see why it plugged up. This may give you a helpful clue. Usually the obstruction will be due to a buildup of sediment inside the catheter.
4. **Type of catheter.** This is one of the least common causes, but for some people a 100 percent silicone catheter will last longer than a latex catheter. However, it is also more expensive, so you must decide which is cheaper in the long run.
5. **Size of catheter.** Catheter sizes are measured in French units (which is 1/3 of a millimeter). The most commonly used size is 16 or 18 Fr. However, what most people do not realize is that this measurement refers to the outside diameter of the catheter, not the inside. There is a wide variation in the size and shape of the inside of catheters, depending on the manufacturer and the catheter material. The inside size and shape can make a big difference in how quickly a catheter can become plugged up. Smaller openings plug up more easily than larger openings. To find out what type of catheter you have, cut an old one open crosswise and see what the inside is like. Any type of "coated" catheter (such as Teflon

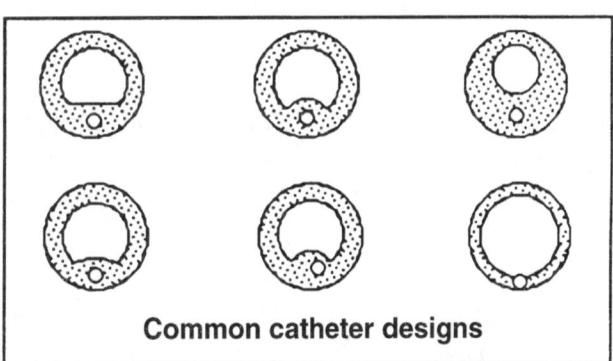

Common catheter designs

continues

continued

coated) will nearly always be smaller than a noncoated type. It is usually not helpful to get a larger catheter because it will plug up for the same reason the small one did and may cause other complications in the urethra.

6. **Bladder stone.** The need to change catheters often may mean that you have bladder stones. You should ask your doctor to see if you have them. Most large stones will show up on an X-ray (a KUB), but small ones often do not. People with catheters are more likely to get stones than people without catheters. Cystoscopy (looking in your bladder) may be advisable even if the X-ray is negative.

7. **Alkaline urine.** Normally the urine is acid (pH 5–6.5) and this tends to discourage the growth of most bacteria and the production of bladder stones. If your urine becomes alkaline, you can tell by the strong urine smell. If you want to be sure, you can buy some pH paper at the drugstore and test it yourself. Alkaline urine is pH 8–9. Certain bacteria can make your urine alkaline, but so can carbonated drinks (Coke, 7-Up, etc.) and certain foods. Sometimes it may be helpful to take an antibiotic for 7–10 days to kill the bacteria you have and hope that the new ones that come back will not do the same thing. In most cases though, the best way to change the urine back to acid is to DRINK MORE WATER!

8. **Bladder irrigation.** If you have tried all of the above (and you are sure you are putting out at least three quarts of urine per day) but nothing works, your doctor may tell you to irrigate your bladder with a solution to make it acid. The least expensive is $\frac{1}{4}$ percent acetic acid. (See the following instructions to make acetic acid at home.) There are more expensive solutions that can be prescribed by your doctor.

INSTRUCTIONS FOR MAKING $\frac{1}{4}$ PERCENT ACETIC ACID

A $\frac{1}{4}$ percent acetic acid solution is frequently recommended for use at home to irrigate a bladder, to use as a wet dressing on wounds, or for some other purpose. This is the procedure for making the solution.

Necessary Materials

- **Water.** Use either distilled water or tap water that has been boiled and cooled.
- **Vinegar.** Use plain white vinegar.
- **Clean container.** An example is a mason jar with lid, preferably boiled (or washed in dishwasher).

The solution should not be kept for more than two (2) weeks, so do not make up more than you will need in that length of time. It is best to keep it in the refrigerator after you begin using it, but be sure to allow it to return to room temperature before irrigating the bladder.

continues

continued

Directions

Decide how much acetic acid you need, then make up **one** of the volumes below:

- To make **about 1 pint** of acetic acid, add 5 teaspoons of vinegar to 1 pint of water.
- To make **about 1 quart** of acetic acid, add 10 teaspoons of vinegar to 1 quart of water.
- To make **about 1 gallon** of acetic acid, add 13 tablespoons of vinegar to 1 gallon of water.

Notes:

Courtesy of Shirley McCluer, MD, Medical Director, Arkansas Spinal Cord Commission, Little Rock, Arkansas, December 1990.

Leg/Bedside Drainage Bag Care

VINEGAR CLEANING METHOD

1. Empty the urine out of the bag.
2. Rinse the bag out with water.
3. Empty the water out of the bag.
4. Put about 1/8 to 1/4 cup of vinegar in the bag.
5. Shake the bag a few times. Lay the bag flat so the vinegar touches all parts of the bag. The vinegar must stay in the bag at least 10 minutes. If vinegar stays in the bag longer, it will not hurt the bag.
6. Empty the vinegar out of the bag. Do not rinse the vinegar out.

BLEACH CLEANING METHOD

1. Empty the urine out of the bag.
2. Rinse the bag out with water.
3. Empty the water out of the bag.
4. Put about 1/8 to 1/4 cup of bleach mixture (see below) in the bag.
5. Shake the bag a few times so the bleach mixture touches all parts of the bag.
6. Empty the bleach mixture out of the bag. You can rinse the bleach mixture out if you want to, but it will not hurt the bag if it stays in.

The bleach mixture you use should be 1 part bleach and 10 parts water. Below is a chart to help you make the bleach mixture. Which one you decide to use depends on how much you want to make up. The bleach mixture keeps well, so make up the amount that will be best for your routines.

Bleach	1 tsp	1/8 c	1/4 c	1/2 c	3/4 c	1 c
Water	2/3 c	1 1/4 c	2 1/2 c	5 c	7 1/2 c	10 c

OTHER CLEANING METHODS

1. If you use soap and water to clean out your bag/bedside drainage bag, do not use a lot of soap. If too much soap is used, it will be very hard to rinse the soap out of the bag.
2. There are other liquids that can be used to clean your bag/bedside drainage bag. They are found at your medical supply store. Follow the directions they give you.

NIGHTTIME DRAINAGE

- You can get the kind of bag that you used in the hospital at a medical supply store.
- You can make your own by using an empty bottle (for example, a Clorox or laundry bottle). You can get the tubing and special bottle cap at the medical supply store.

Source: *Spinal Cord Injury Manual,* University of Rochester, Strong Memorial Hospital Rehabilitation Unit, Rochester, New York, © 1986, rev. 1994.

Selecting Proper Urological Supplies

While you were in the hospital, you were exposed to a limited selection of supplies for your bladder program. On discharge, many more options will be available to meet your specific needs through one of the large medical supply companies. When evaluating various products, you should consider effectiveness, ease of use, comfort, and cost.

External (condom) catheters come in two basic styles: molded one-piece sheath or Texas type with tubing attached to a lighter-weight sheath. These condoms come in various sizes, weights, and construction, with a considerable range in price. One-sided or two-sided adhesive strips are specifically designed to attach the condom, or elastic tape can be used. Each has special characteristics of adhesion, elasticity, ease on skin, and resistance to moisture. Several types of skin adhesives are also available in tubes, cans, or spray applicators. Adhesive removers come in spray, individual wipes, or liquid. Some condoms come with a coating of adhesive on the inner surface and do not require additional adhesive.

Several skin barriers are available to protect the skin from the harshness of frequent taping. Some are packaged with the condoms or can be obtained in spray or wipes. Other skin care products are available to protect, cleanse, and condition skin that is in frequent contact with tape or urine. These products are good preventive measures that you can use before you get skin breakdown.

You will find a multitude of leg bags in various designs. Two basic types are disposable plastic, which can be washed and reused several times, and rubber reusable, which is designed to last for months. Special features to look for are reflux valves, push/pull valves, foam and Velcro straps, or flocked backing. Some companies have accessories that fit only their own leg bags. Make sure you select a total system that is compatible. You may want to have more than one system to meet your varying needs, such as large capacity when you are out for long periods.

Numerous accessories are available that will fit your particular needs. Tubing can be obtained in various sizes and lengths, in clear plastic or more flexible rubber. Connectors are available in many sizes, shapes, and style of clamping apparatus to ease your draining procedure. Special cleansers and brushes are designed to remove sediment, clean, and deodorize your equipment while prolonging the life of your supplies.

Straight or intermittent catheters are also available in plastic or rubber. There may be some difference in flexibility and surface quality from brand to brand. Often catheter manufacturers that sell to hospitals do not sell in the home market, but don't worry—there are excellent catheters available for your use. Numerous kits are available with insertion supplies to meet your particular needs. Two different prep solutions are available—povidone iodine or BZK. Kits will contain sterile gloves, barrier, lubricant, forceps, cotton balls, and a collection device or specimen cup. The kits come without a catheter or with a plastic or red rubber catheter. If you don't need all of this equipment, each of the items is available separately at a substantial savings. Catheters come in 6-inch or 16-inch lengths and can be lengthened by using extension tubing.

continues

continued

Foley catheters come with or without kits similar to the straight catheters. Foleys can be plain latex, silicone or Teflon-coated, or all silicone. Irrigation equipment consists of either a bulb or piston-type syringe that can be bought separately or as part of a kit.

Night drains come in various sizes and shapes. The usual bedside drain bags have various methods to drain or attach to the bed or frame. An expandable plastic tube is available, as are several adapters that can be connected to a container like a Clorox bottle. There are numerous devices to hold the tubing to your leg or to the bed.

Underpads and specially designed absorbing undergarments are available for your convenience and comfort. If you need a little extra protection or if you do not use a catheter procedure, there are some new products for you to consider, such as the Dignity System or Attends.

It is certainly worth a visit to a medical supply center to discuss your particular needs and see what is available. There is no need to "make do" on what you find at your local store. Large companies can give you excellent selection and personalized service when you order over the telephone or by mail. Some of these centers offer a good selection of aids for eating, dressing, hygiene, communication, and recreation. As you progress, and your needs change, these supplies will greatly improve your ability to be independent.

Notes:

Source: Shirley S. Paulson, *Spinal Cord Injury Home Care Manual,* Norman B. Nelson Rehabilitation Center, Santa Clara Valley Medical Center, San Jose, California, © 1994.

BOWEL MANAGEMENT

Bowel Program: Overview

WHAT IS THE BOWEL, AND WHAT DOES IT DO?

The bowel is the last portion of your digestive tract and is sometimes called the large intestine or colon. The digestive tract as a whole is a hollow tube that extends from the mouth to the anus (see illustration below).

The function of the digestive system is to take food into the body and to get rid of waste. The bowel is where the waste products of eating are stored until they are emptied from the body in the form of a bowel movement (stool, feces).

A bowel movement happens when the rectum (last portion of the bowel) becomes full of stool and the muscle around the anus (anal sphincter) opens (see diagram below).

With a spinal cord injury, damage can occur to the nerves that allow a person to control bowel movements. If the spinal cord injury is above the T12 level, the ability to feel when the rectum is full may be lost. The anal sphincter muscle remains tight, however, and bowel movements will occur on a reflex basis. This means that when the rectum is full, the defecation reflex will occur, emptying the bowel. This type of bowel problem is called an upper motor neuron or reflex bowel. It can be managed by causing the defecation reflex to occur at a socially appropriate time and place.

A spinal cord injury below the T12 level may damage the defecation reflex and relax the anal sphincter muscle. This is known as a lower motor neuron or flaccid bowel. Management of this type of bowel problem may require more frequent attempts to empty the bowel and bearing down or manual removal of stool.

Both types of neurogenic bowel can be managed successfully to prevent unplanned bowel movements and other bowel problems such as constipation, diarrhea, and impaction.

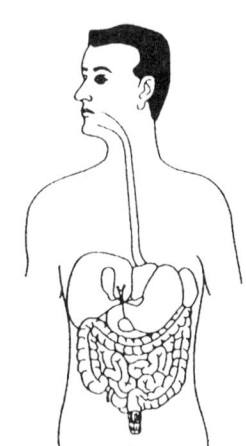

Digestive tract

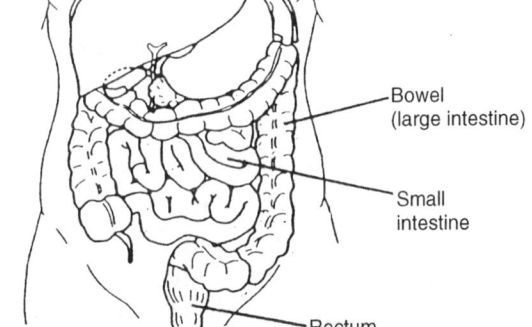

continues

continued

WHAT METHODS CAN BE USED TO EMPTY THE BOWEL?

Each person's bowel program should be individualized to fit his or her own needs. The type of disease or nerve damage (for example, upper or lower motor neuron) should be taken into account as well as other factors (see What Factors Can Affect the Success of the Bowel Program, below). Components of a bowel program can include any combination of the following:

- **Manual removal:** Physical removal of the stool from the rectum. This can be combined with a bearing down technique called a Valsalva maneuver. (Avoid this technique if you have a heart condition.)
- **Digital stimulation:** Circular motion with the index finger in the rectum, which causes the anal sphincter to relax.
- **Suppository:** Dulcolax (stimulates the nerve endings in the rectum, causing a contraction of the bowel) or glycerin (draws water into the stool to stimulate evacuation).
- **Mini-enama:** Softens, lubricates, and draws water into the stool to stimulate evacuation.

WHAT IS A BOWEL PROGRAM?

Most people perform their bowel program at a time of day that fits in with their prior bowel habits and current lifestyle. The program usually begins with insertion of either a suppository or a mini-enema, followed by a waiting period of approximately 15 to 20 minutes to allow the stimulant to work. This part of the program should, preferably, be done on the commode or toilet seat.

After the waiting period, digital stimulation is performed every 10 to 15 minutes until the rectum is empty. To avoid damage to the delicate rectal tissue, no more than four digital stimulations should be performed in any one session. Those with a flaccid bowel frequently omit the suppository or mini-enema and start their bowel program with digital stimulation or manual removal. Most bowel programs require 30 to 60 minutes to complete.

Bowel programs vary from person to person according to their individual preferences and needs. Some people use only half of a suppository, some require two suppositories, and some use no suppository or mini-enema at all. Some choose to do the entire program in bed, while others sit on the toilet from the beginning. Some find that the program works better if they can eat or drink a warm beverage while it is in progress, others find that this is not helpful. What is most important is that you discover what works best for you.

WHAT FACTORS CAN AFFECT THE SUCCESS OF THE BOWEL PROGRAM?

Any one of the factors listed, or a combination of factors, can affect the success of a bowel program. Changing one factor may produce results almost immediately, or it may take several days to see the results. Changing more than one factor at a time makes it difficult to determine

continues

continued

the effects of individual factors, and may increase the time it takes to develop a stable bowel program.

Factors That Can Affect the Success of a Bowel Program

- **Previous bowel history:** What have your bowel habits been in the past?
- **Timing:** Do you do your bowel program in the morning or evening? At the same time every day? After a meal or warm beverage? What is the interval between programs—half a day, one day, or two days? (You should do a bowel program at least every two or three days to reduce your risk of constipation, impaction and colon cancer.)
- **Privacy and comfort:** Does someone else share your bathroom? Do you have enough time to complete your program?
- **Emotional stress:** Has your appetite been affected? Are you able to relax?
- **Positioning:** Where do you do your program—on a commode chair, raised toilet seat, on the toilet, or in bed? It will probably work better when you are sitting up because of gravity.
- **Fluids:** How much and what type of fluid do you drink? (Prune juice or orange juice can stimulate the bowels, or another type of fruit juice may work best for you.)
- **Food:** How much fiber or bulk (such as fruits and vegetables, bran, and whole-grain breads and cereals) do you eat? Some foods (such as dairy products, white potatoes, white bread, and bananas) can contribute to constipation, while others (such as excess amounts of fruit, caffeine, or spicy foods) may soften the stool or cause diarrhea.
- **Medication:** Some medicines (such as codeine, Ditropan, Pro-Banthine, and aluminum-based antacids like Aludrox) can cause constipation, while others (including some antibiotics, such as ampicillin, and magnesium-based antacids such as Mylanta and Maalox) can cause diarrhea. Consult your health care provider for information about the medications you are taking.
- **Illness:** A case of the flu, a cold, or an intestinal infection may affect your bowel program while you are ill. (Even if your digestive system is not directly affected, your eating habits, fluid intake, or mobility may change, which can alter your bowel program.)
- **Activity level/mobility:** How much exercise do you get? How much time do you spend out of bed?
- **Weather:** Hot weather increases the evaporation of body fluids, which can lead to dehydration and constipation.
- **External massage:** Massaging the lower abdomen in a circular, clockwise motion from right to left increases bowel activity.
- **Valsalva (bearing down):** This technique is not recommended for patients with cardiac problems.
- **Assistive/adaptive devices:** Devices such as a suppository inserter, finger extension, or digital stimulator may be required to assist you in establishing a successful bowel program.

Courtesy of the University of Washington Medical Center, Northwest Regional Spinal Cord System, Seattle, Washington, © 1994.

Ensuring Success of Your Bowel Program

WHAT TO AVOID

Regular Use of Stimulant Laxatives

Stimulant laxatives include bisacodyl (Dulcolax) tablets, phenolphthalein (Ex-Lax), cascara, senna, and magnesium citrate. Laxative use on a regular basis will cause your bowels to become dependent on them. When this happens, the bowel will not work well without the laxative, and eventually the "lazy bowel" that results will require more and stronger laxatives to work at all. An occasional small dose of a mild laxative, such as Milk of Magnesia or an herbal laxative, can be used to treat constipation if other measures have not worked. (We recommend that you use no more than three doses per month.)

Enemas

Any full-size enema (such as Fleet's, soap suds, or tap water) is too irritating to the bowel to be used on a regular basis and will cause the same problem with dependence as a stimulant laxative. A "mini-enema," which has only a few drops of liquid stool softener, does not fall into this category and can be used regularly. Occasionally, your health care provider may prescribe a full-size enema as preparation for a medical procedure or for treatment of severe constipation.

Skipping or Changing the Time of Your Program

Your bowels will move more predictably if your bowel care program is carried out on a regular, predictable schedule. Skipping your program can also result in constipation or accidents.

Rushing

The more tense you are, the more difficult it will be for you to empty your bowels. A hurried program will increase the likelihood of an unplanned bowel movement later in the day.

More Than Four Digital Stimulations at a Time

This can cause trauma to the rectum, resulting in hemorrhoids or fissures (cracks or breaks in the skin).

Long Fingernails

Fingernails can damage the rectal tissue and cause bleeding, even through a glove.

continues

continued

WHAT TO DO IF

Stool Is Too Hard (Constipation)

Do your bowel program on a daily basis until constipation resolves. Add or increase the dose of a stool softener (such as DOSS or colace). Add or increase the dose of psyllium hydro-mucilloid (such as Metamucil or Citrucel). Increase your fluid intake (this is essential if you are increasing psyllium). Increase your activity level and your intake of dietary fiber. Avoid foods that can harden your stool, such as bananas and cheese.

Mucous Accidents

If you notice a clear, sticky, sometimes odorous drainage from the rectum, try switching from a suppository to a mini-enema, or using only half of a suppository, or try eliminating suppositories or mini-enemas completely and begin your program with digital stimulation only. Avoid hard stools.

No Results for Three or Four Days

Treat constipation as recommended above. If there are no results in three days, take 30 cc of Milk of Magnesia or a single dose of an herbal laxative at bedtime. Do your bowel program in the morning. If there are still no results, repeat the dose of Milk of Magnesia or herbal laxative the next evening. If there are no results in the morning, consult your health care provider.

Stool Is Liquid or Runny (Diarrhea)

Temporarily discontinue the use of any stool softeners. Continue your bowel program at the regular time and frequency. (If you are having accidents, increase the frequency of your program.) Try adding or increasing the dose of psyllium hydro-mucilloid (Metamucil, Citrucel), which adds bulk to liquid stool. If the diarrhea seems to be related to an acute viral or bacterial illness, change to a liquids only or very bland diet for 24 hours (avoid milk, however). If diarrhea persists for more than 24 hours or if you have a fever or blood in your stool, consult your health care provider.

A frequent cause of diarrhea is a blockage or impaction of stool (liquid stool leaks out around the blockage). Evaluate whether you may have this problem. Have you had small hard stools recently? Or have you had no results from the past several programs? If you suspect impaction, consult your health care provider.

Frequent Bowel Accidents

Be sure your rectum is completely empty at the end of your program. Increase the frequency of your program (some people with a flaccid bowel may need to empty their bowels twice daily).

continues

continued

Try using only half of a suppository. Evaluate stool consistency—if it's too hard or too soft, see above. Monitor your diet for any foods that may overstimulate your bowel, such as spicy foods.

Rectal Bleeding

Keep your stool soft. Be very careful to do digital stimulation gently and with sufficient lubrication, and keep your fingernails short. If you have known hemorrhoids, you may treat them with an over-the-counter hemorrhoidal preparation such as Anusol or Anusol HC. If bleeding persists or is more than a few drops, consult your health care provider.

Excessive Gas

Avoid constipation. Increase the frequency of your bowel programs. Avoid gas-forming foods, such as beans, corn, onions, peppers, radishes, cauliflower, sauerkraut, turnips, cucumbers, apples, melons, and others that you may have noticed seem to increase your own gas. Try simethicone tablets to help relieve discomfort from gas in your stomach.

Bowel Program Takes a Long Time to Complete

Try switching from a suppository to mini-enemas. Increase your intake of dietary fiber and add or increase the dose of psyllium hydro-mucilloid. Try switching your program to a different time, and be sure you schedule it after a meal to help increase intestinal peristalsis.

Autonomic Dysreflexia During Bowel Program

Use xylocaine jelly (available by prescription from your health care provider) for digital stimulation. You may also need to insert some of the jelly into your rectum before beginning the program. Keep your stool as soft as possible. If dysreflexia persists, consult your health care provider. You may need medication to treat or prevent this condition.

Courtesy of Harborview Medical Center, Northwest Regional Spinal Cord System, Seattle, Washington, © 1994.

Digital Stimulation

WHAT IS DIGITAL STIMULATION?

Digital stimulation is gently rotating a finger in a circular motion against the anal sphincter wall to relax the muscle. Remember, the anal sphincter is the opening of the rectum to the outside of the body. This relaxation increases peristalsis (the wave-like contractions that help waste move through the bowel/intestines and be eliminated). This helps people have timely and complete bowel movements.

WHEN IS DIGITAL STIMULATION USED OR NEEDED?

People with the following signs may need digital stimulation:

1. decreased activity
2. weak or paralyzed abdominal (stomach) and/or rectal muscles
3. decreased feeling or lack of feeling in the rectal area

HOW IS DIGITAL STIMULATION USED?

Digital stimulation is used to:

1. Relax the anal sphincter muscle before using a suppository.
2. "Speed up" results by relaxing the anal sphincter and starting peristalsis. (Wait at least 15 minutes after giving the suppository.)
3. Completely empty bowel after suppository results.
4. Start peristalsis without a suppository program.

WHAT EQUIPMENT IS NEEDED?

- Water soluble lubricant (K-Y jelly)
- Chux or protective pad
- Gloves
- Soap
- Water
- Washcloth

continues

continued

STEPS FOR DIGITAL STIMULATION

1. Sit on the commode or toilet:
   - Digital stimulation is best in a sitting position.
   - Gravity helps move stool into and out of the rectum.
   - If doing the procedure in bed, however:
     —Use a Chux or protective pad.
     —Lie on the left side of the body.
2. Glove a hand and lubricate index finger.
3. Find anal opening.
4. Check rectum for stool using gloved finger.
5. Gently remove any formed stool blocking the anal opening. Do this with a circular motion of the finger.
6. After removing any stool, use more lubricant on the fingers if needed.
7. Gently put gloved finger into the rectum about 1/2 to 1 inch.
8. Gently rotate finger using a circular motion against the anal sphincter wall. Do this for about 30 seconds.
9. Allow at least 15–20 minutes for a bowel movement.
10. After the bowel movement, put gloved finger into the rectum to check for stool. If stool is present, remove manually.
11. Thoroughly wash and dry the area.

HELPFUL HINTS

- Breathe deeply if rectal sensation (feeling) is present.
- Use plenty of lubrication.
- Use an anesthetic lubricant (Nupercainal ointment, Anusol cream, hemorrhoidal cream) to:
  —Help prevent autonomic dysreflexia during digital stimulation.
  —Reduce pain with hemorrhoids and/or rectal discomfort.

Source: Kelly B. Wascher, ed., *Patient Education and Discharge Planning Manual for Rehabilitation,* St. Joseph Rehabilitation Hospital and Outpatient Center, Aspen Publishers, Inc., © 1995.

Constipation

WHAT IS CONSTIPATION?

Constipation is hard and infrequent stools that are difficult to pass. It happens when a person's normal bowel pattern changes.

WHAT IS A NORMAL BOWEL PROGRAM?

All people are different in how often they have bowel movements. It is not necessary to have a bowel movement every day. One to three days between bowel movements is NORMAL.

CONSTIPATION	
Causes	**Do**
Most Common Cause: **Poor eating habits/diet** Diet • A low-fiber diet slows the time it takes food to move through the intestines. • When stool remains in the intestines longer: —More water leaves the stool. —Stool gets harder.	• **Do** eat foods high in fiber.
Fluids • Not drinking enough fluid can cause stool to get hard.	• **Do** drink at least eight 8 oz glasses of water each day (if fluids are not limited for medical reasons). • **Do** try different types of fruit juice. Some may act as natural laxatives (prune or orange juice). • **Do** take a full glass of liquid before each meal.
Other habits Exercise • Less activity slows the bowel. • The slower the stool moves through the bowel, the harder it gets. • Weak stomach muscles make it hard to bear down.	• **Do** exercise regularly to: —Improve stomach muscle strength. —Move the stool through the bowel. • **Do** ask the therapist about exercises to use at home.

continues

continued

Causes	Do

Bowel habits
• Normal bowel habits can be changed by travel or lack of privacy.
 	
Laxatives
• Overusing laxatives can cause long-term constipation.
• Strong laxatives completely empty the bowel:
  —The bowel then needs a few days to collect enough stool to have a normal BM.
  —The person may worry about not having another BM and take another laxative.
  —The bowel eventually gets "lazy" and responds only to strong laxatives.
Medications
• Some medications can cause constipation, for example:
  —some antacids
  —pain medications
  —iron pills
  —some cough/cold medications
  —antidepressants
Impaction
• Impaction is very hard stool in the rectum that will not move.
• Liquid stool may ooze around the impaction (diarrhea).
• DIARRHEA CAN BE A SIGN OF CONSTIPATION/IMPACTION.
	• **Do** set an unhurried time for bowel movements.
	• **Do** sit for at least 10 minutes, whether there is a bowel movement (BM) or not.
	• **Do** be patient in adjusting bowel habits.
	• **Do** go to the bathroom when the urge happens.
	
	• **Do** stop taking laxatives.
	• **Do** try natural fiber laxatives (Citracil or Metamucil with lots of water).
	• **Do** try stool softeners (Colace).
	• **Do** try a Fleet's enema for temporary relief.
	• **Do** call the doctor if constipated more than two weeks.
	
	• **Do** talk about medications with a doctor/nurse/pharmacist.
	• **Do** report any changes in usual bowel habits after starting a new medication.
	
	• **Do** try a suppository. You may need to use them a few days in a row.
	• If no results, **do** try an enema.
	• **Do** call the doctor, if unable to get rid of the impaction.

continues

continued

SPECIAL RECIPE TO INCREASE FIBER IN DIET

INGREDIENTS	HOW TO MAKE
1 cup applesauce 1 cup unprocessed bran 1/4 cup prune juice	Mix all three ingredients together.

DIRECTIONS FOR USE

1. Start with 2 tablespoons a day.
2. Follow with a glass of water.
3. After 7 to 10 days, increase by a tablespoon a day.
4. After 3 weeks, may increase up to 4 tablespoons a day.
5. There may be some increase in gas and a bloated feeling when first using. This will go away in a few weeks.
6. Keep the mixture in the refrigerator or freezer.
7. Premeasured servings may be frozen in sectioned ice cube trays and thawed as needed.

Notes:

Source: Kelly B. Wascher, ed., *Patient Education and Discharge Planning Manual for Rehabilitation,* St. Joseph Rehabilitation Hospital and Outpatient Center, Aspen Publishers, Inc., © 1995.

How to Give a Suppository

To give a suppository you will need:

- Gloves
- Lubricant
- Padding for the bed
- Your suppository

WHAT TO DO

1. Pad the bed.
2. Turn on your side and put on the gloves.
3. Lubricate your finger. Check your rectum and take out any stool that is there. If the suppository is put into stool, it will not work.
4. Lubricate the suppository. Put the suppository in as far as you can, and be sure it is against the wall of the rectum.
5. Be sure to digitally stimulate your rectum and disimpact as needed. This is to be sure your rectum is empty. You may need to digitally stimulate your rectum to help you start to have a bowel movement. Also, you need to do it after a bowel movement to be sure your rectum is empty.

ADDITIONAL INFORMATION

With practice you will learn how long you can wait before getting up to a commode, when and how many times you need to digitally stimulate your rectum, and other things about how your body acts after a suppository.

Adaptive equipment is available, such as a suppository gun or digital stimulator if you are unable to use your fingers due to your injury.

To **digitally stimulate** your rectum, you put your gloved finger into your rectum. Next, you rub the wall of the rectum with your finger. This rubbing causes the bowels to empty by reflex action. This usually is done at least two or three times, with a few minutes between each stimulation.

To **disimpact** stool means that you put your gloved finger into your rectum and take out any stool that is in your rectum.

There may be some bleeding when you disimpact. If there is a small amount of bleeding, keep disimpacting, but do it gently. If the bleeding does not stop or if there is a large amount of bleeding, stop disimpacting and call your doctor.

continues

continued

PLACING THE SUPPOSITORY

Before you give your suppository, check your rectum. Take out any stool that is there (disimpaction).

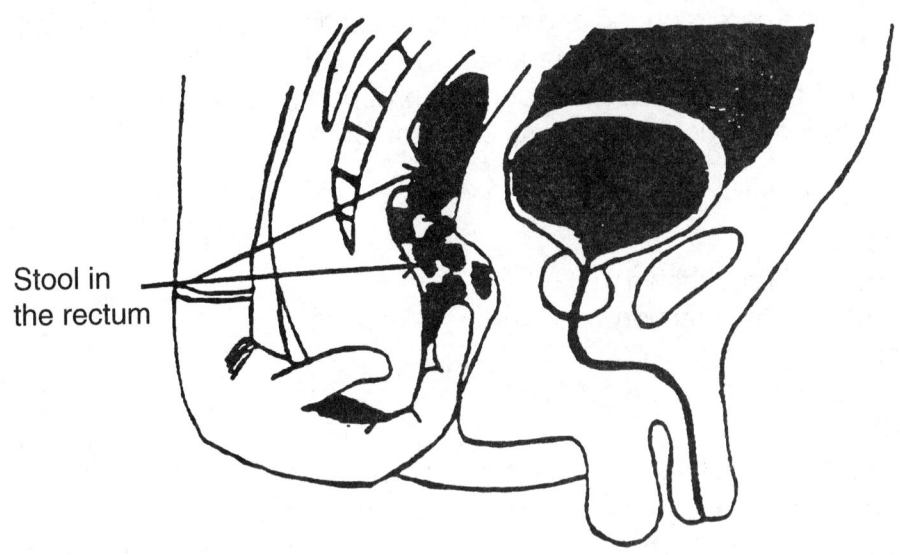

Stool in the rectum

Put the suppository in as far as you can, and be sure it is against the wall of the rectum.

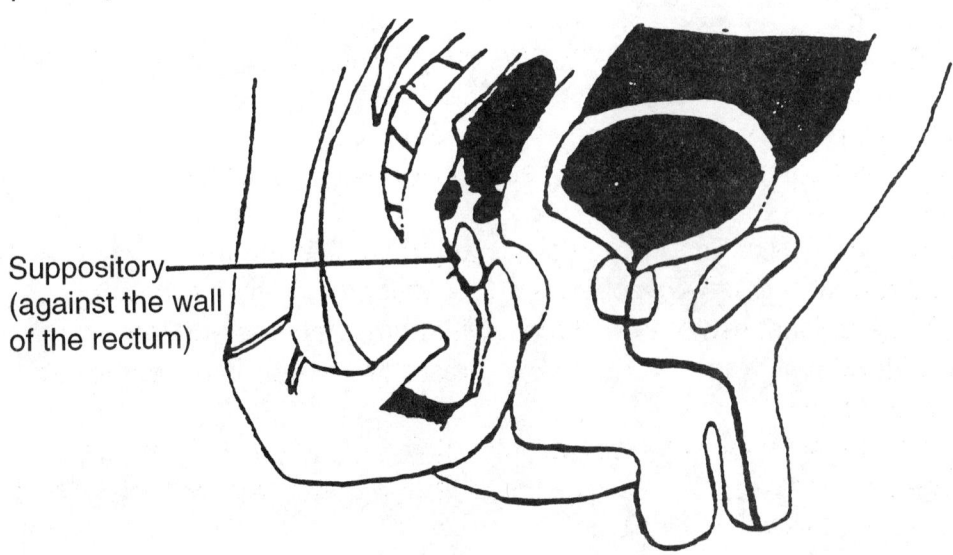

Suppository (against the wall of the rectum)

Source: Wanda Trojanoski, University of Rochester, Strong Memorial Hospital Rehabilitation Unit, *Spinal Cord Injury Manual*, Rochester, New York, © 1986, rev. 1994.

HYGIENE

General Hygiene

Perineal care remains an important part of personal care. It is, therefore, important for you to become familiar with the care required and establish a routine for personal hygiene. Perineal care should be performed twice daily and whenever you experience a bowel or bladder accident. It may be performed on the commode with your feet propped on a wheelchair or a stool, or in bed, using a protective covering such as a plastic sheet or Chux.

- **Objectives:**
  - personal comfort
  - prevention of skin breakdown
  - prevention of bladder infection
- **Equipment:**
  - clean bath towel
  - clean washcloth
  - soap and water
  - gloves (optional)

Notes:

Source: Virginia Spinal Cord Injury System, University of Virginia Medical Center and Virginia Department of Rehabilitative Services, *Virginia Spinal Cord Injury Care and Teaching Manual,* Fisherville, Virginia, © 1980, rev. 1985, 1988.

Male Hygiene

PROCEDURE

1. Wash the penis first:
   - If you have not been circumcised, pull the foreskin back, wash, rinse, and dry the area thoroughly.
   - Push the foreskin back over the head of the penis.
2. Wash outside of the penis, including the posterior (back) side. Rinse well. Dry thoroughly.
3. Wash scrotum thoroughly. Rinse and dry thoroughly. (Erection may occur.)
4. Turn to side, separate buttocks. Wash buttocks, including area around anus. Rinse well. Dry thoroughly.

Notes:

Source: Virginia Spinal Cord Injury System, University of Virginia Medical Center and Virginia Department of Rehabilitative Services, *Virginia Spinal Cord Injury Care and Teaching Manual,* Fisherville, Virginia, © 1980, rev. 1985, 1988.

Female Hygiene

PROCEDURE

1. Wash outer perineum and area between thighs and labia with soap. Rinse well. Dry thoroughly.
2. Separate labia, wash from clitoris over vaginal opening. Wash toward rectum, front to back. Rinse well. Dry thoroughly.
3. Turn to side. Separate buttocks. Wash buttocks, including area around anus. Rinse well. Dry thoroughly.

MENSTRUATION

You probably have many questions regarding your menstrual cycle. Some women may not have a period for up to six months following their injury. Periods may be irregular, lasting only one to two days, or occur more or less frequently than their normal schedule. These changes occur because of the shock to your body at the time of injury. Your change in activity and routines and your adjustment to your injury may also influence your menstrual cycle. If your menstrual cycle does not occur at least once within six months following your injury, you should consult your family doctor or gynecologist.

The signs or signals your body gave to warn you of your period may have changed. However, you will become aware of new signals. Look for signs such as back pain, cramps, or an increase in abdominal or leg spasms. Remember that contractions of your uterus with pregnancy or your menstrual cycle may contribute to autonomic dysreflexia. You will have to give special care to your bowel and bladder routine at these times. If the usual steps followed to resolve autonomic dysreflexia do not relieve the symptoms, contact your doctor immediately.

You may continue to use either tampons or sanitary pads during your menstrual period. Your decision should be based on preference, ease with which you can independently insert tampons or place pads, and comfort. Tampons that come with an applicator may be easier to handle. Also, a mirror may be helpful when inserting tampons. Either tampons or pads should be changed at least every four hours. Complete "peri" care should be done at least twice a day during a menstrual period.

Source: Virginia Spinal Cord Injury System, University of Virginia Medical Center and Virginia Department of Rehabilitative Services, *Virginia Spinal Cord Injury Care and Teaching Manual,* Fisherville, Virginia, © 1980, rev. 1985, 1988.

6
Skin Care

> Most materials in the *Spinal Cord Injury Patient Education Resource Manual* are intended for the health care professional to share with the patient. Materials that are intended solely for the professional are labeled "Exhibit" in the table of contents.

General Skin Care

What Is Healthy Skin?	175
Tips for Maintaining Good Skin	177
Guidelines to Success in Avoiding Skin Problems	178
Additional Guidelines for Skin Injury Prevention	180
Pressure Reliefs to Save Your Skin	182
Steps for Building Skin Tolerance	186
How to Do a Skin Check	187
Common Places Where Skin Breakdown Occurs	189
Other Skin Problems	190

Pressure Ulcers

Pressure Ulcers—Overview	193
Pressure Ulcer Care by Risk Factors	197
Helping Pressure Ulcers Heal	198
Basic Steps of Pressure Ulcer Care	207

GENERAL SKIN CARE

What Is Healthy Skin?

Your skin is much more than an outer surface for the world to see. It protects you from bacteria, dirt and other foreign objects, and the ultraviolet rays of the sun, and contains the nerve endings that let you know if something is hot or cold, soft or hard, sharp or dull. Your skin also plays an important role in regulating your body's fluids and temperature.

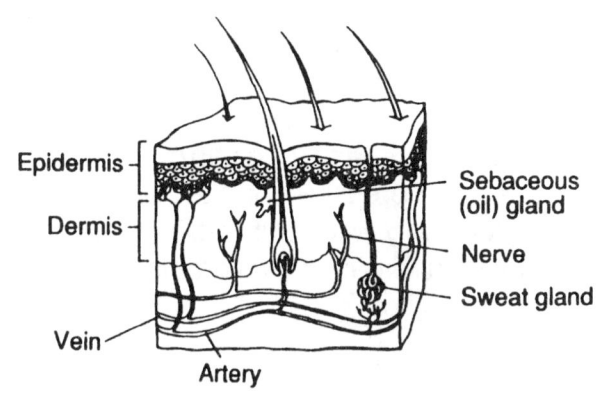

Below the smooth, hairy outer skin, or epidermis, that we see every day is a thick, strong, and elastic layer of tissue known as the dermis. The dermis is richly supplied with blood vessels, sweat and oil glands, and nerve endings.

Healthy skin is smooth, with no breaks in the surface. It is warm (not hot or red) and neither dry and flaky nor moist and wrinkled. Healthy skin is a mirror of a healthy body.

HOW TO TAKE CARE OF YOUR SKIN

Nutrition

To keep your skin healthy, eat a well-balanced diet that includes plenty of protein foods, fresh fruits and vegetables, and liquids. If you are having a skin problem, such as a pressure sore or a healing surgical incision, you should increase your intake of protein (lean meats, dairy foods, and legumes); carbohydrates (breads, cereals); vitamins A, C, and E; and zinc. Extra iron may be needed if you are anemic (see below).

Circulation

The skin is served by a large number of blood vessels, and adequate circulation is needed to maintain skin health. You can help ensure a healthy blood supply by considering the following suggestions:

- **Smoking**—DON'T! Nicotine in cigarettes causes blood vessels to get small (constrict) and prevents blood, oxygen, and nutrients from flowing to the body tissues.
- **Edema**, or swelling caused by fluid collecting in the tissues, usually occurs in a part of the body that is not moved frequently and is below the level of the heart (i.e., the feet, legs, and hands). Skin over areas of edema becomes thin and pale and injures easily because of poor

continues

continued

circulation. Edema can be prevented by elevating your legs and hands frequently, performing regular range of motion (ROM) exercises, and wearing compressive stockings.
- **Anemia** is a decrease in red blood cells. Oxygen is essential for skin health, and it is carried by red blood cells. A decrease in their number means less oxygen gets to the skin, which means that skin cells may become unhealthy or even die. Anemia should be evaluated and treated by your health care provider.
- **Vascular disease**, or a narrowing of the blood vessels, can be caused by diabetes, smoking, high blood pressure, or elevated cholesterol. The result is decreased blood flow to the skin. Work closely with your health care provider to manage conditions that can lead to vascular disease and cause skin problems.

Notes:

Courtesy of the University of Washington Medical Center, Northwest Regional Spinal Cord System, Seattle, Washington, © 1991.

Tips for Maintaining Good Skin

- Keep the skin clean and dry. Wash with soap and water daily, then rinse and dry thoroughly.
- Skin folds or creases (as in the groin area and underarms) need washing more frequently—twice a day, morning and bedtime. Rashes can easily form in these areas because of increased moisture and warmth. Increasing the air circulation to these areas to help prevent rashes can be accomplished by positioning the arms and legs so the skin surfaces are separated. For example, use the "frog" position to air the groin area. Air these areas two times a day.
- Rashes can be caused by tapes, soaps, fabrics, or other irritants. Total body rashes may result from food or drug allergies. Consult your health care provider for treatment of these and any other rashes you may have.
- Avoid using items that may dry the skin, for example, harsh soaps or alcohol-based products such as lotions.
- Lubricate dry skin with moisturizing creams or ointments (such as Eucerin or Aquaphor). Use care in applying creams over bony areas, since they may soften the skin and promote skin breakdown.
- Soiled skin can break down easily. Urine and stool have irritants in them and should be cleaned up immediately to prevent weakening and breakdown of the skin surface.
- Avoid using talc powders, as they may support yeast growth. They can also "cake up" and keep moisture in, causing skin breakdown.
- Calluses may form on your feet and hands. These can be removed by soaking frequently in warm water and toweling briskly to remove dead skin. You can use moisturizing creams to help soften calluses.
- Finger- and toenails require special care. Soak them and rub gently with a towel to remove dead skin and decrease the chance of hangnails forming. Nails are easier to cut after soaking; be sure to cut them straight across to avoid ingrown nails. Keep your nails short for safety.

Notes:

Courtesy of the University of Washington Medical Center, Northwest Regional Spinal Cord Injury System, Seattle, Washington, © 1991.

Guidelines to Success in Avoiding Skin Problems

The best way to **treat** skin breakdown is to **prevent** it. Ways to prevent skin breakdown must become part of your daily routine, just like brushing your teeth or washing your hair.

Good skin care will help you stay out of the hospital for pressure ulcer treatment or surgery. It will also allow you more time for work and recreation.

DO PRESSURE RELIEFS AT LEAST EVERY 30 MINUTES (OR MORE!)

The relief of pressure, especially over bones, is very important for healthy skin. This doesn't mean you relieve pressure **after** you notice signs of skin breakdown. "Pressure reliefs" are a means by which to **prevent** skin breakdown from the very start. Do your pressure reliefs often enough to meet the needs of your skin (every 20–30 minutes, or as prescribed by your doctor).

EAT FOODS THAT FEED YOUR SKIN

A poor diet doesn't give your body enough building blocks to make strong, healthy skin. Drinking enough **fluids** of any kind, along with a good diet full of needed **protein, vitamins**, and **minerals** helps strengthen the basic structure of your skin. Strong skin doesn't break open easily and heals quickly if scratched or cut.

- **Protein**. When you are sick, as with flu or infection, or are losing weight, your skin is more sensitive to pressure. At these times, you should **increase** the amount of **protein** you eat. **Foods high in protein:** fish, lean red meat, milk, cheese, eggs. Keep in mind the effect these foods may have on your bladder program.
- **Fluids.** Drink lots of fluids, but keep in mind that it must be **within the limits of your bladder program**.

KEEP YOUR SKIN CLEAN AND DRY

Unclean skin is a home for germs. Old skin cells may flake off, but not very quickly, so cleansing the skin helps wash away the old cells and the germs before a problem can occur. Wet skin also breaks down more easily because moisture softens the skin.

- Change wet clothing **right away**. This includes clothes wet by sweat, spilled foods, or liquids. Take care to **pat dry** your skin (including skin folds) before putting on dry clothes.
- Follow your bowel and bladder programs. This may prevent soiling from an accident.
- If you have a bowel or bladder accident, change soiled clothing **right away**. Wash your skin with soap and warm (not hot) water. If your skin is red, be careful not to rub it—instead, pat dry. To prevent drying and cracking of skin, apply a lotion or cream on a routine basis.

Caution: NEVER use heat or a hair dryer to dry your skin or clothes. You can get burned without knowing it.

continues

continued

BUILD UP SKIN TOLERANCE

Skin tolerance is how much time your skin can stand to be under pressure before damage starts to occur. Each person's skin tolerance is different. Some people may need to relieve pressure very often, others may not.

Building up skin tolerance is a gradual process. The pinkness of your skin (the FIRST SIGN of a pressure ulcer) and the amount of time it takes for it to clear will tell you whether to increase or decrease your time between pressure reliefs and your sitting time.

CHECK YOUR SKIN

Check your skin twice a day:

- once before you get out of bed
- once before you go to bed

It is not enough to take a quick look at the parts of your skin you can see easily. You will need to use a **long-handled mirror** to see areas that are not easy to see (back, tailbone, heels, groin, buttocks, etc.), or ask someone to check those areas for you.

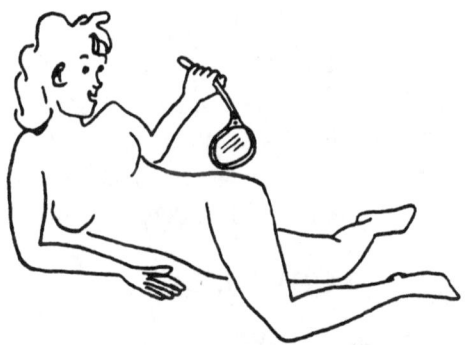

By looking over your skin inch by inch twice a day, you will know if a pressure ulcer is starting, so you can prevent it from getting worse. It will also tell you if you are doing enough pressure reliefs, so you will be able to adjust your routine for better skin care.

BE KIND TO YOUR FEET!

Feet get a lot of abuse: they are banged on furniture, pinched in poorly fitting shoes, etc. Keep an eye on your feet. Pressure ulcers or cuts can be very hard to heal, because circulation is slower there.

IF YOU SMOKE, STOP!

We don't need to tell you much more than that. Smoking decreases the blood supply to your skin. It will slow down the healing process of simple cuts and bruises.

Source: *Spinal Cord Injury Manual*, Kessler Institute for Rehabilitation, West Orange, New Jersey.

Additional Guidelines for Skin Injury Prevention

EQUIPMENT

Are you using the best equipment? Does it fit you properly?

- **Wheelchair:** Does it support your back? Are your footrests the right height? Are you using the best wheelchair cushion?
- **Bed:** Are you using a good mattress?
- **External catheters:** Is the correct size being used? Is it being changed frequently enough?
- **Leg bags:** Are the straps too tight?
- **Splints/Braces:** Do they fit properly? Do you do skin checks after wearing them?

TEMPERATURE

Extremes of temperature call for extra caution in protecting your skin:

- **Heat:** Avoid sunburn by covering up or using sunblock. Don't put plates of hot food on your lap without protecting your skin. When riding in a car, keep your feet away from the heat outlet, and check vinyl seats before you sit on them to make sure they aren't too hot. Any exposed pipes in your kitchen or bathroom sink should be wrapped to protect your legs from burns. When you go camping, protect your feet by sitting a safe distance from the campfire.
- **Cold:** Be sure to dress properly to prevent frostbite if you are out in cold weather for long periods of time. Avoid putting frozen foods on your lap.
- **Fever:** Your skin tolerances can change due to the increased body temperature that occurs with a fever. You may find that you cannot lie in one position as long.

BODY WEIGHT

- **Too much:** Being overweight can cause increased pressure on bony prominences. Delayed healing may occur because there are fewer blood vessels in fat tissue.
- **Too little:** Excess pressure over bony prominences may occur because there is less padding (muscle and fat) over these surfaces. In addition, underweight persons may lack the proper nutrition to maintain healthy skin.

CLOTHING

Proper fit is important. Avoid sitting on seams and back pockets, and always check your skin carefully after wearing new shoes or clothing.

- **Too loose:** Loose clothing can form wrinkles that put pressure on your skin.
- **Too tight:** Overly tight clothing can hinder circulation.

continues

continued

ALCOHOL

Overindulgence in alcohol—or any other drug—may interfere with attention to your personal care needs. For example, while under the influence you might forget to turn yourself or be too weak to transfer yourself properly.

STRESS

Stress and depression can have a similar effect by causing you to lose interest in your personal care and pay less attention to your skin and general health.

SPASTICITY

Spasticity may cause your arms and/or legs to bump against an object, or to fall off your armrest or footrest, and be injured. Spasms may cause your skin to rub against something (for example, the sheets on your bed), which could produce an open sore.

Notes:

Courtesy of the University of Washington Medical Center, Northwest Regional Spinal Cord Injury System, Seattle, Washington, © 1992.

Pressure Reliefs to Save Your Skin

CUSHIONS AND WHEELCHAIRS

- Proper cushions for the bottom and sides of your wheelchair can prevent many skin problems. They evenly distribute pressure and protect you from the edges of your wheelchair. Cushions by themselves DO NOT prevent pressure ulcers.
- The proper fit of your wheelchair is important too. The fit of your wheelchair and how well you can move around in and out of its seat can be the difference between cuts and bruises and healthy skin. See your physiatrist if problems arise.

TURNING AND POSITIONING IN BED

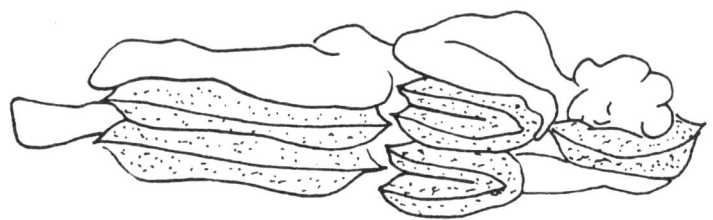

On Your Side

- Position pillows to prevent pressure on your hip bones and the sides of knees.
- Your topside leg should be on a pillow.
- Your drainage bag should be on the side of bed you are facing.

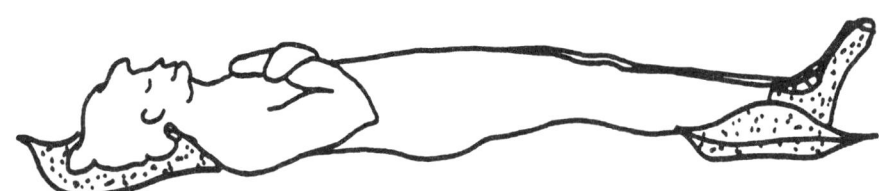

On Your Back

- Watch your lower back (*sacrum*) for signs of pressure.
- To prevent pressure on your heels, be sure you have your protective booties on.

continues

continued

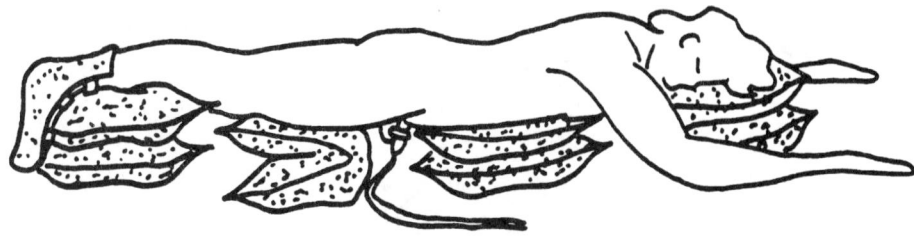

On Your Stomach

This position is good for persons with paraplegia and low-level quadriplegia, but always check with your physiatrist first. Lying on your stomach straightens your hips and prevents tightness. It also helps to decrease leg spasms.

- Place pillows as shown to avoid pressure on your breast bone, genitals, hips, knees, and toes.

CAUTION: You will need to build up tolerance to this position.

SITTING UP IN YOUR WHEELCHAIR

LOCK YOUR WHEELS AND WEAR YOUR SEAT BELT.

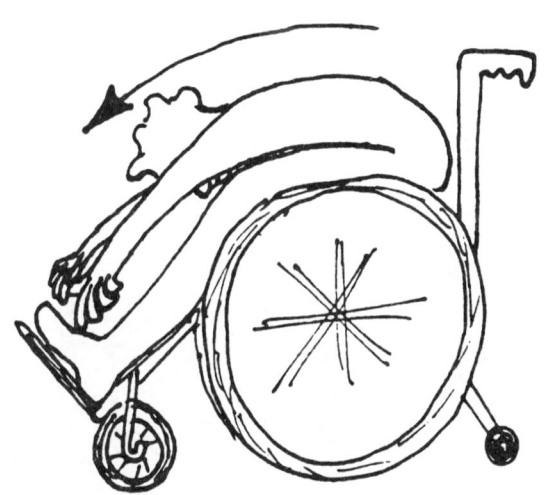

- **Slump over your feet.** Lean forward over your feet (be careful not to tip your chair). Hold that position for **5 minutes**.

continues

continued

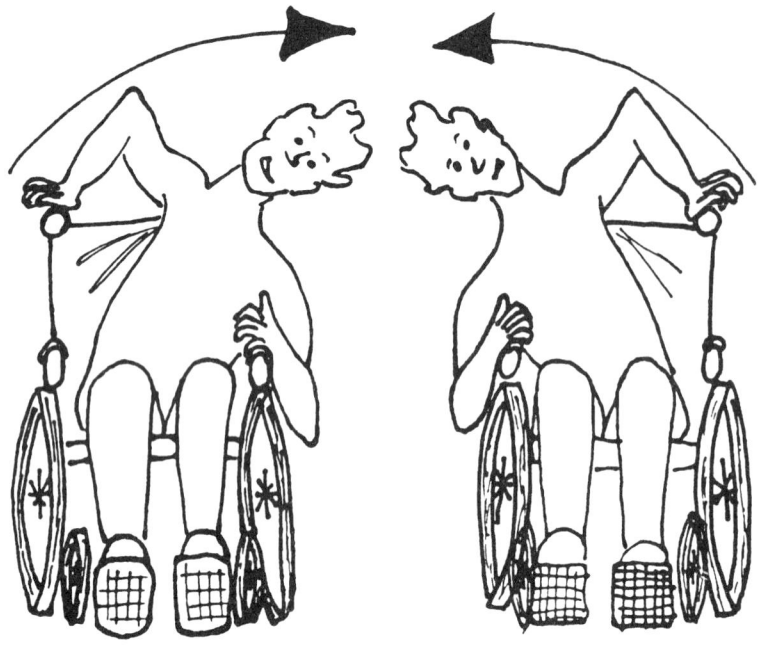

- **Lean to the side.** Lean to one side over your armrail (Be careful not to tip your chair). Hold that position for **5 minutes**. Then lean to the other side over your armrail. Hold that position for **5 minutes**.

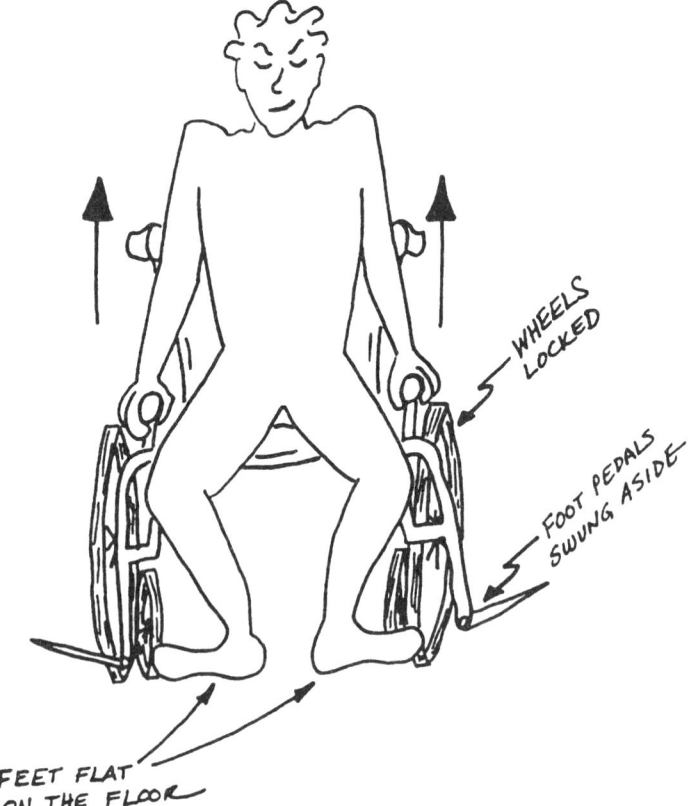

- **Lift yourself up**. This takes good arm strength. Put your hands on your armrails. Lift yourself up until your arms are straight. Hold that position for **1 minute**. GENTLY set yourself down.

- **Wiggle!** Just keep moving. Every time you reach away from yourself, you are shifting the pressure on your seat. Being active will naturally shift your body around so that pressure is relieved.

continues

Skin Care 185

continued

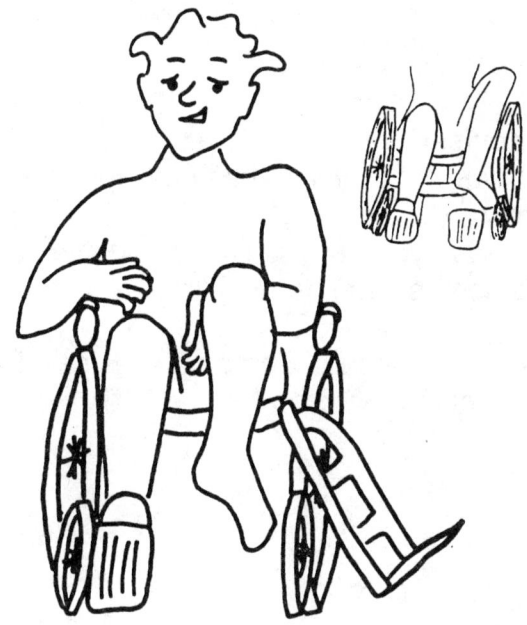

- **Lift your leg.** Hook your arm under one of your legs. Lift it up. Hold it that way for **5 minutes**. Gently put it down. Lift up your other leg. Hold it that way for **5 minutes**. You can also do this type of pressure relief by bringing one foot up onto some part of your wheelchair frame and setting it there. After 5 minutes, switch feet.

Notes:

Source: *Spinal Cord Injury Manual*, Kessler Institute for Rehabilitation, West Orange, New Jersey.

Steps for Building Skin Tolerance

You can build skin tolerance for any position, lying down or sitting:

- **Lie in one position for the amount of time advised by your doctor.**
- **Look at your skin. Test if the pink areas of your skin turn white when touched.**
- **Let the redness or pinkness clear completely.**
  - *If color clears in 15–30 minutes*, you may increase your turning time by 30 minutes.
  - *If color doesn't clear in 15–30 minutes*, don't increase your turning time.

Eventually you may be able to tolerate up to three to five hours. Some sources say that if you lie on your stomach, you can stay that way for eight hours.

Notes:

Source: *Spinal Cord Injury Manual*, Kessler Institute for Rehabilitation, West Orange, New Jersey.

How to Do a Skin Check

LOOK FOR THESE SIGNS

- **ANY** changes in how your skin looks
- **ANY** changes in the color of your skin over bony areas:
  - Pinkness that doesn't go away in 15 minutes
  - Redness that doesn't go away in 15 minutes
  - Redness with a hardened area under it
  - Yellowness
  - Blackness
- **PLEASE NOTE:** You will need to learn what is NOT a normal color for you, based on the color of your skin. Olive, Asian, Black, very tanned, or other kinds of skin coloring may vary from the warning colors listed above. Find out what is normal for you.
- Scrapes or cuts
- Blisters
- Bruises

CHECK THESE PARTS OF YOUR SKIN

- **Over all bones** that you can feel
- **ANY** place over which you have worn a **splint or brace**
- **Skin folds** (genitals, buttocks, breasts, etc.): This is very important. Moisture can build up in these folds and quicken the rate of breakdown. Folds are also a great place for germs.

HOW TO CHECK YOUR FEET

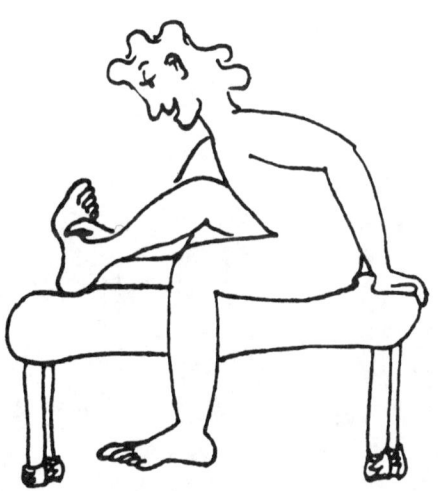

When you do skin checks, you must take a special look at your feet:

- Check for cracks, cuts, calluses, and long toenails, which can lead to sores and/or skin trouble. Look between your toes.
- Check your feet for red areas after you wear shoes and/or stockings for a given amount of time. Depending on the redness, increase or decrease your wearing time. Take special care with new shoes.
- **Please note:** Even if you can't feel the heat or cold, your feet can be sensitive to burns from hot bath water, car heaters, hot sand or pavement, snow, or radiators. Avoid or take care with such sources of heat and cold.

continues

continued

Routine care for your feet should be done **weekly:**

- Soak your feet in a pan of warm soapy water (**not hot water**—test it with your elbow or a place where you can feel first) for 20–30 minutes.
- Gently rub each foot with a washcloth to loosen and remove dead skin.
- Rinse in clear water.
- Pat your feet dry feet with a towel, especially between your toes.
- Massage very dry skin with an **emoulient** (not a moisturizer, which would soften skin and increase your chance of skin breakdown), like cocoa butter lotions.
- If your doctor says it's okay, you can trim nails as needed—otherwise, see a podiatrist (foot doctor). Your toenails should be trimmed with a straight-edged clipper or sharp scissors, cutting straight across and not too short.
- If the nail bed (the area around the nail) becomes red, this could be a sign of an ingrown toenail. See your podiatrist as soon as possible.

Notes:

Source: *Spinal Cord Injury Manual*, Kessler Institute for Rehabilitation, West Orange, New Jersey.

Common Places Where Skin Breakdown Occurs

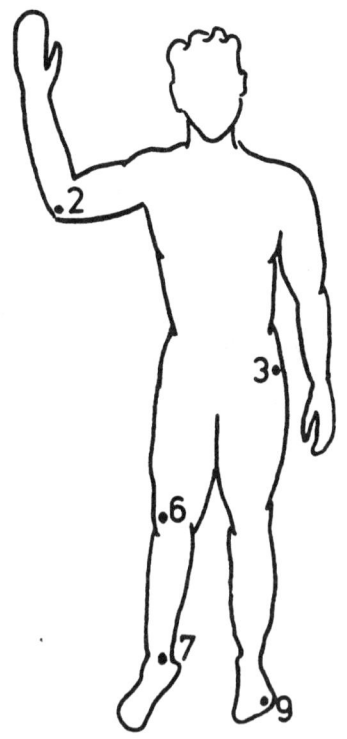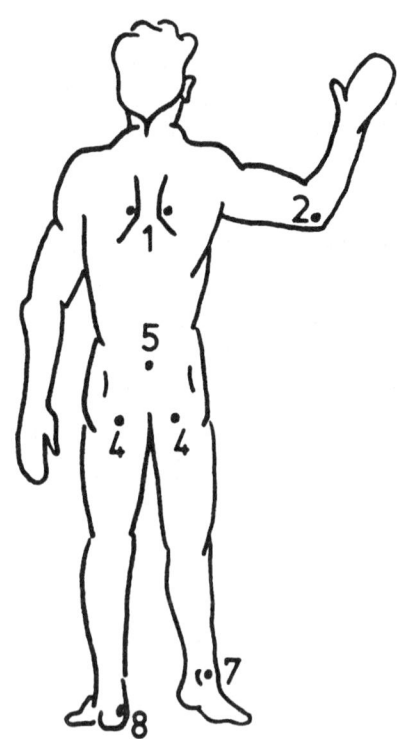

- **Scapula (1):** Caused by halo vests when the skin has not been washed, lining has gotten soiled with flaked skin, or pressure/poor fit of vest.
- **Elbow (2):** Caused by leaning on it or using it to prop up on wheelchair, mattress, or stretcher. Use elbow protectors.
- **Trochanter (*Tro-can-turr*) (3):** Caused by lying on your side too long.
- **Ischium (*ISH-ee-um*) (4):** Because the ischium supports your weight in sitting, skin breakdown in this area is common, caused by not doing weight shifts often enough while sitting, or by setting foot pedals too high (tilts weight of legs onto ischium).
- **Sacrum (and Coccyx) (5):** Caused by lying on your back in a semisitting position too long or sliding forward in your wheelchair.
- **Knee (6):** Caused by bumping knees, hot spills, etc.
- **Ankle (7):** Caused by lying on your side with too much pressure on sides of foot.
- **Heels (8):** Caused by pressure of heels on the bed.
- **Toes (9):** Caused by tight or poorly fitting shoes, elastic stockings, or bumps from not wearing shoes.

Source: *Spinal Cord Injury Manual*, Kessler Institute for Rehabilitation, West Orange, New Jersey.

Other Skin Problems

Problem	Signs	Cause	Do	Do Not
Rashes (Where skin comes in contact with skin, e.g., groin, armpits, under breasts)	Pimples, red blotches	Moisture and lack of air	Keep areas clean and dry. Allow air to reach rash area. If no improvement in couple of days, see doctor.	DO NOT apply ointment or powder unless ordered by your doctor. If ordered by doctor, do not use too much or it will "cake" or clump.
Frostbite (Usually fingers and toes)	Skin turns pale or white then red	Combination of loss of sensation and extreme cold	Wear warm footwear and gloves in cold weather as preventive measure. If it occurs, put part in LUKEWARM water and call doctor immediately.	DO NOT stay out in cold too long. DO NOT rub the part or put in hot or cold water.
Burns (Anywhere)	Redness of skin or possibly blisters	Cigarettes (from ashes you can't feel) Hot water pipes/radiator/car heaters/car upholstery	Always wear shoes in car. Wrap exposed pipes under sink with insulating material. Keep car heating systems in good working order. If car seat is too warm, sit on sheepskin or your own cushion.	DO NOT set ashtray on your lap. DO NOT sit too close to radiators or other heating system (heat can be conducted through wheelchair pedals if they are close to heat source).

continues

Skin Care 191

continued

Problem	Signs	Cause	Do	Do Not
Burns (Anywhere)		Bathing/hot water	Test shower or bath water, or have someone do it for you.	DO NOT leave water running on your body where you cannot feel.
		Just-cooked foods, hot liquids/pans from oven or microwave	Use care in handling hot liquids, foods, and cooking utensils. Use a wooden tray to carry hot objects.	DO NOT carry cups of hot liquid or food on lap or between legs.
		Hot water bottles/heating lamps/electric heating pads		DO NOT use, even on areas with sensation (they could slip down and cause a burn).
			If a burn happens: Call your doctor. Apply cold water for 30 minutes.	DO NOT apply ointments or medicines to burns or sores unless prescribed.
Bruises (Anywhere)	Redness or bluish tinge to skin	Careless transferring and turning (if swelling is present there may be a fracture)	Guard against injury when transferring or turning.	DO NOT go without shoes.
		Spasticity	Guard against injury from spasms.	

continues

continued

Problem	Signs	Cause	Do	Do Not
Friction burn (ischium, sacrum)	Redness—skin scraped off	Sliding down in bed or chair; spasms in bed or chair	Wear clothing when transferring with sliding boards.	DO NOT EVER let anyone pull your bare skin across a sheet.
Blisters (Anywhere)	Raised, fluid-filled areas	Leg bag straps may be too tight; may signal start of pressure sore. Shoes may be too tight or too loose		DO NOT break blister.
Foot problems (Feet are a likely place for problems. They are farthest from the heart, so circulation is less efficient)	Dry, scaly skin	Not enough circulation or air to feet	Keep feet very clean. Soak in warm water, then remove dead skin with pumice stone or gentle brush. Put bath oil in water to help moisturize. Apply lanolin, lotion or corn oil to keep skin lubricated.	DO NOT EVER pick off dry, flaky skin.
Ingrown toenails (Usually on large toe)	Redness, increased warmth, drainage, swelling around toenail	Toenails cut too short or rounded in corners. Tight shoes. Poor hygiene. Trauma. Skin breakdown	Cut toenails straight across.	DO NOT trim or round corners on toenails.

Source: Shirley S. Paulson, *Spinal Cord Injury Home Care Manual*, Norman B. Nelson Rehabilitation Center, Santa Clara Valley Medical Center, San Jose, California, © 1994.

PRESSURE ULCERS

Pressure Ulcers—Overview

WHAT IS A PRESSURE ULCER?

A pressure ulcer is any redness or break in the skin caused by too much pressure on your skin for too long a period of time. The pressure prevents blood from getting to your skin, so the skin dies. Normally the nerves send messages of pain or feelings of discomfort to your brain to let you know that you need to change position, but damage to your spinal cord keeps these messages from reaching your brain.

You may need to learn new ways to change your position to prevent too much pressure. Pressure ulcers can occur, for example, when you sit or lie in one position too long. *Shearing* is also a kind of pressure injury. It happens when the skin moves one way and the bone underneath it moves another way. An example of this is if you slouch when you sit.

Another type of injury, an abrasion, can occur when pulling yourself across a surface instead of lifting. This is an example of a friction injury. In addition, short exposure to high pressure, such as a bump or fall, may cause damage to the skin that may not show up right away.

STAGES OF PRESSURE ULCERS AND HOW TO CARE FOR THEM

Stage One

How to recognize: Skin is not broken but is red or discolored. The redness or change in color does not fade within 30 minutes after pressure is removed.

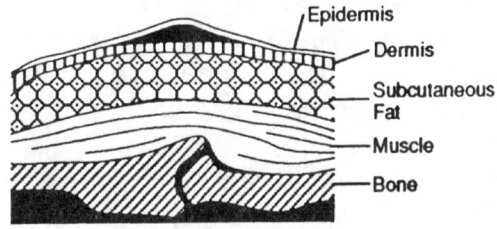

What to do:

1. Keep pressure off the ulcer.
2. Maintain good hygiene. Wash with mild soap and water, rinse well, pat dry carefully (but gently). Do not rub vigorously directly over the wound.
3. Evaluate your diet. Are you getting enough protein, calories, vitamins A and C, zinc, and iron? All of these are necessary for healthy skin.
4. Review your mattress, wheelchair cushion, transfers, pressure releases, and turning techniques for a possible cause of the problem.

continues

continued

5. If the ulcer seems to be caused by friction, sometimes a protective transparent dressing such as Op-Site or Tegaderm may help protect the area by allowing the skin to slide easily.
6. If the ulcer does not heal in a few days or if it recurs, consult your health care provider.

Stage Two

How to recognize: The epidermis or topmost layer of the skin is broken, creating a shallow open sore. Drainage may or may not be present.

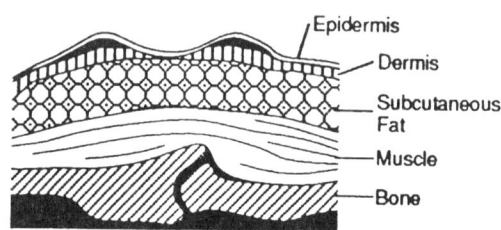

What to do: Follow steps 1 through 4 under Stage One. Further treatment should be determined by your health care provider and may include the following:

1. Cleanse the wound with saline solution only and dry carefully. Apply either a transparent dressing (such as Op-Site or Tegaderm), a hydrocolloid dressing (such as DuoDERM), or saline-dampened gauze. The first two types of dressing can be left on until they wrinkle or loosen (up to five days). If using gauze, it should be changed twice a day and should remain *damp* between dressing changes.
2. Check for signs of wound healing with each dressing change.
3. If there are signs of infection, consult your health care provider for alternative wound care ideas and review of possible causes (see step 4 under Stage One).

Stage Three

How to recognize: The break in the skin extends through the dermis (second skin layer) into the subcutaneous and fat tissue. The wound is deeper than in Stage Two.

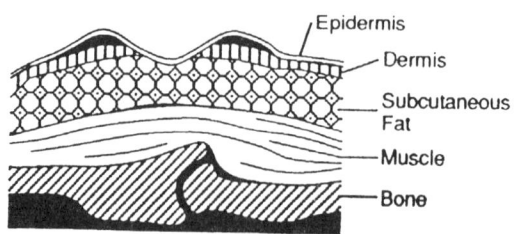

continues

continued

What to do: Follow steps 1 through 4 under Stage One and all steps under Stage Two. **Always consult your health care provider.** Wounds in this stage frequently need additional wound care, such as special cleaning agents (half-strength hydrogen peroxide or dilute Hibiclens), debriding agents (such as Elase), irrigations (forceful cleansing of the wound bed), and/or packing of the wound bed (DuoDERM granules, moist gauze). Occasionally an antibiotic (oral pills or Silvadene cream) may be used. Your health care provider will order what is appropriate for you.

Stage Four

How to recognize: The breakdown extends into the muscle and can extend as far down as the bone. Usually lots of dead tissue and drainage are present.

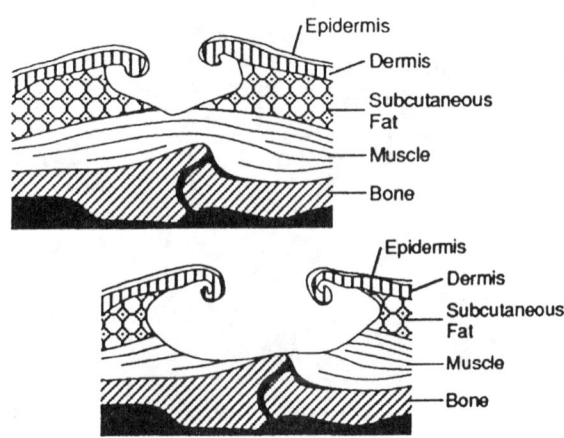

What to do: Consult your health care provider right away. Surgery is frequently required for this type of wound.

HOW DO I KNOW IF THE ULCER IS HEALING?

- The ulcer will get smaller.
- Pinkish tissue usually starts forming along the edges of the ulcer and moves toward the center; you may notice either smooth or bumpy surfaces of new tissue.
- Some bleeding may be present. This shows that there is good blood circulation to the area, which helps healing.

continued

WHAT ARE THE SIGNS OF TROUBLE?

You need to seek help if any of the following occurs:

- An increase in the size or drainage of the sore.
- Increased redness around the sore or black areas starting to form.
- The ulcer starts smelling and/or the drainage becomes a greenish color.
- You develop a fever.

WHAT KIND OF COMPLICATIONS CAN BE CAUSED BY PRESSURE ULCERS?

- They can be life threatening.
- Infection can spread to the blood, heart, or bone.
- They may result in amputations.
- You may need prolonged bed rest.
- They can result in autonomic dysreflexia.

Notes:

Courtesy of the University of Washington Medical Center, Northwest Regional Spinal Cord System, Seattle, Washington, © 1991.

Pressure Ulcer Care by Risk Factors

Risk Factor	Preventive Actions
1. Bed or chair confinement	• Inspect skin at least once a day. • Bathe when needed for comfort or cleanliness. • Prevent dry skin. • For a person in bed: ——Change position at least every two hours. ——Use a special mattress that contains foam, air, gel, or water. ——Raise the head of the bed as little and for as short a time as possible. • For a person in a chair: ——Change position. ——Use foam, gel, or air cushion to relieve pressure. • Reduce friction by: ——lifting rather than dragging when repositioning ——using cornstarch on skin • Avoid use of doughnut-shaped cushions. • Participate in a rehabilitation program.
2. Inability to move	• Persons confined to chairs should be repositioned if they are unable to do so themselves. • For a person in a chair who is able to shift his or her own weight, change position at least every 15 minutes. • Use pillows or wedges to keep knees or ankles from touching each other. • When in bed, place pillow under legs from midcalf to ankle to keep heels off the bed.
3. Loss of bowel or bladder control	• Clean skin as soon as soiled. • Assess and treat urine leaks. • If moisture cannot be controlled: —Use absorbent pads and/or briefs with a quick-drying surface. —Protect skin with a cream or ointment.
4. Poor nutrition	• Eat a balanced diet. • If a normal diet is not possible, talk to health care provider about nutritional supplements.
5. Lowered mental awareness	• Choose preventive actions that apply to the person with lowered mental awareness. For example, if the person is chairbound, refer to the specific preventive actions outlined in Risk Factor 1.

Source: *Preventing Pressure Ulcers: A Patient's Guide,* U.S. Department of Health and Human Services, Public Health Service, Agency for Health Care Policy and Research, Publication No. 92-0048, May 1992.

Helping Pressure Ulcers Heal

Healing pressure ulcers depends on three principles: pressure relief, care of the ulcer, and good nutrition.

PRESSURE RELIEF

Pressure ulcers form when there is constant pressure on certain parts of the body. Long periods of unrelieved pressure cause or worsen pressure sores and slow healing once an ulcer has formed. Taking pressure off the ulcer is the first step toward healing.

Pressure ulcers usually form on parts of the body over bony prominences (such as hips and heels) that bear weight when you sit or lie down for a long time. Figure 1 shows "pressure points" where ulcers often form.

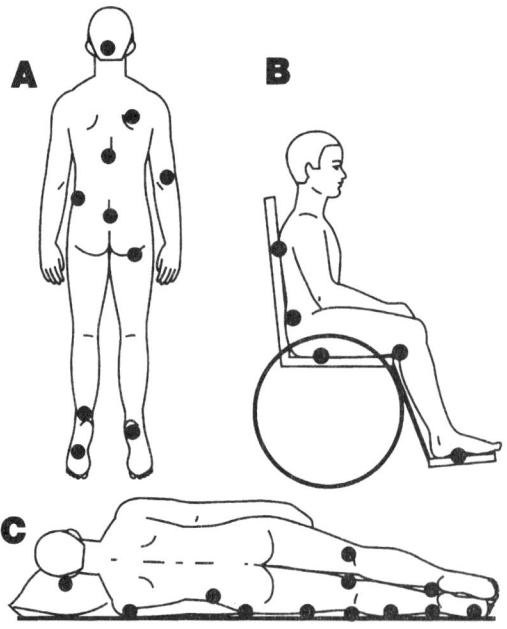

Figure 1. Pressure Points. Dots show pressure points when lying on back (A), when sitting (B), and when lying on side (C).

continues

continued

You can relieve or reduce pressure by:

- using special surfaces to support your body
- putting your body in certain positions
- changing positions often

Support Surfaces

Support surfaces are special beds, mattresses, mattress overlays, or seat cushions that support your body in bed or in a chair. These surfaces reduce or relieve pressure. By relieving pressure, you can help pressure ulcers heal and prevent new ones from forming.

You can get different kinds of support surfaces. The best kind depends on your general health, your ability to change positions, your body build, and the condition of your ulcer. You and your doctor or nurse can choose the surface best for you.

One way to see if a support surface reduces pressure enough is for the caregiver to do a "hand check" under the person. The caregiver places his or her hand under the support surface, beneath the pressure point, with the palm up and fingers flat. If there is less than 1 inch of support surface between the pressure point of the body and the caregiver's hand, the surface does not give enough support. If you need more support, your doctor or nurse will recommend a different support surface.

Caregivers should know that pressure ulcers are often painful, and a hand check may increase pain. Caregivers should ask if it will be okay to do a hand check, which should be done as gently as possible.

Good Body Positions

Your position is important in relieving pressure on the ulcer and preventing new ones. You need to switch positions whether you are in a bed or a chair.

In Bed

Follow these guidelines:

- Do not lie on the pressure ulcer. Use foam pads or pillows to relieve pressure on the sore, as shown in Figure 2.
- Change position at least every two hours.

continues

continued

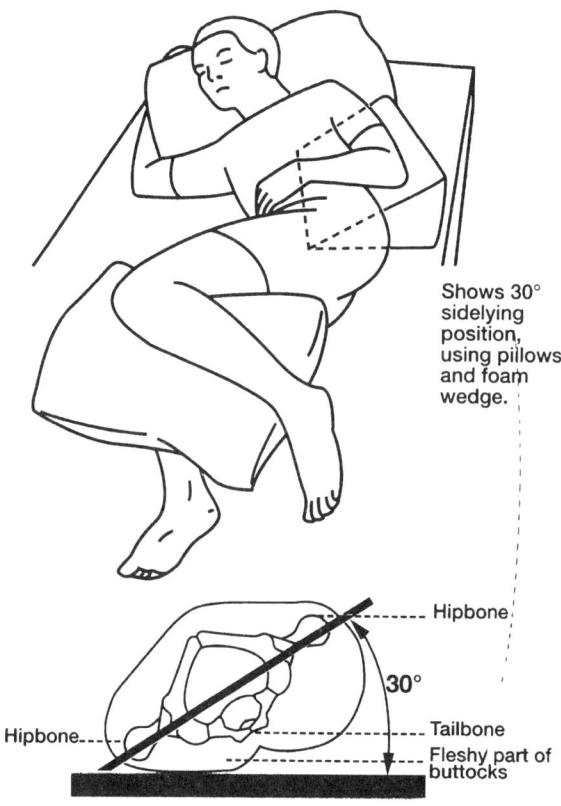

Figure 2. Best Position while on Side*

- Do not rest directly on your hipbone when lying on your side. A 30-degree sidelying position is best (see Figure 2).
- When lying on your back, keep your heels up off the bed by placing a thin foam pad or pillow under your legs from midcalf to ankle (Figure 3). The pad or pillow should raise the heels just enough so a piece of paper can be passed between them and the bed. Do not place the pad or pillow directly under the knee when on your back, because this could reduce blood flow to your lower leg.

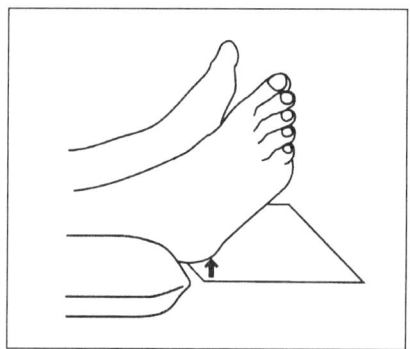

Figure 3. Keep Heels off Bed**

*Source: Reprinted by permission of Medical Economics/RN Magazine/J. Tandy.
**Source: Adapted with permission from *Pressure Ulcers: Guidelines for Prevention and Nursing Management,* Springhouse Corporation, © 1991. All rights reserved.

continues

continued

- Do not use donut-shaped (ring) cushions—they reduce blood flow to tissue.
- Use pillows or small foam pads to keep knees and ankles from touching each other.
- Raise the head of the bed as little as possible. Raise it no more than 30 degrees from horizontal (Figure 4). If you have other health problems (such as respiratory ailments) that are improved by sitting up, ask your doctor or nurse which positions are best.
- Use the upright position during meals to prevent choking. The head of the bed can be moved back to a lying or semireclining position one hour after eating.

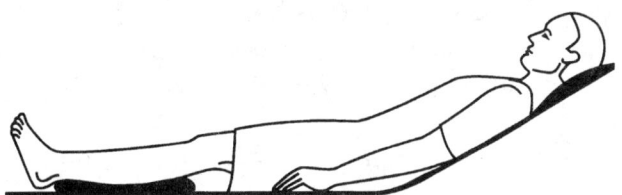

Figure 4. Head of Bed Raised 30°

In a Chair or Wheelchair

When sitting, you should have good posture and be able to keep upright in the chair or wheelchair (Figure 5). A good position will allow you to move more easily and help prevent new sores.

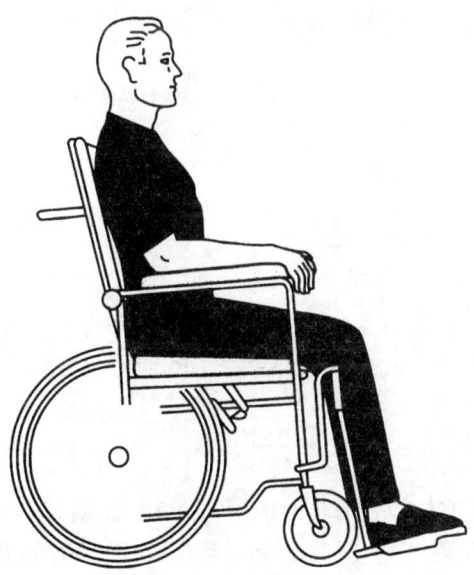

Figure 5. Best Position while Sitting. Ankles should not be flexed or extended. Note position of thighs, hands, and forearms. Use a specially designed 2- to 3-inch seat cushion.

continues

continued

For your specific needs, use cushions designed to relieve pressure on sitting surfaces. Even if pressure can be relieved with cushions, your position should be changed every hour. Remember to:

- Avoid sitting directly on the pressure ulcer.
- Keep the top of your thighs horizontal and your ankles in a comfortable, "neutral" position on the floor or footrest (Figure 5). Rest your elbows, forearms, and wrists on arm supports.
- If you cannot move yourself, have someone help you change your position at least every hour. If you can move yourself, shifting your weight every 15 minutes is even better.
- If your position in a chair cannot be changed, have someone help you back to bed so you can change position.
- Do **not** use donut-shaped or ring cushions, because they reduce blood flow to tissue.

Changing Positions

Change your body position often—at least every hour while seated in a chair and at least every two hours while lying in bed. A written turning schedule or a turn clock (with positions written next to times) may help you and your caregiver remember turning times and positions. You may want to set a kitchen timer.

Be sure your plan works for you. It should consider your skin's condition, personal needs and preferences, and your comfort level.

PRESSURE ULCER CARE

The second principle of healing is proper care of the ulcer. The three aspects of care are:

1. cleaning
2. removing dead tissue and debris (debridement)
3. dressing (bandaging) the pressure sore

You should know about ulcer care even if only your caregiver is caring for the sore. Knowing about your care will help you make informed decisions about it.

Cleaning

Pressure ulcers heal best when they are clean. They should be free of dead tissue (which may look like a scab), excess fluid draining from the sore, and other debris. If not, healing can be slowed, and infection can result.

A health care professional will show you and your caregiver how to clean and/or rinse the pressure sore. Clean the ulcer each time dressings are changed.

continues

continued

Cleaning usually involves rinsing or "irrigating" the ulcer. Loose material may also be gently wiped away with a gauze pad. It is important to use the right equipment and methods for cleaning the ulcer. Tissue that is healing can be hurt if too much force is used when rinsing. Cleaning may be ineffective if too little force is used.

Use only cleaning solutions recommended by a health care professional. Usually saline is best for rinsing the pressure ulcer. Saline can be bought at a drugstore or made at home (see below).

Recipe for Making Saline (Salt Water)

1. Use 1 gallon of distilled water or boil 1 gallon of tap water for 5 minutes. **Do not use well water or sea water.**
2. Add 8 teaspoons of table salt to the distilled or boiled water.
3. Mix the solution well until the salt is completely dissolved. Be sure storage container and mixing utensil are clean (boiled).

Note: Cool to room temperature before using. This solution can be stored at room temperature in a tightly covered glass or plastic bottle for up to one week.

Caution: Sometimes water supplies become contaminated. If the health department warns against drinking the water, use saline from the drugstore or use bottled water to make saline for cleaning ulcers.

Do not use antiseptics such as hydrogen peroxide or iodine. They can damage sensitive tissue and prevent healing.

Cleansing methods are usually effective in keeping ulcers clean. However, in some cases, other methods will be needed to remove dead tissue.

Removing Dead Tissue and Debris

Dead tissue in the pressure ulcer can delay healing and lead to infection. Removing dead tissue is often painful. You may want to take pain-relieving medicine 30 to 60 minutes before these procedures.

Under supervision of health care professionals, dead tissue and debris can be removed in several ways:

- Rinsing (to wash away loose debris).

continues

continued

- Wet-to-dry dressings. In this special method, wet dressings are put on and allowed to dry. Dead tissue and debris are pulled off when the dry dressing is taken off. This method is only used to remove dead tissue; it is never used on a clean wound.
- Enzyme medications to dissolve dead tissue only.
- Special dressings left in place for several days help the body's natural enzymes dissolve dead tissue slowly. This method should not be used if the sore is infected. With infected ulcers, a faster method for removing dead tissue and debris should be used.

Qualified health care professionals may use surgical instruments to cut away dead tissue.

Based on the person's general health and the condition of the ulcer, the doctor or nurse will recommend the best method for removing dead tissue.

Choosing and Using Dressings

Choosing the right dressings is important to pressure ulcer care. The doctor or nurse will consider the location and condition of the pressure ulcer when recommending dressings.

The most common dressings are gauze (moistened with saline), film (see-through), and hydrocolloid (moisture- and oxygen-retaining) dressings. Gauze dressings must be moistened often with saline and changed at least daily. If the dressing is not kept moist, new tissue will be pulled off when the dressing is removed.

Unless the ulcer is infected, film or hydrocolloid dressings can be left on for several days to keep in the ulcer's natural moisture.

The choice of dressing is based on:

- the type of material that will best aid healing
- how often dressings will need to be changed
- whether the sore is infected

In general, the dressing should keep the ulcer moist and the surrounding skin dry. As the ulcer heals, a different type of dressing may be needed.

Storing and Caring for Dressings

Clean (rather than sterile) dressings usually can be used, if they are kept clean and dry. There is no evidence that using sterile dressings is better than using clean dressings. However, contamination between patients can occur in hospitals and nursing homes. When clean dressings are used in institutions, procedures that prevent cross-contamination should be followed carefully.

At home, clean dressings may also be used. Carefully follow the methods given below on how to store, care for, and change dressings:

continues

continued

- Store dressings in their original packages (or in other protective, closed plastic packages) in a clean, dry place.
- Wash hands with soap and water before touching clean dressings.
- Take dressings from the box only when they will be used.
- Do not touch the packaged dressing once the sore has been touched.
- Discard the entire package if any dressings become wet or dirty.

Changing dressings. Ask your doctor or nurse to show how to remove dressings and put on new ones. If possible, he or she should watch you change the dressings at least once.

Ask for written instructions if you need them. Discuss any problems or questions about changing dressings with the doctor or nurse.

Wash your hands with soap and water before and after each dressing change. Use each dressing **only once**. You should check to be sure the dressing stays in place when changing positions. After the used dressing is removed, it must be disposed of safely to prevent spread of germs that may be on dressings.

Using plastic bags for removal. A small plastic bag (such as a sandwich bag) can be used to lift the dressing off the pressure ulcer (Figure 6). Seal the bag before throwing it away. If you use gloves, throw them away after each use.

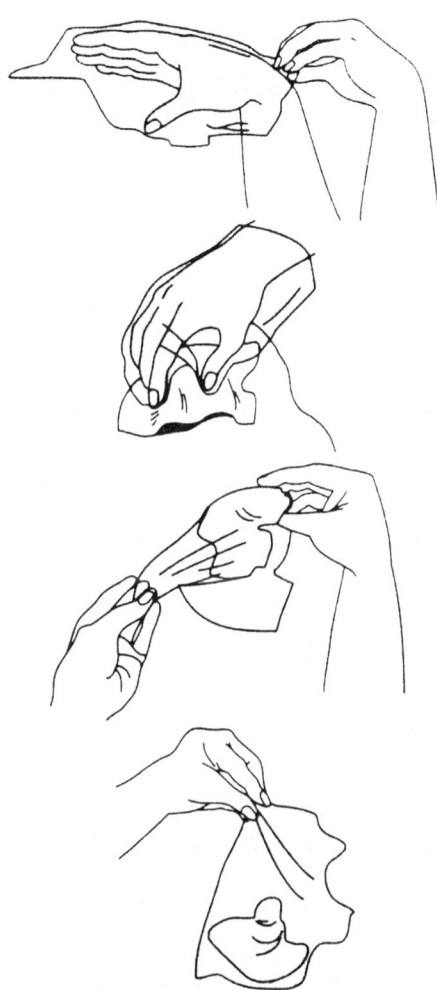

Figure 6. Plastic Bag Method of Removing Bandages. Place small, clean bag over hand like a mitten. Carefully lift dressing off ulcer and turn bag inside out to enclose dressing. Seal before throwing it away.

Adapted from J. Maklebust, M.A. Magnan. Approaches to Patient and Family Education for Pressure Ulcer Management. *Decubitus*, July 1992, pp. 18–26. Copyright, 1992. Used with permission of Springhouse Corp.

continues

continued

GOOD NUTRITION

Good nutrition is the third principle of healing. Eating a balanced diet will help your pressure sore heal and prevent new sores from forming.

You and your doctor, dietitian, or nurse should review any other medical conditions you have (such as diabetes or kidney problems) before designing a special diet.

Weigh yourself weekly. If you find you cannot eat enough food to maintain your weight or if you notice a sudden increase or decrease, you may need a special diet and vitamin supplements. You may need extra calories as part of a well-balanced diet.

Tell your doctor or nurse about any weight change. An unplanned weight gain or loss of 10 pounds or more in six months should be investigated.

Notes:

Source: *Pressure Ulcer Treatment Consumer Guide: Treating Pressure Sores*, U.S. Department of Health and Human Services, Public Health Service, Agency for Health Care Policy and Research, Publication 95-0654, December 1994.

Basic Steps of Pressure Ulcer Care

PREPARE

1. Wash hands with soap and water.
2. Get supplies: saline; irrigation equipment (syringe or other device, basin, large plastic bag); dressings and tape; disposable plastic gloves and small plastic (sandwich) bag; towel; glasses, goggles, and plastic apron (optional).
3. Move patient into comfortable position.
4. Place large plastic bag on bed to protect bed linen.

REMOVE DRESSING

1. Place hand into small plastic bag.
2. Grasp old dressing with bag-covered hand and pull off dressing.
3. Turn bag inside-out over the old dressing.
4. Close the bag tightly before throwing it away.

IRRIGATE ULCER

1. Put on disposable plastic gloves. (Wear glasses or goggles and plastic apron if drainage might splash.)
2. Fill syringe or other device with saline.
3. Place basin under pressure ulcer to catch drainage.
4. Hold irrigation device 1 to 6 inches from ulcer and spray it with saline.
5. Use enough force to remove dead tissue and old drainage, but not damage new tissue.
6. Carefully remove basin so fluid doesn't spill.
7. Dry the skin surrounding the ulcer by patting skin with soft, clean towel.
8. After assessing and dressing the ulcer, remove gloves by pulling them inside out. Throw away gloves properly.

ASSESS ULCER

1. Assess healing. As ulcer heals, it will slowly become smaller and drain less. New tissue at the bottom of the ulcer is light red or pink and looks lumpy and glossy. Do not disturb this tissue.
2. Tell health care provider if the ulcer is larger, drainage increases, the sore is infected, or there are no signs of healing in 2 to 4 weeks.

continues

continued

DRESSING THE ULCER

Place a new dressing over the ulcer as instructed by the doctor or nurse. Remember:

- Use dressings only once.
- Keep dressings in the original package or other closed plastic package.
- Store dressings in a clean, dry place.
- Throw out the entire package if any dressings get wet, contaminated, or dirty.
- Wash your hands before touching clean dressings.
- Do not touch packaged dressings once you touch the sore.

Notes:

Source: *Pressure Ulcer Treatment Consumer Guide: Treating Pressure Sores*, U.S. Department of Health and Human Services, Public Health Service, Agency for Health Care Policy and Research, Publication 95-0654, December 1994.

7

Sexuality and Reproduction

> Most materials in the *Spinal Cord Injury Patient Education Manual* are intended for the health care professional to share with the patient. Materials that are intended solely for the professional are labeled "Exhibit" in the table of contents.

General Sexuality

Sexuality: Overview 211
Common Questions about Marriage,
   Children, and Relationships 213
Preparing for Sex 216
Sexual Excitement 218
Special Concerns 219

Male Sexuality

Male Sexual Anatomy 221
Physical Changes in Male Sexual
   Function 222
Male Reproductive Function after
   Spinal Cord Injury (Exhibit) 226
Sexual Concerns of the Male with
   Spinal Cord Injury 228

Female Sexuality

Female Sexual Anatomy 234
Female Sexual Function after Spinal
   Cord Injury 235
Common Questions about Female
   Sexuality 238

Reproductive Counseling for Women
   with Spinal Cord Injury (Exhibit) 240
Evaluation of Contraceptive Methods
   for Women with Spinal Cord Injury
   (Exhibit) 241
Caring for Women with Disabilities:
   Guidelines for the Gynecologist
   (Exhibit) 242
Caring for Women with Disabilities:
   Guidelines for the Obstetrician
   (Exhibit) 244
Differential Diagnosis: Preeclampsia
   versus Autonomic Dysreflexia
   (Exhibit) 245
Give Yourself a Chance: Reaffirming
   Your Sexuality 246
Spinal Cord Injury and Breast Cancer 248

Sexual Health

Five Steps to a Healthier and Safer Sex
   Life 251
Sexually Transmitted
   Diseases—Counseling Checklist and
   Guidelines (Exhibit) 253
Talking to Your Partner about AIDS 254
The HIV Test 255

GENERAL SEXUALITY

Sexuality: Overview

WHAT IS SEXUALITY?

Sexuality is many different things. It is how you dress, how you feel about your body, and how you relate to others, emotionally and physically. After a spinal cord injury, many people find there are some changes in how they express themselves sexually. This is normal since after a spinal cord injury you need to adjust socially, emotionally, and physically. How you express yourself sexually is in your control and is still an important part of your life. It gives you feelings of closeness, pleasure, self-worth, tension release, and it may help you with some of the pressures and frustrations in your life.

You may think that you cannot have relationships that last, that you cannot get married or stay married, that you cannot enjoy a sexual relationship, or that you can get hurt again during sex. You may also think you have no sexual feelings or needs. These beliefs are not true. You are as sexual as anyone else. Having a physical disability does not get rid of sexual feelings any more than it gets rid of your need for food or drink. You still feel attraction, excitement, desire, and love. How you feel about yourself and how you deal with others will make a difference in how they act toward you.

COMMUNICATION

Expressing what you think and feel is important in all relationships. You do this through talking and body language such as gestures. Depending on how your injury has affected you, you may need to use different body movements and use more talking to express yourself.

Many people do not know how your injury has affected you, so remember that the people close to you or someone you are attracted to may not know how your injury affects your sexuality. You need to find out for yourself and talk with your partner about how you feel about yourself and your relationship. It is also very important that you and your partner talk about your physical abilities, what feels good to you, and what pleases both of you.

SEXUAL ACTIVITY/ORGASM

Intercourse is not the only way to share sexually. Touching, cuddling, massaging, and fantasizing can also give you sexual pleasure.

Orgasm is both physical and emotional. Orgasm is mostly felt in the pubic area. Other areas of your body can also give you feelings of orgasm. Often, areas above your level of injury become extra sensitive to touch. Examples of these areas are your ears, neck, shoulders, armpits, and breasts. Many people with a spinal cord injury have reported feeling orgasm when these areas are touched by their partner. Even below your level of injury there may be areas of your body

continues

continued

where you still have some feeling and you may find it pleases you when these areas are touched by your partner. Orgasm is also emotional. Thinking about sex, your partner, and fantasizing can also give you sexual pleasure. You need to try different things to find out what works best for you and what pleases you most. You need to feel free to try different positions and different ways of getting sexual pleasure, for example, touching, cuddling, massaging, oral sex, and the use of vibrators. What is important is that you and your partner find out what pleases both of you and is not against what you feel is right.

You may need to plan before sharing sexually. You may need help with undressing, transferring, or positioning. You may need to empty your bladder or leg bag. You need to talk with your partner about any help you need. It is important to find out what routines will work best so your time of sharing is easier and more pleasing.

Notes:

Source: *Spinal Cord Injury Manual*, University of Rochester, Strong Memorial Hospital Rehabilitation Unit, Rochester, New York, © 1986, rev. 1994.

Common Questions about Marriage, Children, and Relationships

Q. Why do some marriages with a person who has spinal cord injury fail?

A. Many fail for the same reasons that marriages between able-bodied individuals fail; for example, poor communication, immaturity of one or both partners, unrealistic expectations for marriage, or an unwillingness to seek professional help with problems. In marriages that took place before one partner was cord injured, there may be additional problems: long periods of enforced separation due to hospitalization, financial stress resulting from medical expenses, sexual frustration, changes in lifestyle, guilt, etc. Statistics on the number of divorces among people with cord injuries vary considerably, depending on who reports them.

Q. What are the chances of a man with spinal cord injury having children?

A. Statistics vary with the level of the lesion, the completeness of the lesion, and who is reporting the information. Figures as low as 1 percent and as high as 15 percent have been reported.

Q. What are the major reasons for sterility among men with spinal cord injury?

A. The major causes of sterility are an inability to maintain an erection or ejaculate, retroflux ejaculation into the bladder, degeneration of structures in the testes necessary to produce mature sperm, and alterations in the body's heat-regulating mechanism that affect the production of sperm.

Q. What are the chances of my being able to ejaculate?

A. The lower the lesion, the better the chances are of your being able to ejaculate, provided nerve supplies in the sacral region are intact.

Q. If I am able to ejaculate but cannot maintain an erection long enough for intercourse, can the sperm be used to impregnate my partner?

A. You must first find out if there is enough sperm in your semen and if this sperm is viable. This can be determined by a physician using microscopic examination. If it is viable, artificial insemination might provide a way of impregnating your partner. In this process, sperm is collected and frozen. After sufficient quantities of semen are collected, it is artificially inserted into the vagina by a physician. Few males with spinal cord injury have used this method, since their sperm count is usually low and few are able to ejaculate.

continues

continued

Q. I am able to obtain an erection and experience orgasm, but I am not able to ejaculate. How is this possible?

A. When there is erection and orgasm without ejaculation, it is thought that only the sympathetic fibers along the spinal cord have been damaged. The parasympathetic fibers are still intact and make erection and orgasm possible.

Q. Can a woman with spinal cord injury give birth successfully?

A. As long as you continue to menstruate, you are capable of bearing a child, although you are more vulnerable to certain complications of pregnancy. The chances of your having a malformed child are no greater than for the able-bodied woman unless you were injured while pregnant. Abortion is not always necessary if the injury should occur during pregnancy.

Q. What are some of the complications a woman with cord injury might encounter?

A. Women with cord injury usually carry their babies to full term. However, those injured while pregnant may deliver prematurely, particularly if the lesion is above T10.

Autonomic dysreflexia during labor and delivery involves high blood pressure, sweating, chills, and headache.

Urinary tract problems may also be encountered during pregnancy. For this reason it is important that renal functioning be assessed and any flare-ups of urinary tract infections be treated promptly.

Q. What are the best contraceptive techniques for me to use?

A. A variety of methods of varying effectiveness are available. The best method for you to use can be decided only after consultation with your physician. Such factors as effectiveness, side effects, and practicality must enter into the decision.

Q. Is it difficult for a person with spinal cord injury to adopt a child?

A. The fact that you have a spinal cord injury should not prevent you from being considered as an applicant for adoption. You must, however, be physically and emotionally able to care for the child given to you. The adoption agency ultimately makes this decision based on consideration of your individual case.

Q. From whom can I adopt a child?

A. Many county welfare departments offer adoption services, as do several religious organizations (for example, Catholic Family and Children's Services, Lutheran Children's Aid Society,

continues

continued

and Jewish Children's Bureau). However, religious agencies require that the parents and child be of the same religious background. It is also possible to adopt a child from South America, Europe, Asia, or Africa. You might consider, as an alternative to adoption, taking foster children into your home.

Q. What are the most common things required of a person adopting a child?

A. You must be sufficiently stable emotionally to care for a child and have an income sufficient to meet the expenses incurred in the child's daily care. Most adoption agencies require that their clients be willing to tell the child he or she is adopted, usually before the child reaches the age of five. Since adoption agencies seek to place the child in the most suitable home, they research the applicant's background very carefully.

Q. If a child needs special, expensive care, can I receive financial aid that would help me provide this care?

A. For some children with special needs, subsidized adoption is possible.

Q. Do I have to be married to adopt a child?

A. Not necessarily. A single person may be considered if he or she has an acceptable child care plan and is emotionally mature enough to take on the responsibilities of parenthood.

Q. Are there any special things I should consider before entering into a sexual relationship?

A. Yes, there are a few.

First, sex has many meanings. If you have no genital function, you can still have sex in other forms. A lot more goes into making a sexual relationship work than penile insertion.

Second, don't expect too much too soon from your partner. Give your partner time to adjust and to get acquainted with you. Keep the doors of communication open.

Third, it is sometimes difficult for a spouse to continue seeing you as a sexually desirable partner when he or she must routinely provide bowel and bladder care and nursing needs. If such happens to be the case with your partner, try to obtain outside help in performing these tasks, for example, from a visiting nurse, welfare aide, or part-time attendant.

Finally, don't forget that the most important things for you and your partner to develop are mutual trust, a willingness to discuss each other's needs, and a sincere desire to discover how you can mutually satisfy each other. Sexual relationships can enhance life if they grow out of feelings of mutual respect, love, tenderness, and concern.

Source: M.G. Eisenberg and L.C. Rustad, *Sex and the Spinal Cord Injured: Some Questions and Answers*, 2nd ed., Veterans Administration Medical Center, Cleveland, Ohio.

Preparing for Sex

SETTING THE MOOD

Following spinal cord injury, getting ready for sex can take time. You will need to allow extra time to perform bladder care, to remove your clothes, and get into bed. You may want to use these events as a part of foreplay.

BLADDER AND BOWEL CARE

The same reflex that is triggered during sex also controls bladder activity. To prevent accidents, it's best to plan ahead. If possible, limit the amount of fluids you drink for three to four hours before having sex.

If you use an **intermittent catheter**, catheterize yourself just before sex. (This may be useful since it causes an erection in some men and can be used as a part of foreplay.)

If you have an **indwelling catheter**, place a condom over it to prevent irritation and use extra tubing so you have plenty of room to move.

Condom catheters can either be removed or folded over with a regular condom placed over it.

Sex can also trigger your bowels to move. If you perform regular bowel care, this shouldn't be a problem.

In case of accidents, pad the bed well with a waterproof pad so that if you have an accident you can just remove the soiled linen and keep going.

MEDICATIONS

In general, sedatives, pain relievers, blood pressure medications, muscle relaxants, and major tranquilizers may decrease sexual response. Caffeine, alcohol, and tobacco also affect sexual responsiveness. Talk with your doctor if you have any specific questions.

SPASMS

You may need to experiment to see if spasms interfere or help with positioning or movement during sex.

If your spasms interfere, try a warm tub or shower, warmer room temperature, range of motion, relaxation, whirlpool, and deep breathing.

If spasticity helps with movement, avoid medications used for depression and spasms.

continues

continued

AUTONOMIC DYSREFLEXIA

Although it is rare, sex or stimulation can cause dysreflexia in those who have an injury T6 or above. If it occurs, stop, sit up 90 degrees, and treat as appropriate. After this episode is resolved, you may continue with sexual activity.

CONTRACEPTION

Even though you may have trouble with the mechanics of sex, you could still have fertile sperm and should use a form of birth control. Condoms should be worn to prevent pregnancy and to avoid contracting AIDS, sexually transmitted diseases, and urinary tract infections. You may also wish to consider a vasectomy, a permanent form of birth control.

MOVEMENT AND POSITIONING

To save energy, you will want to try a variety of positions. You might also want to use pillows, cushions, and folded blankets to keep you in place. Couples must be willing to experiment to find out what works best for them. Here are some suggestions to help you get started:

- Place yourself beneath your partner to allow your hands to be free and your partner's hips and pelvis to thrust.
- Try having sex in a wheelchair. Remove the wheelchair arms and have your partner straddle over you.
- Lie side by side or face to face to allow your arms and hands to move freely and to lessen any problems with balance.
- Sit up with your legs wrapped around each other and use pillows to help keep your position.
- Lie on top of your partner with your partner's knees bent to your chest. Rocking movements will provide thrusting motions and let your partner's hips move freely.
- If you have paraplegia and have good arm strength, use this strength to do a push-up to perform a pelvic thrust. Place your knees apart and shift your weight in a rocking motion. It will also give your partner room to move the hips.

Source: Anne Leclaire, *Let's Talk Sex: Learning to Adjust after Spinal Cord Injury*, University of Wisconsin Hospital and Clinics Nursing Department, Madison, Wisconsin, © 1995.

Sexual Excitement

Sex drive is not affected by spinal cord injury; however, spontaneity is. This may be due to concerns about mobility, bowel, and bladder. It is possible to include these issues into foreplay and use this time to increase your excitement.

Depending on your comfort level, beliefs, and values, you may try fantasy, massage, use of sexual toys, oral sex, caressing, holding, and kissing instead of or in addition to intercourse to enhance your sexual pleasure and mutual gratification.

Using light and mirrors helps you to watch your partner's reactions. Don't forget to include all areas of your body even if you can't feel them. Use your eyes to follow the movements. Use the memory of how those areas used to feel, the sights, the sounds, and erotic fantasy to heighten sexual excitement. Talking to one another about sensations may intensify them.

After spinal cord injury, you may not feel the same pleasureable feelings from your genital area that you felt before your injury. Concentrate on feelings you get from your erogenous zones (nipples, earlobes, neck, underarms, area just above level of sensation) while caressing and amplify it mentally to increase its intensity. You also may be able to transfer a sensation from a less sensitive area to an area of retained sensation and intensify it in your mind. Using imagination and fantasy may increase sexual sensations and experiences.

EJACULATION AND ORGASM

Ejaculation is not the same as orgasm. They are two separate functions of the body. If you are able to orgasm, it may be somewhat different from the orgasms you had prior to your spinal cord injury. Orgasm is the mind's interpretation of physical sensations. It has been described as a warm sensation, either above or below your level of injury and rated to be either the same as or stronger than it was preinjury. You can also orgasm from stimulation of your erogenous zones. Regardless of whether you are able to ejaculate, you should be able to orgasm.

Experimentation and creativity will be needed to discover and enjoy alternative areas of sensation. You can achieve much sexual gratification.

Source: Anne Leclaire, *Let's Talk Sex: Learning to Adjust after Spinal Cord Injury*, University of Wisconsin Hospital and Clinics Nursing Department, Madison, Wisconsin, © 1995.

Special Concerns

Both men and women have many concerns about their sexual functioning and what problems could happen. It is important that you know what problems could happen so that you can keep some of them from happening and be ready if they do happen. It is very important that your partner knows about these things, too.

HYPERREFLEXIA

This can happen if your spinal cord injury is above T6. During sexual activity you may get a pounding headache. If this happens, you need to stop and rest until it goes away. Sitting up a little will also help. Be sure the bowel and bladder are emptied prior to sexual activity to decrease your chance of hyperreflexia.

URINARY TRACT INFECTION (UTI)

You cannot get a UTI or give a UTI to your partner, even if you are incontinent.

INCONTINENCE

Incontinence does not happen a lot if you do the things that help make it less. It is important that you and your partner know that it can happen. It happens because of the touching and pressure to the pubic area. To help make the chance of bladder incontinence less, empty your bladder before sex. To help make the chance of bowel incontinence less, it is best not to have sex near your usual bowel program time or when you are having bowel problems. You may want to put a pad under you or have a towel within reach so that you are ready if there is any incontinence.

FOLEY CATHETER

The Foley can be taken out or left in during sex. If it is taken out, be sure you put it back in. Put the Foley back in as soon as you can. You can wait for one to two hours if you do not have a problem with incontinence. In men, if the Foley is left in, it can be folded back over the penis. You may wish to place a prophylactic condom over the Foley to decrease friction.

Leave the Foley loose enough so an erection does not pull it. In women, if the Foley is left in, it can be taped to the abdomen or moved to the side out of the way. Be careful not to pull the Foley. If the Foley causes problems from rubbing, extra lubrication may help.

SPASMS

You may have more spasms because of all the touching to your body. You may find the spasms are less if you change your position.

continues

continued

SAFE SEX

Safe sex means being smart and staying healthy. It means showing love, concern, and respect for your partner and yourself. Safe sex means enjoying sexual relations without transmitting or acquiring sexually related infections. Having a spinal cord injury does not change your chances of receiving or passing on a sexually transmitted disease. To reduce your chances of acquiring a sexually transmitted disease, it is important to use safe sex practices with every sexual experience. Use the same precautions you would have used prior to your spinal cord injury.

Notes:

Source: Wanda Trojanoski, University of Rochester, Strong Memorial Hospital Rehabilitation Unit, *Spinal Cord Injury Manual*, Rochester, New York, © 1986, rev. 1994.

MALE SEXUALITY

Male Sexual Anatomy

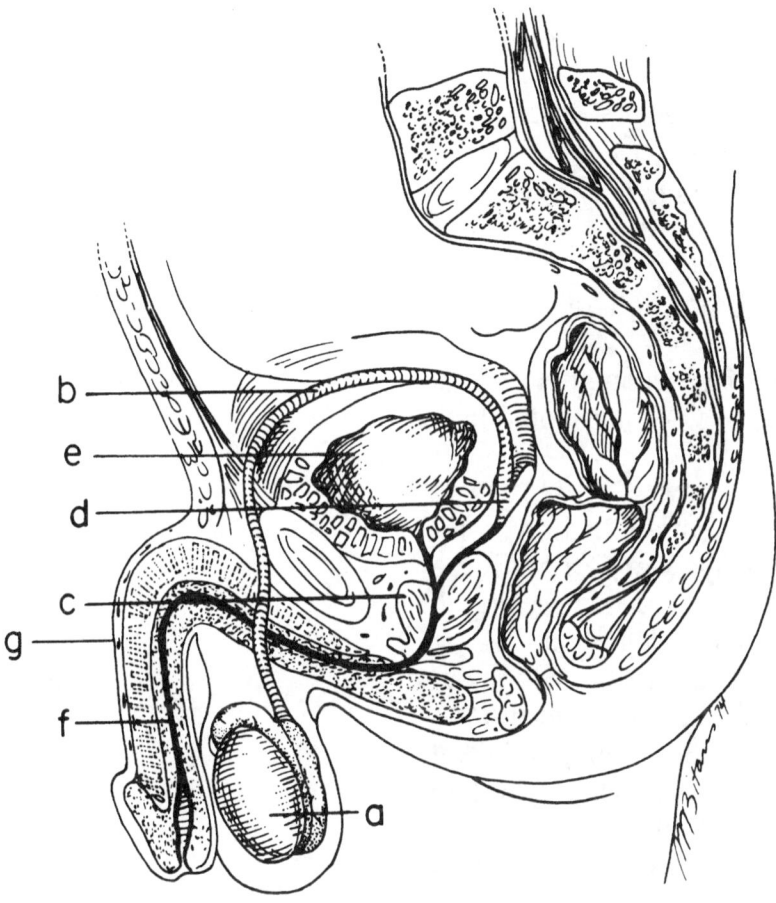

Male Sexual Anatomy
(a) testes, (b) sperm duct, (c) prostate, (d) seminal vesicle, (e) urinary bladder, (f) urethra, (g) penis.

Source: M.G. Eisenberg and L.C. Rustad, *Sex and the Spinal Cord Injured: Some Questions and Answers*, 2nd ed., Veterans Administration Medical Center, Cleveland, Ohio, © 1984.

Physical Changes in Male Sexual Function

After spinal cord injury, it may be harder to move or position yourself. You may have trouble getting or keeping an erection and ejaculating. During sex, you may have less of a rise in your blood pressure, pulse, and breathing rates, and you may have less feeling in your genitals.

TYPES OF ERECTIONS

Understanding types of erections helps you to know how your body may respond after a spinal cord injury. There are two types of erections:

1. **Reflexogenic:** the kind you get by touching the penis.
2. **Psychogenic:** an erection that results from fantasizing or watching something erotic.

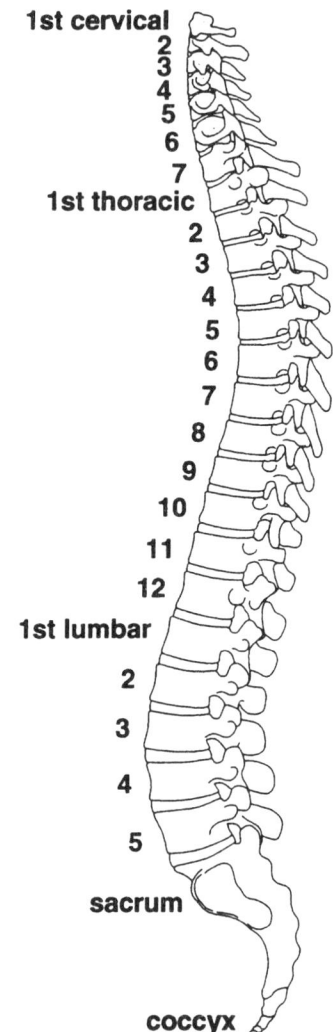

The level of injury affects your body's response. A man with an **injury at T12 or above** is most likely to get an erection by touching. If you have had a *complete* injury at T12 or above, it is unlikely that you will be able to get an erection from fantasizing or watching something erotic. But, if the injury is *incomplete*, it may be possible to be aroused mentally and have some feeling in the genitals.

A man with an **injury at T12 or below** is most likely to respond to mental arousal, but not to touch. Also, there is a chance that he will be able to ejaculate. And, if your injury is incomplete, there's a chance that you may have some genital feeling.

continues

continued

OBTAINING AND MAINTAINING ERECTIONS

Many men have trouble getting and keeping an erection during sex. Here is a list of options to help you deal with these problems. You may also want to talk with your doctor to find specific ways to solve your particular problems.

Nonsurgical Treatments

Self-Injection of Medication

Self-injection is a common and inexpensive treatment. A medication such as Prostaglandin E1 is injected into the penis to dilate the blood vessels. This can cause an erection to last up to four hours. Though this treatment can be very helpful and can be used 1–2 times a week, it also may cause bruising, infection, or scarring. You can learn about this method at a clinic visit. The amount of medicine needs to be prescribed by a doctor. Be sure to follow the instructions carefully since too much medication can cause a painful erection that will not go away. This condition is called priapism. The blood is unable to drain from the penis and may clot. This is a medical emergency that needs to be treated quickly. Priapism and the treatment for it may cause permanent damage to the penile tissue.

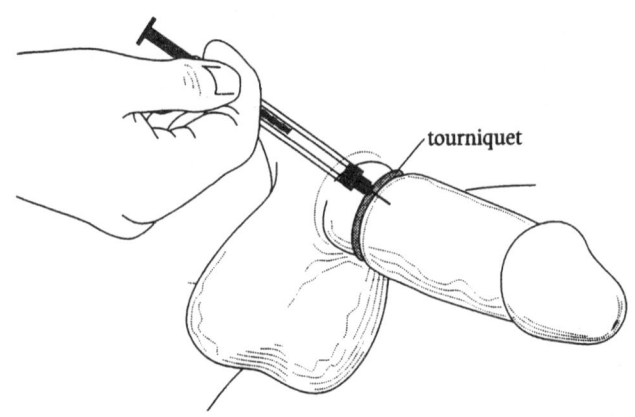

Penile injection testing ("Papaverine" test)

Sex Toys and Aids

Sex toys such as penis stiffeners, rings, dildos, and vibrators may be used to help build erections and assist with vaginal penetration. Many of these toys often require good hand strength.

Vacuum Device

The penis is placed into a vacuum cylinder and pumped up to get an erection. A ring is wrapped around the base of the penis for no longer than 30 minutes to keep the erection. The vacuum can cause bruising. Though there are various vacuum models, you need to look carefully since some require good hand strength. A rubber ring can also be used alone for those who are able to get

continues

continued

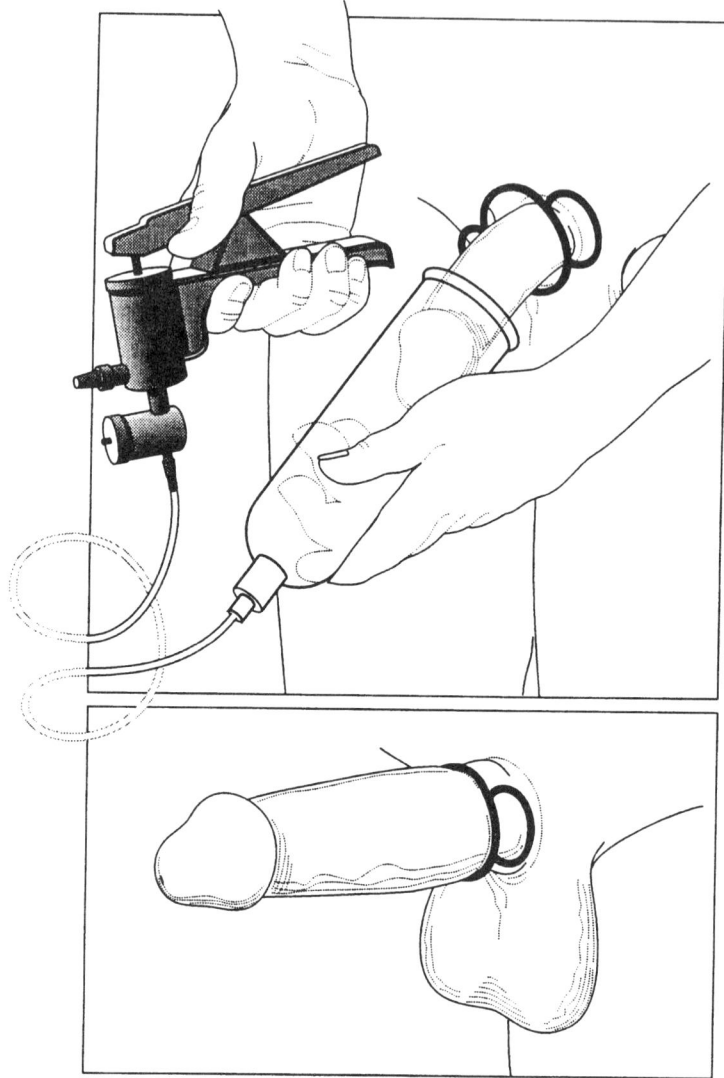

an erection, but need help to keep it. A tight band is placed at the base of an erect penis. This method is easy to use. Battery-operated pumps are also available. Ask your doctor which method is best for you.

Surgical Penile Implants

When simpler treatments do not work, surgical implants may be considered. Implants will not improve one's ability to ejaculate; however, they are useful in keeping catheter condoms on.

continues

continued

Inflatable Implants

Inflatable implants closely mimic normal activity. A small pump in the scrotum is used to create an erection. After sex, the penis is returned to its soft, resting state. Of the three implants, the inflatable one is the most expensive. Also, there are chances that the pump may leak or pressure sores could form inside the penis.

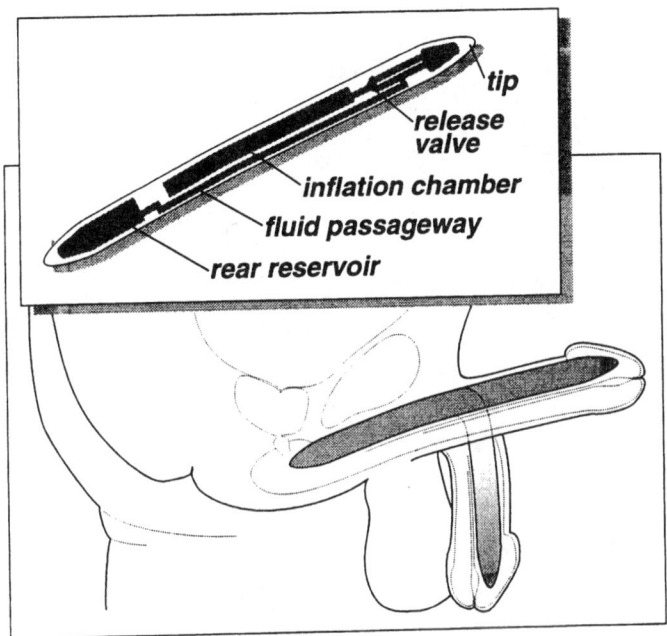

Self-Contained Implant

A self-contained unit is placed in the penis and becomes firm when squeezed or bent. After sex, the penis returns to its soft, flaccid state. While it is safe and simple to use, some men don't feel it is as natural as other methods.

Semirigid Implant

A semirigid implant is a bendable rod placed in the penis. The penis is constantly semierect. Though this approach is less costly, it may cause pressure sores or scar tissue inside the penis.

Other

Erections may be achieved by pulling on pubic hairs; stroking the scrotum, thigh, or rectal area; or using the "stuffing technique" (stuffing a flaccid penis into the vagina). Gentle or vigorous massage of the penis or use of a vibrator may also produce an erection.

Source: Anne Leclaire, *Let's Talk Sex: Learning to Adjust after Spinal Cord Injury*, University of Wisconsin Hospital and Clinics Nursing Department, Madison, Wisconsin, © 1995.

Exhibit
MALE REPRODUCTIVE FUNCTION AFTER SPINAL CORD INJURY

INTRODUCTION

There are approximately 10,000 people who survive a spinal cord injury every year, 80 percent of whom are male. Most are young and in what is considered their "reproductive years" or, perhaps, looking forward to entering them. Although an injury to the spinal cord may affect the male's ability to achieve conception, there are numerous strategies available to help a couple to have children if the man has a spinal cord injury.

UNDERSTANDING EJACULATION

Ejaculation can be divided into three distinctive phases. The first phase is termed *emission* and describes the deposit of the fluid that makes up semen into the *posterior urethra*. The semen comes from the *seminal vesicles* (glands that make most of the fluid found in the ejaculate), the *vasal ampulla* (the end of the sperm transport tube that contains most of the sperm present in the ejaculate), and the prostate. The posterior urethra is the tube that urine comes through on the way from the bladder to the tip of the penis during normal urination or the tube through which a catheter is inserted into the bladder. The second phase occurs concurrent with emission and involves enclosure of the bladder neck so that semen cannot travel backward (retrograde) into the bladder during ejaculation. These two phases are controlled by the sympathetic nervous system originating from spinal segments T10–12. The third phase of the ejaculatory event involves the contraction of the muscles surrounding the urethra to forcefully expel the semen in a forward (antegrade) direction out through the end of the penis. The nerves connecting these muscles exit through the sacral segments (S2–4) of the spinal cord. There are also sensory nerves that travel from the penis back to the sacral spinal cord. These nerves then go up the spinal cord to an ejaculation reflex coordination center, which is located somewhere around T12.

The ejaculation center is responsible for proper neurological coordination of emission, closure of the bladder neck, and antegrade ejaculation. It is a reflex center that is controlled by the brain (thoughts, emotions, etc.) and receives genital input (sensations from the penis and scrotum). When a spinal cord injury occurs at the level of T10–12, then either the ejaculatory center or the sympathetic nervous system in this region will be damaged. If the injury occurs below T12, then the ejaculation center and the sympathetics may be intact, but the pathways back from the penis and out to the muscles around the urethra may not be "connected" to the ejaculatory center. An understanding of this neuroanatomy is important to appreciate the therapies available and why they work.

SPERM PRODUCTION AND TRANSPORT

Sperm are produced in the *testicles*. The testicles work best at a temperature slightly cooler than the inside of the body. Many mechanisms involved in the regulation of testicular temperature may be impaired in a man with a spinal cord injury. The sperm leave the testicles and enter the *epididymis*, which is a gland located behind the testicle. The sperm travel through the epididymis and into the *vas deferens*. The vas transport the sperm up and out of the scrotum into the pelvis and finally into the ejaculate.

Due to numerous improvements in the care and, consequently, the health of men with spinal cord injuries, testicular function is typically quite well preserved; unfortunately, a minority of men experience a significant and severe depression of sperm production and/or sperm quality. The reasons for this are not always evident in a particular individual, but excess heat, prior infections of the reproductive tract or testicle, overall poor health, and chronic use of certain medications probably all combine to lower the efficiency of sperm-producing cells within the testis. However, the ability of the sperm to fertilize an egg is independent of many other factors, and sperm count and motility alone are not good predictors of how well the sperm will work. Therefore, in general, sperm production and quality are adequately maintained in the majority of men with SCI. What makes spontaneous fertility a problem, for the most part, is ejaculatory dysfunction.

The most important part of a therapeutic strategy for a man with SCI and his partner is to define how to retrieve the sperm from him. Once that is done, an appropriate technique to help the couple achieve pregnancy is selected and pursued.

SPERM RETRIEVAL TECHNIQUES

Penile Vibratory Stimulation

Penile vibratory stimulation (PVS) involves placing a powerful vibrating unit on the undersurface of the head of the penis, the site of greatest sensation. The sensory nerves are stimulated and transmit this information back to the sacral spinal cord and up to the ejaculatory reflex center. If the stimulus is enough, the ejaculatory center will be triggered to activate the sequence of ejaculation and semen is delivered through the penis in the usual fashion. Obviously, for PVS to be effective, the nerves traveling from the penis to the spinal cord, the spinal cord itself below T10, the ejaculatory reflex at T12, and the sympathetics from T10–12 must all be intact and functional. Therefore, not all males with SCI will respond to PVS. PVS is a simple technique and does not involve anesthesia of any type. For men with injuries above T6, it may cause autonomic dysreflexia and should always be attempted first in a monitored office setting. If PVS works, the individual and his partner are taught how to do it and how to

continues

continued

collect the semen. This eliminates the need for a physician to be present to help obtain a semen specimen, as is the case for electroejaculation. Once the couple is proficient in capturing the semen, a host of therapies can be tried, depending on the count and motility of the male's sperm. Many couples can be taught self-insemination, where the specimen is retrieved with PVS and then deposited on the cervix. This is as close as possible to copying what takes place during traditional intercourse and does result in some couples becoming pregnant. If this fails or the sperm situation is poor, adjunctive, or high-tech techniques that many couples use to assist in getting pregnant can be employed. These include insemination of the partner's sperm into the uterus or in vitro fertilization, for example.

Electroejaculation

In this procedure, a probe is inserted into the rectum and electrical current is applied. Possible problems with electroejaculation include autonomic dysreflexia, particularly in cases where the individual has a high spinal cord lesion, or damage to the rectal area if the probe becomes too hot. Despite these possible side effects, researchers in the United States and England have reported success with the technique.

FERTILIZATION*

Artificial Insemination: For individuals who can ejaculate with masturbation or vibration but not with intercourse, it is fairly easy to have a sperm count done (to confirm the number and quality of the sperm) and learn how and when to do artificial insemination at home. However, when electrical stimulation is done, the sperm is collected by a physician and preserved until the insemination can be done (usually in a gynecology fertility clinic).

In Vitro Fertilization: This involves collecting sperm by one of the above procedures, collecting an egg from the female partner, combining the two in a test tube in the laboratory until fertilization occurs and then reimplanting the egg in the uterus. This is probably the most successful and reliable method, but is also the most difficult and expensive.

*Courtesy of Shirley McCluer, MD, Medical Director, Arkansas Spinal Cord Commission, Little Rock, Arkansas, July 1992.

SUMMARY

A man with SCI who is interested in fathering a child should first consult a urologist well-versed in SCI to obtain a complete urological exam. Once factors such as erectile and ejaculatory function and sperm viability have been determined, the individual and his urologist should determine the appropriate method of proceeding to improve fertility. For some, intercourse may be all that is needed. For others, medical intervention may be required. In all cases where outside assistance is needed, however, it is essential that the physician have a solid background in the sexual and reproductive function of individuals with SCI and that he or she be familiar with possible complications associated with the different methods available to achieve ejaculation.

Courtesy of the National Spinal Cord Injury Association, 545 Concord Avenue, Suite 29, Cambridge, Massachusetts, 02138. For more information, call (800) 962-9629 or (617) 441-8500.

Sexual Concerns of the Male with Spinal Cord Injury

Q. I've been concerned about my loss of sexual functioning. Is it normal to be preoccupied in this way?

A. This is not at all unusual, especially among the newly injured.

Q. Will I be able to have a sex life?

A. Although you may have to modify or change some of your sexual activities, you can still have a meaningful sex life and continue to be a sexually active human being.

The need to love and be loved is important to most of us. One way of expressing this love is physical contact. With or without an erection or orgasm, physical contact can provide a profound sense of well-being and intimacy and bring pleasure and excitement to you and your partner.

Q. Why should I even think of having a sex life if I can't get an erection?

A. Even though you may be unable to get an erection, sex can add a valuable dimension to your life. People engage in sex for many reasons, not only for the physiologic release that is normally achieved through orgasm, but, more importantly, to help develop and maintain a relationship with another person and to provide a form of communication. Participation in sexual activities helps us develop a sense of personal worth and significance. Through sex we also express affection and love.

Q. Can I still be attractive even though I am confined to a wheelchair?

A. You certainly can be. Whether or not you are depends heavily on your attitude. It is important that you have confidence in yourself and not sell yourself short. If you take advantage of opportunities to meet new people, you will increase your chances of finding someone you will like who will take a personal interest in and be concerned about you.

Q. How do I go about meeting women?

A. Obviously, there is no quick and easy solution to this problem. Your personality style and the way you interact with others, as well as your interests and motivation, are important factors.

Since most women will be found outside of the hospital, perhaps the first step in the right direction involves your making a sincere effort to leave the hospital rehabilitated. Once home, it is important that you not stay there, or the chances of your meeting someone will be very slim. If you pursue interests and activities that you find enjoyable, you are more likely to find someone who shares your interests. The greater the variety of activities in which you

continues

continued

participate (for instance, parties, church groups, volunteering, organizations, etc.) and the more people you get to know, the greater your chances of meeting someone with whom you can talk. You should not become discouraged if you do not meet with success immediately. The results of your injury may require finding a new lifestyle, and adjusting to these changes will take time. Nevertheless, the successes of many individuals with spinal cord injury strongly suggest that formulating a new and satisfying lifestyle is a reasonable goal. It is only after you have achieved this goal that you can be relatively certain that you will find the companionship for which you are looking.

Q. Since I have been injured, my body has changed considerably. Will a woman be surprised when she sees me nude?

A. It is important to remember that if your relationship is a good one, the woman didn't pick you just for your body. It will probably ease your mind and help to prepare your partner if you explain to her what happens to the body when a spinal cord injury is sustained. Mutual exploration of each other's body before you undress or have intercourse would also lessen any surprise your partner might experience. You may feel somewhat awkward and tense initially, but this feeling should soon disappear. Here again, it is important that you be able to communicate openly and honestly with each other.

Q. How can I still consider myself a man if I am not able to perform sexually the way I used to?

A. Unfortunately, for many people in our culture, masculinity is defined as how long a man can maintain an erection or how many times he can accomplish intercourse in an evening. Such a definition of masculinity is extremely narrow. The ability to make commitments and accept responsibility and the ability to give love as well as receive it are just a few of the qualities that contribute to a man's masculinity.

Of course, satisfying your partner's sexual needs is undeniably important. Yet even this does not depend on being able to get or maintain an erection, because you can bring pleasure and excitement to your partner by using other techniques. There is an adage that perhaps bears stating here—it is not the tool that makes the worker but how he uses it.

Q. I'd still like to have a sex life but since I've been injured, my wife seems to have lost all interest in physical intimacy. What should I do?

A. It's difficult to give a pat answer to this question without knowing more about your relationship with your wife. How well did you get along with her before you were injured? Have you both really accepted your disability? How does she feel about it? What are her attitudes toward sex generally? Are you able to openly discuss problems that arise? Are you both willing to make some adjustments to work out a solution?

continues

continued

If you are not able to work out a solution between yourselves, don't hesitate to seek professional counseling from someone with whom you both feel comfortable talking. Counseling at an early stage can often prevent more serious problems from developing later.

Q. As I grow older, will my sex drive diminish?

A. Your sex drive remains basically intact as you grow older, but it might take more time for you to become aroused and to stimulate your partner. Regular sexual expression now will enhance your enjoying sex even in later years.

Q. If I can't get an erection now, does that mean I can never get one?

A. This has to be determined on an individual basis. Just as you may regain function in previously paralyzed parts of your body for up to a year after injury, so you may regain sexual function as time passes and your body adjusts and recovers from the effects of the injury. Most men, however, do not regain sexual function if they lose it following injury and continue to be unable to ejaculate or maintain an erection for a year after their injury.

SOME COMMON PROBLEMS

Q. How does the drug Valium affect my sex drive?

A. Valium and many other psychotropic drugs may diminish sex drive in *some* people. However, we are not suggesting that you discontinue your Valium if you have found it to be essential in controlling spasms.

Q. What do I do with my catheter while engaging in sex?

A. The catheter may be left, lubricated, folded over the penis, and covered with a condom for up to 30 minutes at a time. You may also remove your catheter. If your bladder is empty, it is safe to be without a catheter for three to six hours. Be sure never to force the catheter while removing or replacing it so that you don't cause bleeding. It's a good idea to train your partner in removing and replacing this device in the event that you are unable to do so. If you or your partner need to be shown how to perform this procedure, ask the nurse for instructions.

Q. Can suprapubic and ileo loop drainages be left in place?

A. Both of these drainages can be left in place and taped to the abdomen for a short period. This will avoid traction being placed on the drainage tube and should in no way interfere with your sexual activities.

continues

continued

Q. I sometimes notice a secretion from my penis. What is this and what does it mean?

A. It is difficult to tell without examining it. You should keep a glass laboratory slide by your bedside and make a smear of this discharge for examination by your physician. He or she will usually be able to determine its nature.

Q. What do women with indwelling catheters do?

A. Opinion on this topic varies. It is probably safest to remove the catheter before engaging in sex. Whether she does or not depends to a great extent on the size of her vagina and the position she assumes in intercourse. If the man enters from behind the woman, it may be unnecessary to remove the catheter. You will need to experiment to find what is most comfortable for both. You may also consult with your physician.

Q. Should women use a lubricant before engaging in sexual activity?

A. Some women do use lubricants before engaging in sexual activity. This can make intercourse more comfortable. It is suggested, however, that women use a lubricant that dissolves in water, such as K-Y or surgical jelly. They should *not* use petroleum jelly (Vaseline), because it does not dissolve in water and can be a vehicle for vaginal infections.

Q. Is engaging in oral sex dangerous?

A. With ordinary hygienic precautions, the chance of either you or your partner becoming ill through this kind of sexual contact is no greater than through intercourse.

Q. What if I should urinate or have a bowel movement in bed?

A. This has happened to many persons with spinal cord injury at one time or another. Although you may find this situation embarrassing, if you have explained your physical condition to your partner, this may not come as too great a shock, and she is likely to understand.

Some precautionary measures may be taken. You should empty your bladder and avoid drinking water for a few hours before engaging in intercourse. If possible, you should also try to evacuate your bowels sometime during the preceding day.

Q. Is it possible for me to be accidentally hurt by my partner while engaging in sexual activities?

A. This is highly unlikely if ordinary precautions are observed, including avoiding any unnecessarily rough or harsh handling. Also remember that prolonged pressure on any part of your body that has lost feeling can cause pressure ulcers. If your partner is concerned about hurting you, you should reassure her that injury is not likely. It is important to remember that

continues

continued

people who are frightened do not function at their best and that fear can dampen even the greatest sexual desire.

SOME ALTERNATIVES

Q. You say there are ways I can satisfy my partner other than intercourse?

A. There are many alternative ways of satisfying your partner. Oral and manual stimulation are used as a normal part of foreplay by many couples with spinal cord injury, and they may be used as a way of bringing your partner to orgasm. Vibrators can also be used. In addition, prosthetic devices are available that can aid in maintaining rigidity of the penis or even substitute completely for an erect penis. If, after speaking with your partner about oral or manual sex, you find she does not wish to participate and you cannot seem to find a satisfactory solution to your problem, counseling by a physician or psychologist may be of value.

Q. How can my partner arouse and satisfy me physically?

A. Experimentation is the key. What is effective and satisfying for one couple may not be for another. If you have an open relationship with your partner, you will discover what areas of sensitivity, if any, remain and what types of stimulation you both find pleasing.

If you think you can be aroused only by having your penis stimulated, you are ignoring the fact that sexual arousal, excitement, and gratification come from a variety of sources. You are likely to find stimulation of the lips, nipples, and ears just as erotic as anywhere else. Many men with lesions in the mid-thoracic region find that they have a sexually responsive area just above the point where their loss of sensation begins.

When you touch your partner, try to "feel" the surface of her body touching yours. Don't become so overconcerned in your attempts to arouse and stimulate your partner that you forget to experience and enjoy the sensations you are receiving, for you are stimulating yourself at the same time you are stimulating her. Don't think of it as work. Enjoy it, and you will be communicating joy and increasing her pleasure as well as your own.

Q. How can I best prepare myself for sexual activity?

A. If at all possible, it is best to plan sexual activities for the time of day when you are least tired and have the fewest distractions. Since relaxation heightens sexuality, it is best to loosen up before sexual activities. You may find that taking a warm shower or bath, listening to music, having a drink, being massaged, or using a vibrator can help you to relax.

Q. What positions can we assume for intercourse?

A. Most frequently, the male with spinal cord injury assumes the bottom position for intercourse. This allows your partner the mobility needed to position your penis. From this position you

continues

continued

may also roll over to either side. You and your partner will need to experiment to see what is most comfortable for you.

Q. What intercourse positions can the woman with a spinal cord injury assume?

A. There are any number of positions you can use that may be as comfortable or more comfortable than the missionary position (where the woman lies flat on her back with legs apart). Some women lie on their backs with pillows beneath the knees and buttocks. Others have found that a side position, either facing the partner or with the back toward him is comfortable. Still others prefer lying on the stomach with the man above. You will have to experiment to find which positions are best for you.

Q. My partner seems to enjoy penile insertion. If I can't get an erection how can this be accomplished?

A. The "stuffing" technique has been used by some couples, with many women achieving orgasm. To do this, the man usually assumes the bottom position with the woman on her knees above him. She then gently "stuffs" his penis into her vagina and rotates her pelvis. You might also consider using a prosthetic device.

Q. What areas of my partner's body can I stimulate to help her reach orgasm?

A. The most sensitive area on a woman's body is the genital area, particularly the clitoris and the inner lips. Because it is so sensitive, however, harsh or prolonged direct stimulation of the clitoris may be irritating rather than arousing. A variety of other areas of the body, such as the breasts, ears, mouth, or thighs may also play an important role in arousal. Indeed, any area of the body that contains nerve endings can be potentially arousing. It is important to experiment with your partner to find out where her most sensitive areas are.

Source: M.G. Eisenberg and L.C. Rustad, *Sex and the Spinal Cord Injured: Some Questions and Answers*, 2d ed., Veterans Administration Medical Center, Cleveland, Ohio.

FEMALE SEXUALITY

Female Sexual Anatomy

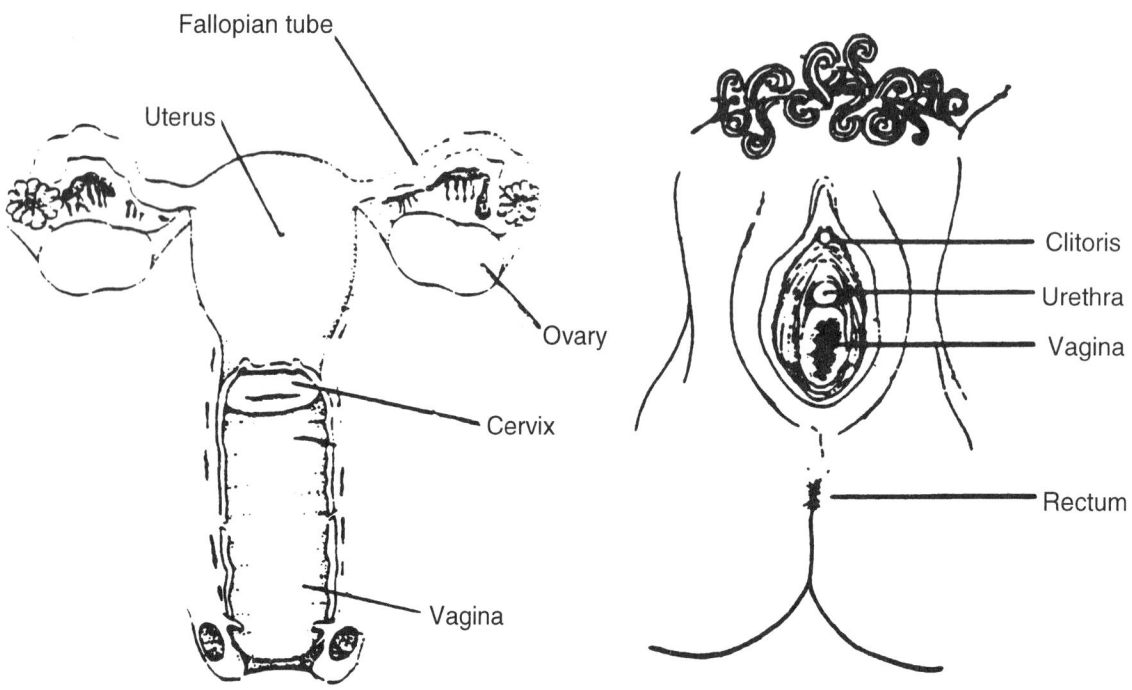

Figure 1. Internal Anatomy

Figure 2. External Anatomy

Courtesy of Shirley McCluer, MD, Medical Director, Arkansas Spinal Cord Commission, Little Rock, Arkansas, May 1992.

Female Sexual Function after Spinal Cord Injury

In women, the ability to be sexually active is mostly the same as before a spinal cord injury. A spinal cord injury causes a change in your feeling and movement, but there is no effect on fertility.

VAGINAL LUBRICATION

Lubrication happens by thinking about sex (psychogenic) or by touching of the pubic area (reflexogenic). Whether lubrication will happen and how much there will be depend on the amount of injury to the spinal cord. Psychogenic lubrication can happen only if the injury to the spinal cord is incomplete. Reflexogenic lubrication can happen if the injury to the spinal cord is above the reflex area. The injury to the spinal cord keeps the message from getting to or from the brain, but lubrication happens because of reflex action. If your body does not make enough lubrication, you will need to use something else to lubricate your vagina before sex. It is best to use a lubricant that is water soluble (melts in water). An example is K-Y jelly.

MENSES

In some women, when there has been a sudden injury to the spinal cord, menses stops for a while. This is because of the stress your body has gone through. Usually, menses starts again within six months, but it can take longer. If you are near menopause when you have your injury, your menses may not start again.

FERTILITY

Your ability to have a child is not changed. If you are sexually active and do not want to become pregnant, you need to think about birth control.

BIRTH CONTROL

You need to choose the kind of birth control that you feel will work best for you. Your doctor can talk to you about different kinds of birth control. You can use the same kinds of birth control as women without a spinal cord injury. Some examples of birth control methods are the pill, Norplant, IUDs, diaphragm and/or condom with spermicidal foam, contraceptive sponge, cervical cap, rhythm method (this kind of birth control does not work as well as other kinds), and having your tubes tied or the man having a vasectomy (these two kinds of birth control are usually permanent). Because of your spinal cord injury, you need to be more careful when using some kinds of birth control. Some kinds of birth control and what to watch for are as follows:

continues

continued

- **The pill.** This kind of birth control works best to prevent pregnancy, but it can cause problems. If you are taking the pill, your chance of getting thrombophlebitis (blood clots) is higher than usual because of less movement in your legs. Women who smoke have even a greater risk for thrombophlebitis. You need to watch for the warning signs of thrombophlebitis: swelling in the leg, redness and hardness in the leg, pain in the leg, and the leg feels hot. You need to contact your doctor if you have any of these symptoms.
- **Norplant.** The timed-released capsules contain hormones that are implanted under your skin and are effective for several years. The side effects are similar to those of the pill. Reports have shown that there are problems for women in the general population using Norplant.
- **Intrauterine device (IUD).** A problem that can happen with IUDs is a higher chance of infections of the uterus. You need to watch for these warning signs: pain in the pubic area, cramps, fever, a change in vaginal discharge, changes in menstrual periods, spotting (light vaginal bleeding), and you may have more spasms. This kind of birth control may require assistance from your partner, because the IUD needs to be checked for placement.
- **Diaphragm/condom.** This kind of birth control causes the fewest problems. It prevents pregnancy 88 percent of the time.
  - The diaphragm may be hard to put in, but practice may help make this easier. Also, there are inserters that can help you put it in, or you can have your partner do it. Before sex, you should check to be sure it is in the right way, since it may have moved, for example, if you push on your bladder to empty it. The diaphragm needs to be refitted if you have lost or gained weight. The diaphragm can also cause urinary tract infections with prolonged placement.
  - Condoms are easy to use. When using the diaphragm and/or condom, remember to use a spermicidal foam or jelly. **Note:** When a condom is used and you have a Foley that stays in during sex, you need to be careful. There is a chance that the Foley could tear the condom.
- **Contraceptive sponges and cervical caps.** These methods of birth control are fairly effective; however, they require adequate hand function to insert.

PREGNANCY

Pregnancy is much the same as that of a woman without a spinal cord injury. Some problems pregnant women have are anemia, thrombophlebitis, swelling in the legs, blood pressure changes, urinary tract infections, and constipation.

Some special problems you may have because of your spinal cord injury are additional skin problems because of added body weight and hyperreflexia, if your injury is above T6. Hyperreflexia may happen especially during labor. Make sure your doctor knows about hyperreflexia. The doctor could think you are having other problems and not know you are having hyperreflexia. Make sure your doctor knows what medications you are on, because many of them may go across the placenta and affect the baby.

continues

continued

You may not know when you go into labor because of the changes in feeling in your abdomen/trunk area. You can have a normal delivery, but you may need help from the doctor if you cannot push down.

Your having a spinal cord injury does not hurt the baby in any way. The chances of the baby having any birth defects are no higher than if you did not have a spinal cord injury. You can have a healthy pregnancy and a healthy baby. You can still breastfeed if you want, even if you have a cervical injury. The baby's sucking action causes a reflex to bring down milk. Since you can have special problems that will need to be watched closely, you should be seen early in your pregnancy by an obstetrician.

Notes:

Source: *Spinal Cord Injury Manual*, University of Rochester, Strong Memorial Hospital Rehabilitation Unit, Rochester, New York, © 1986, rev. 1994.

Common Questions about Female Sexuality

Q. I am a 25-year old woman with a recent T12 complete spinal cord injury. Can I still have sexual intercourse and orgasms even though I am paralyzed and have no sensation below my injury? Can I still get pregnant? If I can, what type of birth control should I use? Can birth control pills cause problems for women with SCI?

A. Your questions are good ones. Many women with spinal cord injury are concerned about sexuality and fertility. Though much of the research concerns men, there is a growing body of literature dedicated to the practical and physiological issues of interest to women with spinal cord injury.

You can indeed engage in sexual intercourse despite your injury. Orgasm, per se, is often impaired after spinal cord injury. Nonetheless, some women can perceive orgasm even in the absence of normal genital sensation. Research is currently underway to better understand this process. In any event, it's important to explore alternate erogenous zones to compensate for sensory losses. Your present or future partner should explore mutually agreeable ways of satisfying your sexual needs.

Questions often arise about the possibility of bowel or bladder incontinence during sexual activity. With adequate preparation you can greatly reduce anxiety related to continence. You can also use water-based lubricants if vaginal lubrication is compromised following a spinal cord injury.

Female fertility is not affected by spinal cord injury. Although your menstrual cycle may be interrupted after the initial injury, it usually returns to normal in a few months. Therefore, you should practice contraception if you don't wish to become pregnant.

Finding an optimal method of birth control after spinal cord injury can be a challenge. Oral contraceptives are not recommended because of the risk of deep vein thromboses, better known as clots, due to decreased mobility. IUDs (intrauterine devices) are contraindicated after a spinal cord injury as a woman may not feel the pain in her uterus should the IUD cause a perforation or become dislodged. Diaphragms, spermicidal sponges, and cervical caps are all reliable, although they may be hard to insert due to a lack of sensation, mobility, or hand dexterity. Tubal ligation and abstinence are other options. Barrier methods, such as gels and condoms are useful and safe. The safety of the recently available contraceptive implants needs to be explored. In the spirit of safe sex, always use condoms until a monogamous relationship is well established.

If you do become pregnant, remember these key points:

- As your weight increases and ease of movement decreases, the risk of pressure ulcers, or friction-induced breakdown, rises. You may wish to rent a wider wheelchair to accommodate your extra weight, or if you find your skin is being pinched in your usual wheelchair.
- Women with injuries at the level of T10 and above may not sense labor. Thus it is important that the date of conception and the expected due date are accurately monitored.

continues

continued

- In women with levels of injury at T6 and above, autonomic dysreflexia may be brought on by labor. Autonomic dysreflexia is a response to painful stimulation below the level of injury and is characterized by dangerous elevations in blood pressure, headache, flushing, and a low pulse. Be sure your obstetric team understands these risks. They can then deal with any problems should they arise.
- Vaginal delivery is feasible and appropriate in most cases.
- Think about your child care needs well ahead of your baby's arrival. If you require personal assistance, you may need to adjust the hours of care you receive.

Q. I am a 36-year-old woman with T6 complete paraplegia. Sex is exciting, but it's not the same as it was before my injury. Sometimes when I'm sexually active, I feel as if I'm going to have an orgasm, but it just doesn't happen. This frustrates me and makes me not even want to try anymore. Other times, I get pounding headaches when I'm having sex. Is there anything I can do to feel better?

A. You are clearly frustrated. After spinal cord injuries, it usually takes a longer time to achieve orgasm and only about half the people with spinal cord injuries say they can have them. The good news is it doesn't matter if you have a complete injury or an incomplete injury; there is no greater or lesser chance of having an orgasm. You seem fixated however, on that issue and are also becoming frustrated and possibly also suffering from autonomic dysreflexia with your sexual activity.

Take a step back. Rather than focusing on having an orgasm during sexual activity, try just to have fun. For a while, limit the scope of your sexual activity and try to enjoy the basics again, such as kissing, hugging, and touching. Try not to focus on having an orgasm, because if you spend your time trying too hard to have an orgasm, it may backfire on you. Focus instead on enjoying yourself and feeling pleasure. Feeling pleasure may involve using techniques that you have not used in the past. For instance, using a vibrator or experimenting with various lotions or oils can improve your sensation. Stimulation in new areas can also be a source of pleasure after spinal cord injury. Many people feel their breasts or their ears or their lips are much more sensitive than before their injury for example. You should also consider self-stimulation to discover what feels good and what doesn't. This way, you can learn to direct your partner and in that way feel better yourself.

Concerning your headaches, it sounds like you may be getting autonomic dysreflexia during sexual activity. This results in excessively high blood pressure, and the treatment is generally to stop the activity. If it is a repetitive problem, consider seeing your doctor and asking for some medication to take against dysreflexia during sexual activity. Then you can relax and enjoy yourself.

Source: "Common Questions about Sexuality," *Spinal Cord Injury Life*, National Spinal Cord Injury Association, Cambridge, Massachusetts, © 1995. *SCI Life* printing courtesy of Eastern Paralyzed Veterans Association. For more information, contact NSCIA at 545 Concord Avenue, Suite 29, Cambridge, MA, 02138.

Exhibit
REPRODUCTIVE COUNSELING FOR WOMEN WITH SPINAL CORD INJURY

SEXUALITY COUNSELING

The rehabilitation specialist and the obstetric/gynecologic specialist may both lack experience dealing with the need for sexual information of women with spinal cord injury. For many such women, the information they receive deals only with reproductive functions, ignoring their inner feelings and desires, which may be in turmoil.

Sexuality is difficult to define and is thought of as a very personal subject. Much of our sexuality is defined by society's expectations, with motherhood still a societal ideal for many women. Given the media's focus on the perfect woman, it is understandable that many women feel anxious and resentful about their own sexuality. A broad definition of sexuality is especially important when supporting or taking care of a woman whose spinal cord is injured. What the disability means to her sexuality cannot be overemphasized.

Some women with spinal cord injury who are contemplating sexuality counseling are afraid of criticism, of being treated as an "oddity" or as "an interesting case." The woman's self-esteem may be lowered by general alienation, dislike for her body, and anxiety. In addition, she may be subjected to some of the following myths: Women with disabilities are asexual. The more perfect a woman's body is, the more desirable she is as an intimate partner. Women with disabilities are only desirable to men with disabilities. If an able-bodied man is dating a woman with a disability, it is because he can't get anyone else or he feels sorry for her. A nonjudgmental, in-depth discussion is necessary to dispel myths about sexual function and expression.

For some, the problems of sexual functioning may be more imaginary than real. If genital sex is not possible, alterations in position, stimulation, and penetration need to be explained. It must be remembered that the disability does not necessarily limit the scope of sexual and reproductive options for women with spinal cord injuries.

CONTRACEPTION

Closely related to sexual expression is a discussion of the woman's reproductive abilities and plans. The woman needs to be supported in the belief that decisions about contraception are hers to make and her only obligations are to herself and to her partner. However, not all contraceptives are easily used or safe for all women with spinal cord injuries, and some may be contraindicated. (See the following exhibit for an outline of specific contraceptives and advantages and disadvantages of each.)

When evaluating contraceptive methods, it is necessary to look at the following:

- the quality of circulation, especially in the lower extremities
- loss of sensation
- manual dexterity
- the condition, whether stable or progressive, and whether a particular type of contraceptive would aggravate the condition
- history of abnormal clotting
- medication that may interact with a hormonal contraceptive
- depression
- problems with menstrual or genital hygiene

The effectiveness and safety of contraceptive methods are heavily influenced by the woman's understanding. Involving the partner in the decision-making process is beneficial.

Women with spinal cord injuries must be given the same opportunities for health care and health education as other women. Like all women, they have concerns about sexuality and contraception. The gynecological exam, conducted with care and sensitivity, is an excellent setting in which to approach these topics, to remind the woman, and her partner, that she is valued and entitled to the full expression of her sexuality in the broadest sense.

Source: Copyright 1993, The American Journal of Nursing Company. Reprinted from *The American Journal of Maternal/Child Nursing*, Vol. 18, No. 5. Used with permission. All rights reserved.

Exhibit
EVALUATION OF CONTRACEPTIVE METHODS FOR WOMEN WITH SPINAL CORD INJURY

Method	Lowest Expected Failure Rate	Intervention/Evaluation with Spinal Cord Injury
Spermicidal jellies, creams, and foams	3%	Need manual dexterity. More able partner may be needed to assist with insertion.
Diaphragm	6%	Need manual dexterity. More able partner may be needed to assist with insertion.
Sponge	Parous women 9% Nulliparous women 6%	Need manual dexterity. More able partner may be needed to assist with insertion. Sponge is more effective for women who have not delivered a baby (nulliparous).
Cervical cap	6%	Need manual dexterity. More able partner may be needed to assist with insertion.
Condom	2%	Male takes the role.
Combination pills	0.1%	Contraindicated with spinal cord injury due to decreased or impaired sensation in lower extremities. Thrombophlebitis could go undetected.
Progestin-only pills	0.5%	May be considered. Need to be taken at same time each day to maintain consistent hormone levels.
Progestagen injections (Depo-Provera)	0.4%	Intramuscular injection provides protection for 90 days.
Subdermal implants (Progestin)	0.04%	Alternative to long-term sterilization. Can remain in place for five years.
Intrauterine device (IUD)	Copper bearing 0.8% Progesterone releasing 2.0%	Contraindicated because of increased risk for infection if menstrual hygiene is difficult to maintain. Increased bleeding is a concern. Due to decreased sensation, a pelvic inflammatory disease could go undetected. The woman or her partner would have to check the string.
Tubal ligation	0.2%	Should be considered permanent.

Source: Copyright 1993, The American Journal of Nursing Company. Reprinted from *The American Journal of Maternal/Child Nursing*, Vol. 18, No. 5. Used with permission. All rights reserved.

Exhibit
CARING FOR WOMEN WITH DISABILITIES: GUIDELINES FOR THE GYNECOLOGIST

Women with disabilities are living longer and more productive lives because of improved medical technology. According to The National Institute of Disability and Rehabilitation Research, there were 43 million people with disabilities in the United States in 1992, one-third of whom are women. Employment figures seem to indicate that women with disabilities are at a greater disadvantage than men with disabilities and nondisabled men and women; only 23 percent of women with disabilities are in the work force compared with 42 percent of men with disabilities. These findings suggest the need for new strategies—including obstetric and gynecologic care—to enhance quality of life for women with disabilities.

Obstetrician-gynecologists have the opportunity to interact with all patients in a personal and supportive manner. When the patient is a woman with a disability, it is important to consider certain specific problems during the gynecologic visit: body image, self-esteem, vulnerability, sexual needs, sexually transmitted diseases, contraception, prenatal diagnosis, obstetric care, infertility, and adoption.

Without knowing it, clinicians may create basic obstacles to women seeking care who have a disability. For example, offices may be inaccessible. Ramps and elevators make a world of difference to many women. Many emotional obstacles impede care as well. The woman with a disability may be extremely sensitive to subtle impressions, and an unwelcoming attitude from a rushed office staff member may cause her to feel that her disability is an imposition. In some cases, it may be more convenient for both the patient and the staff to schedule her as the last appointment.

Being able to handle the physical limitations of a woman with a disability is important. When the physician enters the examination room, his or her choice of words can be crucial to an open interaction with any patient. Instead of saying, "I'm sure you need help undressing and getting on the table, don't you?" clinicians should try a nonjudgmental approach, for example, "Is there any way I can be of help?" This question gives the patient the opportunity to request help gracefully or decline assistance if not required.

Tables in which the foot end drops in a graduated fashion are used to assist in transferring a patient from her wheelchair to the examination table. With staff assistance or a transfer board, this allows the patient to move to the examination table from a level that is almost equivalent to her wheelchair. The table can also drop to a lower level for easier transfer.

Two situations present special problems. During the examination of patients with spinal cord lesions above T4–T6 (above the outflow of the splanchnic nerves), physicians should be aware of precipitating factors causing autonomic hyperreflexia. This serious complication of spinal cord injury is precipitated by distended bladder, impacted bowel, pelvic examination, or labor. Because it usually occurs when the woman is supine, the patient should assume a semisitting position for pelvic examination. For both pelvic and rectal examinations of patients with disabilities, make sure a staff member is able to assist with leg positioning and leg spasm.

For patients who are so physically or mentally disabled that they are institutionalized, the pelvic examination can be a special challenge. In one approach, physicians combine the gynecologic examination with dental procedures in which the patient requires sedation. The dentist works on her mouth while the gynecologist obtains a Papanicolaou smear and performs an adequate pelvic examination. For institutionalized patients, the pelvic examination is particularly important because it may highlight signs of sexual abuse.

BODY IMAGE

Body image—or an internalized sense of body self—can be distorted for many reasons, including physical impairments. Because a young girl's body image is based on comparisons with her peers and surrounding adults, it is especially important for young girls with physical disabilities to interact with other similarly impaired people. This exposure will help them realize that a physically disabled body is not undesirable, unusual, or unacceptable and will give them confidence to interact positively with nondisabled children and adults.

For the woman who became disabled later in life, body image adjustments can be extremely difficult. A woman with a recent disability often feels that she has not changed and, on an emotional level, she may not accept that her body has changed. She will either accept her condition and seek support, or she will deny her condition and withdraw from personal interactions with others. If her family, physical therapist, physician, or social worker identifies the denial-grief reaction, immediate intervention may be successful.

SELF-ESTEEM

Self-esteem refers to a person's judgment of her own worth. Some young girls who are physically disabled from a very early age accept challenges with a positive outlook and strive for excellence within their capacities. Others feel they will never be able to aspire to the achievements made by their unaffected counterparts. This view may lead to unnecessarily low aspirations and goals and hinder creativity and enthusiasm.

In some cases, a self-defeating cycle may develop. If the girl feels inadequate and isolates herself, potential friends may think she is aloof and unfriendly. Further, her obvious physical difference can make it easy for her peers to rationalize rejecting her. This social interaction pattern usually begins at a very early age. Physicians should be alert to this pattern so it can be addressed promptly.

continues

continued

For teenagers or adults who have poignant memories of not being physically limited, self-esteem adjustments may be much more difficult. Unfortunately, this may be exacerbated by other adults and teenagers who frequently feel uncomfortable around the individual with a disability. They seem to fear that the affliction is, in some way, contagious. This can lead to blatant rejection by long-standing friends and coworkers, which may result in severe isolation and depression. Again, family support and understanding medical care are essential. Often, the woman must overcome her own self-consciousness and discomfort and try to win a new circle of friends who will not be threatened by her disability.

SEXUALITY

If a teenager or woman with a disability feels undesirable, she may become vulnerable to exploitation, particularly in sexual relationships. This can be dangerous to her health and well-being. For example, before the woman became disabled she may have refused to participate in unprotected sexual intercourse; now she may feel that if she does not consent, no one else will approach her. These are fears she may hesitate to discuss with her clinician. It may be useful to give her an opportunity to express her concerns.

Open communication is especially important when dealing with sexual difficulties so that problems can be clearly identified and solutions explored. However, the Sex and Disability Project survey indicates that less than 5 percent of the respondents ever received sex education or counseling. It is common practice for gynecologists to discuss sexual issues with all patients, and they should follow this example with patients who have disabilities as well. Physicians should not guess what the patient needs—they should ask. A careful history may differentiate between an impairment in genital functioning and a situational dysfunction.

Loss of innervation to the vaginal area can make it difficult for a woman to obtain adequate lubrication, making intercourse uncomfortable. Vaginal accommodation may be reduced because of anatomic changes; orgasmic sensation may be delayed, reduced, or absent. A woman with a disability may experience anxiety about her ability to satisfy her partner. Her sexual partner, who may perceive her as fragile, may be afraid to touch her or to find ways to achieve mutual satisfaction.

SEXUALLY TRANSMITTED DISEASES

Detecting and managing sexually transmitted diseases (STDs) in women with disabilities present many obstacles. Spinal cord lesions below the level of T10–T12 will obliterate all sensation from the uterus to below the perineum. For a woman with this type of injury, symptoms of early infection—pain, low-grade fever, and vaginal discharge—are difficult to detect. This is combined with her reluctance to seek help because of concerns that the pelvic examination for the woman with limited lower body mobility can be difficult. Without proper treatment, these issues may result in prolonged infection, which can lead to some serious sequelae.

Most individuals with disabilities like to control their lives as much as possible, and physicians should be open to their needs. Many women are self-conscious about volunteering information about special problems. Patients with vision problems may be unable to monitor their temperature; patients with a hearing impairment may require written instructions to comply with follow-up. Some neurologic conditions involve dysphagia, which can make swallowing pills difficult. Find out whether the patient will have problems with monitoring her infection and taking the prescribed antibiotics. Prescription orders should specify easy-open packaging or liquid forms of medication as required.

CONTRACEPTION

Obstetrician-gynecologists commonly ask reproductive-aged women if they need contraception. The same procedure should be used when caring for a woman with a disability. However, her contraceptive choice may be somewhat different. For instance, barrier methods may not be suitable because a loss of range of motion and impaired finger dexterity can make inserting a diaphragm or cervical cap difficult.

Although oral contraceptives are not usually recommended for patients with spinal cord injuries—because of the possible increase of thrombotic events—they may be appropriate for other women with disabilities. Packaging may create a variety of problems. Certain products require women to push and turn a dial as well as puncture a seal to get to the pill. This is not suitable for a woman whose precision of hand movement is altered. A 21-day regimen is better for patients who have imprecise finger control. This will prevent patients from inadvertently taking an inert pill. In general, ensure that the patient is comfortable with the mechanics of her medication.

Also, some women with disabilities live with family or in settings that limit their privacy. In these situations, a woman may have difficulty concealing her contraceptive use. Open dialogue between all concerned parties can avoid an unpleasant confrontation.

In some cases, medroxyprogesterone acetate (Depo-Provera) may be a good contraceptive alternative. This method requires one injection approximately every three months. The levonorgestrel implants (Norplant) have a contraceptive efficacy of at least five years.

An intrauterine device is another alternative, but it is not a good choice for a patient with spinal cord injury because she cannot easily detect infection.

Source: Sandra L. Welner, "Gynecologic Care of the Disabled Woman," *Contemporary Ob/Gyn*, Vol. 38:1, Medical Economics Publishing, Montvale, New Jersey, © 1993.

Exhibit
CARING FOR WOMEN WITH DISABILITIES: GUIDELINES FOR THE OBSTETRICIAN

PRENATAL DIAGNOSIS

Many women with disabilities feel that when they make an appointment for prenatal care, the physician assumes they want to terminate the pregnancy. Often, the physician and staff are so uncomfortable with a woman's disability that they ignore her special needs and treat her like any other patient. Alternatively, they sometimes assume that the pregnant woman with a disability does not have the same obstetric needs as other pregnant women.

Screening for neural tube defects, Down syndrome, and physical congenital malformations is standard care. A couple that has grown to accept a physical congenital disability may not necessarily want to terminate a pregnancy when a fetus is diagnosed with a similar deformity. Such patients may feel that the suggestion of abortion implies that their physical differences make them unacceptable members of society. A sensitive, accepting approach to counseling couples with disabilities is essential.

SPECIAL PROBLEMS DURING PREGNANCY

Managing the pregnancy of a woman with a disability requires special attention: continuous monitoring for urinary tract infections, overcoming problems in weighing patients with spinal cord injury using standard office equipment, and difficulties in detecting premature labor. The pregnant patient will also need assistance in adjusting to increased physical limitations. To prevent premature delivery, patients with spinal cord injury may need more frequent examinations during the third trimester to evaluate cervical change.

The changing physical condition of the pregnant woman may also require evaluations by a physiatrist and physical therapist. For example, a pregnant woman using a straight cane may want to switch to a quad cane or walker for more stability. Pregnant women with disabilities need to make similar adjustments to pregnancy as nondisabled women do. These include accepting the new role of childbearing and the impending responsibilities of parenthood; accepting extra nurturing and assuming a more dependent role; seeking a less active lifestyle to cope with fatigue; and maintaining self-esteem, body image, and confidence about sexuality. A pregnant woman with a disability must understand the relationship between her pregnancy and her disability to make the necessary lifestyle modifications.

LABOR AND DELIVERY

Delivery in the patient who has suffered a spinal cord injury can be straightforward, but there is the risk of muscle spasms and autonomic dysreflexia. Autonomic dysreflexia occurs mainly with lesions above T4–T6 and is a response to noxious sensory output arising from the bladder, bowel, and other pelvic organs in which the supraspinal influence over the major part of the sympathetic outflow has been lost.

The clinical manifestations of autonomic dysreflexia include paroxysmal hypertension, fluctuating heart rate, sweating forehead, severe headache, blotchy skin, and piloerection above the level of the lesion. This condition has been confused with pre-eclampsia (see following exhibit) and a number of cases of intracranial hemorrhage and death due to misdiagnosis have been reported. During labor and delivery of a woman with spinal cord injury, the usual signs of pain may be replaced by other, less clearly defined symptoms such as abnormal heart rate, hyperventilation, and increased spasticity.

An epidural is usually the anesthesia of choice. Carefully monitor oxytocin induction, because it has been associated with increased incidence of severe autonomic dysreflexia. Promptly treat elevated blood pressure from autonomic dysreflexia with improved pain control and antihypertensive agents.

For patients with lesions above T4–T6, use a birthing bed or chair so that the woman can sit for labor and delivery. Autonomic dysreflexia is more likely to occur when the woman is supine. Prolonged positioning in stirrups may be uncomfortable; using straps to control leg muscle spasms may injure the patient's skin. Occasionally, forceps may be required for ineffective pushing efforts. Caesarean section is not always necessary, but, in some cases, it is the safest route.

POSTPARTUM CONCERNS

In patients with spinal cord injury, decreased circulation and muscle tone in the perineal area may lead to a predisposition for episiotomy breakdown. Because of the patient's immobility, she may be subject to complications from the hypercoagulability of pregnancy and the puerperium. This exacerbates her risk of developing serious complications such as thrombophlebitis and pulmonary embolus. The physician and the postpartum nursing staff should provide as much preventive intervention as possible.

INFERTILITY

Individuals with disabilities may experience problems in finding a specialist willing to help them with their unique needs. Female factors are similar to those addressed in nondisabled women: ovulation irregularities, sperm-mucus interaction abnormalities, and lack of tubal patency. Any abnormality identified should follow established protocols. Refer male partners who have disabilities to a urologist.

ADOPTION

When infertility treatments are not successful, some couples try adoption. Here, too, they may face prejudice. Often, people who are not disabled cannot perceive that a couple with disabilities could care for a child as well as a nondisabled couple. Couples with disabilities are often more creative in coping with

continues

continued

adversity and approach obstacles with great patience. These qualities may make couples with disabilities well suited for the challenge of becoming adoptive parents.

EQUIVALENT CARE

The fundamental concept surrounding care of the woman with a disability is that she is a woman and she has a disability. All the issues associated with the female patient apply. If physicians combine sensitivity, creativity, acceptance, and a nonjudgmental attitude in caring for the woman with a disability, she will receive the best possible care.

Source: Sandra L. Welner, "Gynecologic Care of the Disabled Woman," *Contemporary Ob/Gyn*, Vol. 38:1, Medical Economics Publishing, Montvale, New Jersey, © 1993.

Exhibit
DIFFERENTIAL DIAGNOSIS: PREECLAMPSIA VERSUS AUTONOMIC DYSREFLEXIA

	Preeclampsia	Autonomic Dysreflexia
Etiology	Cause uncertain; central nervous system becomes stimulated	Distension of visceral organs (bladder, bowel, uterus) results in activation of the autonomic nervous system
Manifestations	Hyperactive reflexes, spasm of small blood vessels	Lack of spinal input to central nervous system results in autonomic nervous system overactivity: muscle spasms, dilation of large blood vessels, and visceral organs
Target vessels	Works on small blood vessels in brain, eyes, kidneys, liver	Works on aorta, large blood vessels in brain
Distension of organs	None	Visceral organs (bladder, bowel, uterus)
Target muscles	Skeletal muscles (hyperactive reflexes)	Visceral smooth muscle
Symptoms and findings	Proteinuria, edema, headache	Profuse sweating, headache, severe muscle spasm, piloerection
Worst scenario if mismanaged	Kidney failure, blindness, seizures, stroke	Seizures, hemorrhagic stroke
Risk of death	Rare	Significant

Source: Sandra L. Welner, "Gynecologic Care of the Disabled Woman," *Contemporary Ob/Gyn*, Vol. 38:1, Medical Economics Publishing, Montvale, New Jersey, © 1993.

Give Yourself a Chance: Reaffirming Your Sexuality

Here is a scenario that happens too frequently: I go out with my girlfriend to a blues club on Friday night. The man on the next stool strikes up a conversation with me and of course the conversation gets around to "what kind of work do you do?" I say I am "retired." The man says "you look too young to be retired," and I keep trying to sidestep the issue that I am disabled and live on SSD. I am afraid of scaring him off "again" or having him start trying to discreetly find out what my disability is, as it is not that visible.

Learning to handle the social scene is one thing, but it is much more difficult to communicate the following message to the other sex: Just because you are disabled in some way, you are not completely incapacitated or celibate!

Grappling with this problem has led many people with disabilities to ignore the sex side of their being and not look for companionship with the opposite sex or to deny that they can be attractive and loving to someone else.

How do you solve this problem? I have a few ideas that people with disabilities should think about.

1. Don't think that you should limit yourself to looking for just "abled" persons for boy or girl friends. There are many persons with disabilities who would love to have a relationship with someone that has some understanding of what it is to live with pain; someone who needs time alone, or needs help from someone else, might want to have household help and/or have fun when you are feeling downright wonderful for a change. I have known men with heart problems that think they shouldn't burden a woman with their problem and become recluses. Did they ever stop to think that there are women out there with similar problems who would be thrilled to be with them and love them? Why must people be so selfish as to think that what time they have is better spent with loneliness and boredom, rather than spending special time with someone who needs them and wants to love them and is not concerned about "time"?
2. A person with a disability can have and enjoy sex! Sex is a many-faceted experience. There are many different ways to physically love a person besides the sex act, such as cuddling and just plain touching. Every human being has the ability and right to experience, want, and have love.
3. Get out and make yourself available. I find myself looking around a gathering, bar, or restaurant, and any other place to meet people, for someone with a cane, wheelchair, or indication of a disability. We all sort of have a tendency to feel an empathy with a fellow "disabled." However, I look to see if I am attracted and, if so, look for a wedding ring or to see if he has a date. I have been so disappointed that I don't see more people with disabilities going out on Friday "Singles Night." I know they are out there.
4. Join singles' groups, special interest groups, support groups, clubs, and/or any other group you can physically handle. If one group does not meet your expectations (after you give it

continues

continued

a chance to work), drop it and try another one. Don't be shy, make yourself important, and decide which group works best for you and put your heart into it and enjoy.

People with somewhat "hidden" disabilities like mine (I limp when I walk and have trouble with stairs) are even afraid to get out and meet others. However, you can and must take the initiative—stop being shy, stop being self-defeating, and try.

Notes:

Source: Ann Whiting, "Give Yourself a Chance," *ABLED*, Fondren, Texas, © Summer 1995.

Spinal Cord Injury and Breast Cancer

Breast cancer is the most common cancer among women, accounting for more than 30 percent of all of their cancers. While spinal cord injury itself does not place women at higher risk of breast cancer, some of the results of spinal cord injury—reduced sensation, less likelihood of bearing children—can place women with spinal cord injury in higher risk categories.

WHAT IS BREAST CANCER?

Cancer is really a number of diseases caused by the abnormal growth of cells. Often the cells grow out of control, divide more than they should, and form masses known as tumors. Malignant, or cancerous, tumors not only invade normal tissue, but their cells can travel to other parts of the body to form more malignant tumors. This spreading is called metastasis.

Breast cancer most often begins as a painless lump or thickening in the upper outer portion of the breast; it can, however, occur anywhere in the breast, including the nipple. Breast cancers may spread to the lymph nodes in the armpit and then throughout the body.

WHAT ARE THE RISKS?

Because the cause of breast cancer is unknown, there is no way to truly prevent it. However, several things put women at higher risk of developing breast cancer:

- a personal or close family history of breast cancer—mother, sister, aunt, grandmother
- never giving birth, having your first full-term pregnancy after the age of 30, or experiencing an abortion during your first pregnancy
- obesity
- early onset of menstruation—before age 12
- late menopause
- cigarette smoking
- high-fat diet
- alcohol consumption

Risk also increases dramatically with age: at age 25 the odds are 1 in 20,000; by age 50 the odds are 1 in 50; by age 85 the odds are 1 in 8.

DOES SPINAL CORD INJURY INCREASE THE RISK?

Spinal cord injury does not place women at greater risk of developing breast cancer, but some of the consequences of spinal cord injury may increase risk and interfere with prevention and early detection. Women injured young may be less likely to bear children. Inactivity may lead to weight gain. Reduced hand function and sensation can interfere with self-exams. And living in a chair may make positioning for mammographies challenging or impossible.

continues

continued

HOW CAN I DECREASE THE RISKS?

Several basic steps keep your risk as low as possible. Avoid obesity—cut fat intake to 25 percent to 30 percent of your total calories, less than 50 grams of fat per day. Eat high-fiber foods like whole-grain cereals, fruits and vegetables, foods rich in vitamins A and C, and deep green vegetables, such as broccoli, cauliflower, or other foods from the cabbage family. Limit salt-cured, smoked, and nitrate-cured foods: cold cuts, ham, hot dogs, and sausage. If you have fluid-filled sacs or small cysts in the breasts (called fibrocystic breasts), cut down or eliminate caffeine. Reduce your alcohol use to two or fewer drinks per day. Quit smoking!

The most common sign of breast cancer is a lump or thickening, especially one that does not go away and does not change the way it feels. Other signs include swelling, puckering or dimpling, discoloration, or soreness of the skin; a fixed inversion of the nipple that is a change from before; skin ulcers; and scaling, crusting, or drainage from the nipple or areola.

Monthly Exams Are a Must

The American Cancer Society recommends:

- monthly breast self-examination for women over age 20
- a baseline mammogram by age 40 with a repeat every one to two years for women in their 40s then yearly starting at age 50
- clinical breast exam by a health care professional every three years from ages 20 to 40, yearly after age 40

The American Cancer Society also strongly recommends the biopsy of *all* suspicious lumps!

Monthly breast self-exams are recommended because breast cancer can develop between clinical exams or mammograms. Actually, most breast lumps are found by women themselves or by their sexual partners. For your monthly exam, first use a mirror to look for lumps, changes in breast shape, pain, or discharge from the nipple. Then palpate, using your fingers to feel your breasts in overlapping areas about the size of a dime. Remember to also check the underarm and upper chest areas.

Quadriplegia and Decreased Sensation

Changes in your risk factors if you have quadriplegia or decreased sensation make these self-exams even more important. You can still do your own visual inspections, but if your sensation is at all impaired, get help to do a proper and complete exam. Have your husband, lover, or friend help. Ideally, you should do your self-exam four to seven days after your menstrual period. However, you may wish to combine these exams with a monthly catheter change and have your nurse or caregiver help you at that time. Be sure to have whoever helps you write down any questions or changes they feel so that the changes can be rechecked by your doctor.

continues

continued

Remember: do these exams faithfully every month. Your spinal cord injury has changed some of the risks, so exams are even more important.

WHAT IF I FIND SOMETHING?

This is the dreaded question, often the one that prevents self-exams in the first place. Remember that 80 percent of lumps—four out of five—are benign, but they feel the same as cancerous lumps. If you find a lump or notice a change, see your health care professional immediately.

IS THERE ANY GOOD NEWS?

YES! A new, large core biopsy technique has been developed that can be done in the doctor's office. This procedure has a shorter recovery time, doesn't leave a scar, and costs much less than a surgical biopsy. It's available in about 100 U.S. hospitals. Also, over 600 Contour Mammography Systems are now available in nearly all 50 states to serve women with spinal cord injury. This system allows you to remain in your chair while a tilt arm conforms to your position. Ask your doctor or call Bennett X-ray Technologies at 516-691-6100 to locate one in your area.

The best news of all is that breast cancer treated at its earliest, noninvasive stage has an almost 100 percent survival rate.

RESOURCES

American Cancer Society: 1-800-ACS-2345
Y-ME: 1-800-221-2141
Susan G. Komen Breast Cancer Foundation: 1-800-462-9273
National Cancer Institute: 1-800-422-6237
For accredited mammography centers: 1-800-4-CANCER

Source: The Rehabilitation Research and Training Center on Aging with SCI, a joint project of Craig Hospital and the Department of Rehabilitation Medicine at the University of Colorado Health Sciences Center. Funded by the National Institute on Disability and Rehabilitation Research. For more information about the "SCI & Aging" publications, contact the RRTC at 800-5-REHAB-8.

SEXUAL HEALTH

Five Steps to a Healthier and Safer Sex Life

1. Use a condom every time!

- Condoms offer the best protection against sexually transmitted infections (STIs) for people having sexual intercourse.

2. Talk with your partner before sex:

- Partners should care about each other and be interested in one another's pleasure, comfort, and health.
- Be open. Let your partner know your health concerns and sexual health history, and encourage your partner to be open, too.
- Be direct. Talk about your sexual needs and expectations.
- Be persistent. Don't let your partner remain silent on these issues.

3. Keep medically fit:

- Have a checkup for STIs every year.
- Protect your immune system. Eat well, get enough rest, and limit your use of alcohol, tobacco, and other drugs.

4. If you think you or your partner has an STI:

- See a clinician for testing, diagnosis, and treatment.
- Find out if your partner(s) needs to be examined and treated too.
- Use **all** the medication that is prescribed. Symptoms often disappear before an infection is cured.
- Do not take anyone else's medicine, and do not share yours.
- Do not have sex until your infection is under control.

5. Stay in charge:

- Alcohol and other drugs weaken good judgment and self-control. Don't let them jeopardize your self-control.

Source: "Sexually Transmitted Infections—The Facts," Planned Parenthood® Federation of America, Inc., © 1995.

Exhibit
SEXUALLY TRANSMITTED DISEASES—COUNSELING CHECKLIST AND GUIDELINES

CHECKLIST FOR SEXUALLY TRANSMITTED DISEASE COUNSELING

____Help the client to relax and to express concerns or fears.
____Reassure client that he or she has assumed responsibility for personal well-being and is better off knowing diagnosis and receiving treatment than going undiagnosed.
____Without imparting guilt, help client understand how his or her specific sexual behavior relates to the sexually transmitted disease (STD) or to other STDs.
____Help client understand the specific disease, its transmission, and its clinical picture.
____Help client understand how the disease is treated and what is involved with the treatment protocol.
____Explain any medication, dosage, administration routine, side effects, and rationale for adherence to routine.
____Assist client with partner notification strategies—role playing, rehearsing, or script writing may be indicated.
____Provide written information to client on diagnosis, treatment, follow-up, partner notification, and supportive services.
____Discuss contraceptives in terms of STDs. Discuss contraceptive strategies to reduce future exposure to and risk of STDs.
____Remind the client to avoid intercourse until cured.

BEHAVIORAL COUNSELING MESSAGES WITH SPECIFIC SEXUALLY TRANSMITTED DISEASES*

Disease	Behavioral Counseling Message
Chlamydia	Condom use; refer partner(s) for evaluation.
Cytomegalovirus	Condom use; refer symptomatic partner(s) for evaluation.
Human papillomavirus	Weekly or biweekly treatment until lesions resolve; early treatment to reduce sequelae; examine partner(s) for warts; abstain from sex or use condoms during treatment; women should have annual Pap smear.
Gonorrhea	Avoid sex until patient and partners are cured; return for evaluation 2 to 3 days after treatment; take medications as prescribed; ensure examination of partner(s) as soon as possible; return early if symptoms persist or recur.
Hepatitis B	Condom use; refer partner(s) for evaluation.
Herpes	Keep lesion area clean and dry; abstain from sexual contact in areas of lesion while symptomatic; realize undetermined risk for transmission during asymptomatic intervals; use condoms for further protection during asymptomatic periods; women should have annual Pap smear.
Syphilis	Return for follow-up serologies 3, 6, 12, and 24 months after treatment; refer sexual partner(s) for evaluation and treatment; avoid sexual activity until patient and partner(s) are cured; use condoms to prevent future infections.

*For all STDs, voluntary, confidential HIV-antibody testing, coupled with pretest and posttest counseling, and evaluation should be routinely offered when the results may contribute either to the clinical management of the person or to the prevention of further disease transmission.

Source: Reprinted by permission of the publisher from "Sexually Transmitted Diseases: Perspectives on This Growing Epidemic" by Linda L. Alexander, RNC, PHD, *The Nurse Practitioner: The American Journal of Primary Healthcare*, Vol. 17:10, © 1992 by Springhouse Corporation.

Talking to Your Partner about AIDS

Following are some ideas to keep in mind when talking with your partner about avoiding risks of human immunodeficiency virus (HIV) infection and AIDS.

- Both you and your partner are responsible for protection against infection with HIV/AIDS.
- Your partner probably has many of the same feelings that you do.
- If you are going to have sex with someone, you should be able to discuss protection with that person.
- You should be concerned about your own and your partner's health and happiness.
- Your concern does not mean that you distrust your partner.
- Both you and your partner should know how to avoid getting infected with the AIDS virus (HIV).
- If there are any doubts about faithfulness in your current relationship, or concerns about the safety of past sexual behavior since 1977, both of you should consider being tested for the AIDS virus (HIV) and get HIV/AIDS counseling.
- If you are concerned that you may already be infected, don't take any chances with your partner's health. Treat your partner as you would like to be treated—with sensitive and loving concern for each other's health and well-being.
- You have a right to ask questions about your partner's past. If you do not like the answers, you may decide not to have sex with that person. If someone doesn't care enough about you to take precautions, maybe you don't know that person well enough and should rethink having sex.
- Talk about AIDS before you have sex. Do not wait until you have already had sex with the person—by then, it may be too late. If possible, do not have the talk in the bedroom or after you are already in a sexual mood.
- If you are in an abusive or violent relationship, it may be hard to talk about protection with your partner. Sensitive subjects, such as AIDS, might increase feelings. If you cannot talk about AIDS or using protection without having a fight, consider seeking help from a counselor or someone else who can help with relationship problems. Check your local Yellow Pages directory or call your local public health department for information about shelters for battered or abused women in your area.
- Call an AIDS hot line if you have questions about HIV/AIDS and sex.
  - AIDS Information Hot Line (toll free): 1-800-342-AIDS
  - For Spanish-speaking persons, Linea Nacional de SIDA: 1-800-344-SIDA
  - For hearing-impaired persons, TTY/TDD Hot Line: 1-800-AIDS-TTY
- You can also get help and information from:
  - your doctor or health care worker
  - your local or state public health department
  - your local AIDS service organization

Courtesy of the American Red Cross, © 1992. All Rights Reserved in all Countries. Permission of publisher required to reprint.

The HIV Test

SHOULD YOU HAVE THE HIV TEST?

HIV stands for human immunodeficiency virus. It is the virus that causes AIDS. To help you decide if you should have the HIV test (sometimes called the AIDS test) to learn if you have been infected with HIV, answer the following questions.

- Have you had sex without knowing *for sure* if the person or persons you had sex with do not have HIV?
- Have you had sex with someone you know has HIV or AIDS?
- Have you had a disease passed on by sex, such as genital herpes or syphilis? (Having these diseases makes it easier to get HIV.)
- Have you had sex with many men or women or had sex with someone who has had sex with many men or women?
- Have you had sex with someone who has used needles to take drugs?
- Have you shared needles or works to take drugs?

If you answer "yes" to any of these questions, you should think about having the HIV test.

HOW CAN HIV TESTING HELP YOU?

If tests show that you don't have HIV, you can learn how to stay HIV-free. (Someone who does not have HIV is called HIV negative.)

If tests show that you do have HIV, you can get medical care right away to help you:

- stay healthy longer
- avoid getting some illnesses caused by HIV
- get early treatment for illnesses that do occur

Testing is the only way to know if you have HIV—and testing is the first step in getting medical care, counseling, and support if you need them.

WHAT STEPS SHOULD YOU TAKE BEFORE HAVING THE TEST?

The HIV test is important, but it is a big step. You should think about how having HIV could affect your life. These following three steps can help you to prepare for the test:

1. Consider telling someone you trust that you are having the HIV test. Support of a family member or a friend can mean a lot.
2. Find out how private your test results will be. Ask the clinic if anyone but you can learn your test results.

continues

continued

3. Set a time to get your results. Don't put it off. The test can help you only when you find out what it shows.

HOW DOES THE HIV TEST WORK?

The HIV test shows if you have signs in your blood of the virus that causes AIDS. HIV testing has four steps:

1. You go to the clinic or doctor's office. A nurse or counselor tells you about the test. You can ask questions and talk about your fears and concerns.
2. You decide to have the test. A nurse or aide uses a needle to take some blood from your arm.
3. Your blood is tested for signs of HIV. If the first test (called ELISA) is positive (shows signs of HIV), the blood will be tested again. If the second test is positive, another kind of test (called a Western blot) will be done to confirm the result.
4. Test results come back to the clinic. A nurse or counselor tells you when to come in, what the results mean, and how to help yourself.

HOW DO YOU GET MORE INFORMATION?

To learn more about HIV and where to get the test in your city or town, call:

- 1-800-342-AIDS (1-800-342-2437)
- your local health department

People at these numbers can answer your questions about HIV. They also can send you booklets that have more information.

REMEMBER: If the HIV test is positive, it will mean that you have the HIV virus that causes AIDS. It also will mean that you can get medical care and support services to help you if you need them.

Source: *Taking the HIV (AIDS) Test: How to Help Yourself*, U.S. Department of Health and Human Services, Public Health Services, National Institutes of Health, September 1992.

8

Psychosocial Adjustment

> Most materials in the *Spinal Cord Injury Patient Education Manual* are intended for the health care professional to share with the patient. Materials that are intended solely for the professional are labeled "Exhibit" in the table of contents.

General Emotional Health

    Emotional Adjustment 259
    Emotional Adjustment Worksheet 262
    Self-Care 263

Depression

    Overview of Depression 264
    Diagnosis of Depression 267
    Treating Depression 270

Additional Mental Health Concerns

    Stress 273
    Effects of Fatigue on People with
        Spinal Cord Injury 275
    Locating Your Fatigue Trouble Spots 280

Alcohol and Substance Abuse

    Facts about Alcohol 283
    Definition of Alcoholism 284
    Are You a Problem Drinker? 285

    What Can I Do about My Drinking? 286
    Alcoholics Anonymous: Basic
        Information 289
    Symptoms of Substance Abuse by
        Adolescents with Spinal Cord Injury 291
    Substance Abuse Symptoms Checklist 294
    Substance Abuse: Suggestions to Help
        You at Home 296

Adapting to Spinal Cord Injury

    Examining Your Feelings Toward
        Disabilities 298
    "Normal" Feelings 299
    Learn to Let Others Know What You
        Need Without Being Rude 301
    Family and Friends 303
    Being a Parent 305
    Accepting New Help as the Years Go By 306

The Caregiver

    Tips for the Long-Term Caregiver 309

GENERAL EMOTIONAL HEALTH

Emotional Adjustment

You may have already been through a lengthy period of hospitalization or other efforts to correct your spinal cord injury. Or your spinal cord injury may have come about suddenly following an accident or a rapidly progressing condition. Your experience involves you as a whole person—mind, body, and spirit. You are entitled to help in recovery emotionally as well as physically. In rehabilitation all of your needs are considered to be very important. The rehabilitation team will encourage you to address the emotional aspects of recovery as well as the physical.

Take a few minutes now and realize how you have been feeling since you learned about the spinal cord injury. Your feelings may have a broad range, or it may seem that you have felt numb or empty inside. Depression, anger, fear, sadness, anxiety, hopelessness, overwhelming fatigue, confusion, powerlessness, and resentment are a few of the feelings people have dealt with following this injury. You may also experience a sense of relief, hope, or confidence that you are succeeding in dealing with a difficult life situation. You may also have a series of mood swings from high to low that may leave you with the feeling that you're losing your marbles. By the way, your family and close friends are probably experiencing many of the same feelings. As you go through this recovery together, you may feel closer or you may find that there are more arguments and stress between you. Stress tends to bring out the best and the worst in all of us, so take it easy, a day at a time, and you'll make it.

Give yourself a break here. Stop and take a look at what you have been through. Of course this has been an emotional event! So much has changed over a short period of time. The pain you may have had or continue to have, fear of the unknown, questions, guilt, or blame may have taken up a good deal of your time and energy.

What can you do to handle all of this? Here are a few suggestions that have helped others through tough times and may get you thinking about your own situation.

- **Attitude.** Develop a win/win attitude. Every time you say "I can't" you give yourself that message and pretty soon you'll be convinced that you can't before you give it a try. Believe in yourself and trust your rehabilitation team's belief in you. Develop a sense that there is always something for you to gain in a situation, exercise, or challenge. Substitute phrases like "that's worth a try" or "I don't see why not." Anyway you want to say it is fine, as long as you give yourself a positive message.
- **Take one day at a time.** Thinking of having pain or numerous limitations for the rest of your life would be very overwhelming. In fact, dealing with any situation forever would be hard to take. So break it down to small, manageable segments—a few minutes, an hour, a day—and you find anything easier to handle. Can I take another five minutes of therapy? Sure.
- **Take advantage of your resources.** Some resources are family, friends, staff, and support groups. Talk to someone who has been there. Another person who has had the same

continues

continued

experience would be ideal, and your nurse or social worker may help introduce you to the right people.

- **Talk about it.** Discussing your feelings doesn't change the situation, but it will help to lighten your burden. When a sorrow is shared it becomes half, and when joy is shared it doubles. Talking things out with someone who cares makes it much easier to keep going. We all need a kind ear and a word of understanding.
- **Be good to yourself.** Do something good for yourself each day. For example, take a long, relaxing shower at the end of the day, dress up in a favorite outfit, spend time reading, listen to music, or watch an enjoyable TV show. Also make sure you rest at night and eat a healthy diet.
- **Easy does it.** Set your goals so that they can be achieved in the time you have. Don't expect to be running a marathon in your first week. Your team members can help you to set realistic, achievable goals. Remember, don't try to be perfect!
- **Develop a sense of humor.** Everyone has a sense of humor, but when we are under stress we sometimes forget to take advantage of one of our greatest and most healing powers. So share a funny story or a joke. Get involved with recreation programs, play games, and have fun just for the fun of it.
- **Relax!** As crazy as it may seem, relaxing can be hard to do. There are some simple exercises and relaxation techniques that can be done. Practice relaxing every day.
- **Practice.** With time and practice, your new skills will become more natural, your confidence will increase, and you will begin to feel more like yourself again. Give it some time and do your prescribed treatments. Pretty soon you'll see results.
- **Work on accepting life on its terms.** Change is change. Don't attach judgment to it. When we experience a change, quite often we tend to say it's "bad" or "good" when in fact its just different. So avoid attaching judgments and look for what you need in each change you experience. Look for the opportunities for growth in this situation.

These are just a few suggestions. You can look to family, friends, other people with spinal cord injury, and your rehab team for a few other ideas.

Every person has his or her own way of dealing with people and with the events that happen from day to day. After a spinal cord injury, this does not change. There are changes in your life that you will have to deal with, changes that can cause stress. Being in the hospital, the changes caused by your spinal cord injury, learning new ways to do things, and worrying about what it will be like after you go home can all cause stress. Stress can cause many feelings. Some of these feelings are:

- *anger* at the injury, its cause, what you may have done or may not have done to cause the spinal cord injury
- *frustration* when things are hard to do or do not happen the way you want
- *depression* when things seem very bad and as if they will never be better

continues

continued

- *fear* about what the future will be like
- *helplessness* when others are doing things for you

You may not have all these feelings, or they may be very strong. These feelings often come and go. Most people find ways to deal with these feelings, but it takes time. There will be good days and bad days. Having these feelings is normal. If you have these feelings, it is because of what has happened to you, not because something is wrong with your mind.

The support of family and friends is important. You need to be aware that those close to you face a lot of stress, too. They may have many of the same feelings that you do, but for different reasons. For example, they may feel angry or helpless (or both) that they could not have prevented the spinal cord injury, or worried that they will not do all the "right things" to help you. You may be able to help them just by talking openly.

You need to know that it is common for family and friends to try to overprotect you and do things that you could do for yourself. This often gets better over time as you practice things and are more sure of yourself. You may need to tell others what you can do and what they should *not* do. If someone close to you is having a hard time adjusting and you think that it gets in the way of your doing what you need to, you may want to see a family counselor.

Problems you may have in adjusting after your spinal cord injury, like all problems, are often easier to solve when talked out with another person. You will probably find that family and/or friends are enough. A professional can also help. Some people feel that professional help is an insult, is only for extreme cases, or is just not for them. But a professional has the skills and experience to help you in ways your family and friends may not be able to help. A professional can help you find new ways to deal with stress or problems, whether on your own or with someone's help, so you can put all your energy back into other parts of your life.

Source: Wanda Trojanoski, University of Rochester, Strong Memorial Hospital Rehabilitation Unit, *Spinal Cord Injury Manual*, Rochester, New York, © 1986, rev. 1994.

Emotional Adjustment Worksheet

Think about or write out your thoughts. Writing things down works best. Discuss your results with someone—family, nurse, social worker, group, or anyone you trust. If this is difficult, your rehabilitation team can suggest further professional guidance.

When I first learned about my condition and all of its complications I felt _____

_____

This is what I did to cope_____

These people helped me_____

My greatest strength has been _____

The hardest part of this was/is/will be _____

I'm proud of my ability to _____

The changes in my activities are_____

The changes in my attitudes toward myself are _____

                about my life in general are _____

                about my body are _____

My fears about my spinal cord injury are_____

My thoughts and feelings about social/sexual/recreational/employment/relationships

_____

_____

What I have today that I didn't have before my spinal cord injury _____

Source: Wanda Trojanoski, University of Rochester, Strong Memorial Hospital Rehabilitation Unit, *Spinal Cord Injury Manual*, Rochester, New York, © 1986, rev. 1994.

Self-Care

Self-care is an attitude. It is the attitude of being responsible for yourself. You can be active in caring for yourself even if you need help with all of your care needs.

You need to know how to take care of yourself. When you do your own care or when you need help from someone else, knowing your care is important. If you do not know your care, you cannot help someone else by telling them what to do for you or how to do it. Also, you will not know if what they are doing is what they *should* be doing or if they are doing it right. Another reason to know all about your care is for your safety and the safety of the person helping you.

Self-care is doing all you can by yourself, to give you more control over your life. It helps lessen your need for others to take care of you, and it helps you adjust to changes that have happened in your life. It is important that you do all that you can do by yourself. *Anything* you do for yourself is something you do not need someone else to do.

While you are in the hospital, you are helped with insurance and Social Security papers, and you are set up with vocational rehabilitation and home care/aide services. After you are discharged, there may be other papers to fill out or you may have problems or questions about your home care/aide services. It is best that *you* take care of these things, for example, by making phone calls. You know what your care needs are, so you are the best person to let the agencies know what kind of help you need.

If you have aides to help you with your care, you may need to teach them about your routines and any special care needs you have. You know what you need done and how to do it, so let them know. If you have any problems, be sure to call the aide service and let them know.

Just because someone else may be doing part or all of your care does not mean you should not pay attention to what is done. For example, ask about your skin condition, ask to have range of motion done, or let them know how you like to be positioned in bed and in the wheelchair.

Your life may be changed in many ways, but you still need to be in control of what happens to you. You are still important and it is *your* life.

Source: Wanda Trojanoski, University of Rochester, Strong Memorial Hospital Rehabilitation Unit, *Spinal Cord Injury Manual*, Rochester, New York, © 1986, rev. 1994.

DEPRESSION

Overview of Depression

WHO GETS DEPRESSED?

Major depressive disorder—often referred to as depression—is a common illness that can affect anyone. About 1 in 20 Americans (over 11 million people) get depressed every year. Depression affects twice as many women as men.

WHAT IS DEPRESSION?

Depression is not just "feeling blue" or "down in the dumps." It is more than being sad or feeling grief after a loss. Depression is a medical disorder (just like diabetes, high blood pressure, and heart disease are medical disorders) that day after day affects your thoughts, feelings, physical health, and behaviors.

Depression may be caused by many things, including:

- family history and genetics
- other general medical illnesses
- certain medicines
- drugs or alcohol
- other psychiatric conditions

Certain life conditions (such as extreme stress or grief) may bring on a depression or prevent a full recovery. In some people, depression occurs even when life is going well.

Depression is not your fault. It is not a weakness. It is a medical illness. Depression is treatable.

HOW WILL I KNOW IF I AM DEPRESSED?

People who have major depressive disorder have a number of symptoms nearly every day, all day, for at least two weeks. These always include at least one of the following:

- loss of interest in things you used to enjoy
- feeling sad, blue, or down in the dumps

You may also have at least three of the following symptoms:

- feeling slowed down or restless and unable to sit still
- feeling worthless or guilty
- increase or decrease in appetite or weight

continues

continued

- thoughts of death or suicide
- problems concentrating, thinking, remembering, or making decisions
- trouble sleeping or sleeping too much
- loss of energy or feeling tired all the time

With depression, there are often other physical or psychological symptoms, including:

- headaches
- other aches and pains
- digestive problems
- sexual problems
- feeling pessimistic or hopeless
- being anxious or worried

WHAT SHOULD I DO IF I HAVE THESE SYMPTOMS?

Too often people do not get help for their depression because they don't recognize the symptoms, have trouble asking for help, blame themselves, or don't know that treatments are available.

Family practitioners, clinics, or health maintenance organizations are often the first places that people go for help. These health care providers can do the following:

- Treat the depression.
- Refer you to a mental health specialist for further evaluation and treatment.

HOW WILL TREATMENT HELP ME?

Treatment reduces the pain and suffering of depression. Successful treatment removes all of the symptoms of depression and returns you to your normal life. The earlier you get treatment for your depression, the sooner you will begin to feel better. As with other medical illnesses, the longer you have the depression before you seek treatment, the more difficult it can be to treat.

Most people who are treated for depression feel better and return to daily activities in several weeks. Because it takes several weeks for treatment to work fully, it is important to get treatment early before your depression gets worse.

As with any medical condition, you may have to try one or two treatments before finding the best one. It is important not to get discouraged if the first treatment does not work. In almost every case, there is a treatment for the depression that will work for you.

continues

continued

WHAT TYPE OF TREATMENT WILL I GET?

The major treatments for depression are:

- antidepressant medicine
- psychotherapy
- antidepressant medicine combined with psychotherapy

In some cases of depression, other treatments, such as electroconvulsive therapy (ECT) and light therapy, are also useful.

WHO SHOULD SEE A MENTAL HEALTH SPECIALIST?

Many people with depression can be successfully treated by their general health care provider. However, some people need specialized treatment because the first treatment does not work, because they need a combination of treatments, or because the depression is severe or it lasts a long time. Many times, a second opinion or consultation is all that is needed. If the mental health specialist provides treatment, it is most often on an outpatient basis (not in the hospital). If you think you need to see a mental health specialist, tell your health care provider.

Thoughts of suicide or death are often a part of depression. If you have these thoughts, tell someone you trust now. Ask that person to help you find professional help right away. Once your depression is properly treated, these thoughts will go away.

Notes:

Source: *Depression Is a Treatable Illness: A Patient's Guide*, U.S. Department of Health and Human Services, Public Health Service, Agency for Health Care Policy and Research, 1993.

Diagnosis of Depression

SYMPTOMS OF DEPRESSION

When someone is depressed, that person has several symptoms nearly every day, all day, that last at least two weeks.

You can use this list to check (✓) off any symptoms you have had for two weeks or more:

- ☐ loss of interest in things you used to enjoy, including sex.*
- ☐ feeling sad, blue, or down in the dumps*
- ☐ feeling slowed down or restless and unable to sit still
- ☐ feeling worthless or guilty
- ☐ changes in appetite or weight loss or gain
- ☐ thoughts of death or suicide; suicide attempts
- ☐ problems concentrating, thinking, remembering, or making decisions
- ☐ trouble sleeping or sleeping too much
- ☐ loss of energy or feeling tired all the time

Other symptoms include:

- ☐ headaches
- ☐ other aches and pains
- ☐ digestive problems
- ☐ sexual problems
- ☐ feeling pessimistic or hopeless
- ☐ being anxious or worried

If you have had five or more of these symptoms, **including at least one of the first two symptoms marked with an asterisk (*)**, for at least two weeks, you may have major depressive disorder. See your health care provider for diagnosis.

If you have some depressive symptoms, you should also tell your health care provider. Sometimes a few symptoms can go on to become major depressive disorder. Some forms of depression are mild, but persistent or chronic. Chronic symptoms of depression also need treatment.

Another Form of Depression

Some people with depression have mood cycles. They have terrible "lows" (depression) and inappropriate "highs" (mania) that can last from several days to months. In between the highs and

continues

continued

lows, they feel completely normal. This condition is called bipolar disorder or manic-depressive disorder.

Bipolar disorder affects about 1 in 100 people. Just as eye or hair color are inherited, bipolar disorder, in most cases, is inherited. It can also be caused by other general medical problems, such as head injury or neurologic or other general medical conditions.

You can use this list to learn the symptoms of mania and to check (✓) off any you might have:

- ☐ feeling unusually "high," euphoric, or irritable*
- ☐ needing less sleep
- ☐ talking a lot or feeling that you can't stop talking
- ☐ being easily distracted
- ☐ having lots of ideas go through your head very quickly at one time
- ☐ doing things that feel good but have bad effects (spending too much money, inappropriate sexual activity, foolish business investments)
- ☐ having feelings of greatness
- ☐ making lots of plans for activities (at work, school, or socially) or feeling that you have to keep moving

If you have had four of these symptoms at one time for at least one week, **including the first symptom marked with an asterisk (*)**, you may have had a manic episode. Tell your health care provider about the episode. There are effective treatments for this form of depression.

CAUSES OF DEPRESSION

Major depressive disorder is not caused by any one factor. It is probably caused by a combination of biological, genetic, psychological, and other factors. Certain life conditions (such as extreme stress or grief) may bring out a natural psychological or biological tendency toward depression. In some people, depression occurs even when life is going well.

Drinking too much alcohol or using drugs can sometimes cause depression. When the drug and alcohol use is stopped, the depression usually goes away. Talk to your health care provider if you have a problem with drugs or alcohol. It can be treated.

Remember, major depressive disorder is not caused by personal weakness, laziness, or lack of willpower. It is a medical illness that can be treated.

DIAGNOSING DEPRESSION

Before depression can be treated, it must be accurately diagnosed. Your health care provider will:

- Ask about your symptoms.

continues

continued

- Ask about your general health.
- Ask about your family history of general medical and mental disorders.
- Give you a physical examination.
- Conduct some basic laboratory tests.

Preparing for Your First Visit

You can help your health care provider diagnose and treat you by giving as much information as possible about your health. Information that you share with a health care provider is confidential.

If your depression is causing you to have a hard time talking and remembering, take a family member or friend along on your first visit to help.

A general medical history, physical examination, and basic laboratory tests can help find out if a general medical disorder is the cause of your depression. About 10 to 15 percent of all depressions are caused by general medical illness (such as thyroid disease, cancers, or neurologic diseases) or medicines. Once the condition is treated or the medicines are changed or adjusted, the depression will usually go away.

If you have a general medical illness and feel depressed, it is important to tell your health care provider. Sometimes depression is a reaction to a life-threatening condition. Getting help during a difficult time in your life may help you to cope with your general medical illness.

If your first episode of major depressive disorder occurred after age 40, a very thorough medical evaluation is important.

Severe? Moderate? Mild?

The terms *severe, moderate,* and *mild* are used to describe depression:

- **Severe depression** is present when a person has nearly all of the symptoms of depression, and the depression almost always keeps him or her from doing regular day-to-day activities.
- **Moderate depression** is present when a person has many symptoms of depression that often keep him or her from doing things that need to be done.
- **Mild depression** is present when a person has some of the symptoms of depression and it takes extra effort to do the things that need to be done.

For each type of depression, there is a treatment that works best. You should talk with your health care provider about your depression and the best treatment for you.

Source: *Depression Is a Treatable Illness: A Patient's Guide*, U.S. Department of Health and Human Services, Public Health Service, Agency for Health Care Policy and Research, 1993.

Treating Depression

Depression is usually treated in two steps: (1) acute treatment and (2) continuation treatment. The aim of acute treatment is to remove the symptoms of depression until you feel well. Continuation treatment (continuing the treatment for some time even after you are well) is important because it keeps the episode of depression from coming back. Depending on the type of treatment you have, your chances of staying well for six months on continuation treatment are extremely good.

In cases of recurrent depression (three or more episodes), a third step, called maintenance treatment, is used to treat the depression. In maintenance treatment, you stay on the treatment for a longer period of time. The purpose of maintenance treatment is to prevent a recurrence of the depression. With maintenance treatment, the chances of staying well are also extremely good.

TYPES OF TREATMENT

The major types of treatment for depression are:

- antidepressant medicine
- psychotherapy
- antidepressant medicine combined with psychotherapy
- other treatments, including electroconvulsive therapy (ECT) and light therapy

For severe depression, research studies show that medicine is very effective. Psychotherapy has not been well studied for the more severe forms of depression.

HOW TREATMENT WORKS

Treatment for depression works gradually over several weeks. With medicine, most people see some benefits by three or four weeks; with psychotherapy alone, it can sometimes take longer. There is a very good chance that your first treatment will work well for you. If treatment is not effective after a certain amount of time, it can be changed or adjusted. There are other treatments to try, and your chances for effective treatment are still very good.

CHOOSING A TREATMENT

You and your health care provider can work together to find the best treatment for you. In choosing which acute treatment is best for you, you should weigh the chances of getting better (benefits) against the chances of possible harms, as well as the expense of the treatment offered and the costs of the depression (time from work, effect on personal relationships, etc.). There are several questions you may want to ask when discussing treatment:

continues

continued

- What are the chances of getting better with this treatment?
- What are the possible risks and side effects of treatment?
- What are the costs of treatment?

ABOUT HOSPITALIZATION

Most people with depression get their treatment through regular outpatient visits to a health care provider. However, sometimes treatment in the hospital is needed. This is because other medical conditions could affect your treatment. Another reason is that people with severe depression may need hospital care (for example, to adjust medicine). Also, people who are at great risk for suicide are hospitalized until those feelings pass and treatment begins to work.

If you must go to the hospital for treatment, it is often only for a few days or a week or two. Early treatment, before the depression becomes severe or chronic, can lower the chances of hospitalization.

WHY DEPRESSION MUST BE TREATED

Without treatment, a major depressive episode can last 6 to 12 months. In between the episodes, most people feel better or are completely well (without symptoms).

Even though some people are able to struggle through an episode of depression without treatment, most find that it is much easier to get some help for their pain and suffering. It is important to get treatment for your depression for several reasons:

- Early treatment may help to keep the depression from becoming more severe or chronic.
- Thoughts of suicide are common in depression, and the risk of suicide is increased when people are not treated and the depression recurs. When depression is successfully treated, the thoughts of suicide will go away.
- Between episodes, about one out of four people with depression will still have some symptoms and trouble doing their daily activities. These people, if not treated, have a greater chance of having another episode of depression.
- Treatment (especially medicines) can prevent recurrences of depression. The more episodes of depression you have had, the greater the chance that you will have another. About half of the people who have one episode of depression will have a second. Without treatment, after two episodes, the chances of having a third episode (recurrent depression) are even greater. After three episodes, the chances of having a fourth are 90 percent.

IF YOU HAVE CONCERNS ABOUT YOUR TREATMENT

If at any time you are worried about your treatment or you don't think that things are going well, tell someone about your concerns:

continues

continued

- Talk to your health care provider.
- Ask for a second opinion.
- Talk to someone you trust.

Health care providers are interested in your concerns and will help you. This may mean getting a second opinion or even finding another health care provider.

Notes:

Source: *Depression Is a Treatable Illness: A Patient's Guide*, U.S. Department of Health and Human Services, Public Health Service, Agency for Health Care Policy and Research, 1993.

ADDITIONAL MENTAL HEALTH CONCERNS

Stress

WHAT IS STRESS?

Stress is tension felt in the body (physical) and mind (mental). There are several signs of stress.

Body (Physical)	Mind (Mental)
Cold hands	Anxiety
Fast breathing	Forgetfulness
Pounding heart	Confusion
Shakiness	Inability to concentrate
Headaches	Irritability
Muscle tightness	Depression
Over/undereating	
Dizziness	
Inability to relax	

Stress is a normal reaction to ALL change, good and bad. Changes and events in life are sources of stress. They may include:

- Present illness/injury
- Emotional upsets
- Family
- Money
- Relationships
- Job

YOUR CAUSE(S) OF STRESS ARE: _____

_____

The way stress is handled can affect health and happiness. Learning how to manage stress can give the body the extra energy and strength it needs to deal with changes.

continues

continued

HOW TO MANAGE STRESS

- Be aware of stress.
- Identify cause of stress.
- Set doable goals.
- Identify what is important:
  - Do important activities first.
  - Let go of less important activities.
- Take time out for yourself.
- Talk about needs.
- Get support.
- Learn about the illness/injury.
- Learn relaxation exercises and do them regularly (follows).
- Have a sense of humor.

HOW DO YOU MANAGE STRESS?_____

_____

RELAXATION EXERCISE

Follow these steps:

1. Go to a quiet place.
2. Sit comfortably, with arms and legs supported.
3. Relax arms and legs.
4. Close eyes.
5. Focus on breathing.
   - Take a deep breath (INHALE) through the nose.
   - Let breath out (EXHALE) through the mouth.
   - With each EXHALE:
     - Think about breathing out tension.
     - Think RELAX.
     - Let your muscles go.
6. INHALE through the nose while slowly counting to five.
7. EXHALE through the mouth while slowly counting to five.
8. Repeat all of the above.
9. Do for 10 to 20 minutes.

Source: Kelly B. Wascher, ed., *Patient Education and Discharge Planning Manual for Rehabilitation*, St. Joseph Rehabilitation Hospital and Outpatient Center, Aspen Publishers, Inc., © 1995.

Effects of Fatigue on People with Spinal Cord Injury

Many people with spinal cord injury (SCI) can be deeply affected by chronic fatigue. It not only hinders their physical abilities but also affects their mental health. Chronic fatigue may make people with SCI too weak to perform their activities of daily living. It can also keep them confined at home because they have no energy to get out in the world. As their daily life becomes more difficult, they may feel depressed, bored, hopeless, and helpless. These feelings will add to their exhaustion and begin a cycle of fatigue and depression that is hard to break.

Fatigue also can affect their self-esteem. Already limited by their injuries, they find they can do even less. If they have a job, they may become too tired to go to work. Their chronic fatigue will affect how much energy they can give to spouses, children, and friends. They may start to feel alone and isolated and too dependent on others for their care. Left untreated, their exhaustion could set up a downward spiral of helplessness and depression.

NONDRUG TREATMENTS

Often the best treatments for easing chronic fatigue come when people make changes in their daily routine and lifestyles. People can ease fatigue if they:

- reduce the amount of daily activities
- try to finish only what has to be done
- find someone to help them with their tasks
- let family members know how they can help
- take more frequent breaks
- find equipment or devices that can help with daily living tasks such as a shower seat or long-handled shoe horn
- increase exercise
- learn relaxation techniques
- meditate
- look into muscle conditioning
- keep a sense of humor

The suggestions in this list fall into three basic groups.

Change or Reduce the Day's Tasks

People who live with chronic fatigue must limit what they can do during the day and focus on how to complete those tasks. They might drop those things that don't have to get done because a smaller workload may leave them with more energy.

continues

continued

Get Help from Other People and Assistive Technology

Help from Others

People living with fatigue should talk to the people they live with and their friends or caregivers about how they can help with some of the daily tasks. Some people, even those who are close to the person with SCI, may not know he or she needs help unless the person asks for it. Some people believe that a person with SCI indicates a sense of security and acceptance of his or her limitations when that person can ask others for help. When a person with SCI reaches out to others for help, he or she gives friends and family members a chance to feel positive and useful.

Help from Assistive Devices

Many adaptive tools or devices can help reduce the effort it takes to get things done. A reacher is an example of a tool that can help a wheelchair user reach things more easily. Peers with disabilities or an occupational therapist could suggest many ways to adapt living spaces and ways to use one's personal energy more efficiently.

A window or central air-conditioner is one piece of equipment that can help a person fight off fatigue during hot weather. Except in the coolest climates, heat and humidity from the spring through late fall can sap a person's energy.

Help from Muscle Conditioning

Studies show that the muscles of people with SCI and multiple sclerosis have greater fatigue than the muscles of nondisabled people. Their muscles go through long periods of disuse or altered use, and they become shorter and weaker with time. Some studies have shown that these changes can be reversed somewhat or halted when the muscles are conditioned through exercise and stretching. Some studies have shown a method called functional electrical stimulation (FES) also can make unused muscles more resistant to fatigue. FES uses electrical signals to condition the muscle. People who have limited use of their muscles should talk to a physical therapist about the things they can do to help improve their muscles' condition.

Self-Help

Many of the things suggested to help ease chronic fatigue can be done by the person living with that fatigue. Getting enough rest, learning relaxation or meditation techniques, and adding some light exercises to the daily routine are things people can learn and manage for themselves.

continues

continued

Rest

Frequent, short rest periods work better than long ones to refresh the body. At the start of a rest period, the heart rate slows quickly and then evens out the longer a person rests. Many short rests give the heart more chances to benefit from a quick slow down.

Relaxation Techniques

Some people have great success using one or a combination of relaxation methods. Some of these activities include yoga, meditation, deep breathing, and guided mental imagery. These methods often are referred to as holistic healing because they work to help the body by using the person's whole self—mind and body—to improve health.

These techniques help fight fatigue because they bring oxygen into the body, they include mild exercise, they help the body relax, and they reduce stress. All of these help restore energy to a body that's tired. These methods also have the added benefit of helping people fight their fatigue by using their own powers of breathing and imagination.

- **Yoga:** Yoga uses simple stretching exercises, steady breathing, and the mind to relax the body and make it feel refreshed. Traditional yoga works on moving the entire body, but yoga exercises also can focus on the muscles in one part of the body, such as the face, neck, shoulders, hands, and arms. Yoga includes exercises and relaxation techniques for everyone, regardless of their physical limitations.
- **Meditation and breathing:** When a person meditates or does deep breathing exercises, he or she becomes quiet and consciously tells the body to relax. These methods can be used by anyone, even people with limited movement. They can help relax the body even when practiced as little as 15 minutes a day. What's important is that a person practice some each day.
- **Guided mental imagery:** Thinking about positive things makes people feel happy and helps them cope with things that are hard or unpleasant. When someone uses visualization, he or she imagines something pleasant, and these thoughts help the person relax. People can also imagine a part of the body that is causing trouble. People who live with fatigue might imagine their tired arms and shoulders or how heavy their head and neck feel. Thinking of these parts of the body causes more blood to flow there. The person holds his or her mind to the spot and then imagines something good happening to that area. For example, the person might imagine warm water washing over the muscle or bright light wrapping around it. These thoughts can help the body feel refreshed and relaxed.

Each of these holistic methods has been used for hundreds of years. Often classes in one or all of these techniques are offered through adult education classes at a local high school, YMCA,

continues

continued

college, or recreation center. In some parts of the country, people skilled in relaxation therapy are licensed to offer help with these methods.

Exercise

Light exercise helps to tone muscles, it boosts energy by increasing the level of oxygen in the body, and it can reduce the muscle spasticity or contractions that affect some people with SCI.

The extent of the spinal lesions will determine the types of exercise best suited to each person. At first, fatigue may limit what a person can do. Some people with SCI can use their chest, arms, and shoulders for aerobic exercise. They can also increase their muscle mass and strength by lifting weights.

People with higher-level spinal cord injuries can use simple deep breathing exercises to increase the oxygen levels in their blood. They may be able to perform simple stretching or isometric exercises to develop and keep some muscle tone and to reduce spasticity. Some people with SCI may need someone else to stretch their arm and leg muscles and extend their joints through a full range of motion.

Where available, aquatic fitness programs have been shown to reduce fatigue and improve strength and work capacity. Pushing a wheelchair for a set distance can improve cardiovascular health, and lifting weights can increase strength and flexibility.

MEDICATIONS

Some doctors prescribe mood-altering medications to fight chronic fatigue. While medicines won't cure the fatigue, some can make a person feel more energetic. Success with these drugs depends on how well the person can talk to his or her doctor. The person must let the doctor know when the drug causes good or bad changes in the body or state of mind. This information will help the doctor adjust the dosage to the right level.

These prescription drugs also can have side effects. They may cause sleepiness and low blood pressure. Because they draw water from the body's tissues, they may also cause dry mouth, constipation, and fluid retention. Problems with fluid retention and elimination are critical to people with SCI who must be watchful of their fluid intake, constipation, and stress on the bladder.

Some medications also can reduce muscle spasticity, which can cause fatigue. Some of these drugs can deepen a person's fatigue, impair thinking, and cause depression.

Before trying prescription medicines, a person living with fatigue should be sure to try nondrug treatments first and use medications as one of the last methods to fight their fatigue.

TERMS YOU MAY HEAR

Carbohydrate (car-bo-hi'-drate): Sugars, starches, and plant fibers that give the body a steady source of energy.

continues

continued

Cardiovascular (car-dee-o-vas'-qu-ler): The system in the body that is made up of the heart and blood vessels.

Depression (de-pre'-shun): The state of feeling blue or sad that can include prolonged sleepiness and often an inability to think. Depression can come from something that has happened in a person's life, such as death of a loved one, or other drastic change. It can also come from chemical changes in the body or the body's reaction to alcohol or medications.

Glucose (gloo'-kos): A colorless to yellowish syrupy mixture that the body makes from the tissues of plants and animals.

Glycogen (gli'-ko-gen): A white, sweet-tasting substance that the body makes from digested food and glucose then stores in the liver for future energy.

Health care worker: This broad term can refer to a number of professionals who work in the health care field—doctors; nurses; physical, occupational, and relaxation therapists; and psychiatrists.

Hypochondriac (hi-po-kon'-dree-ak): A person who is obsessed with the idea that he or she is ill or will become ill. The person may have real pain even when no illness is present.

Immune (im-yoon') **system**: The system within the body that defends a person against the bacteria and viruses that cause illness.

Isometric (i-so-met'-rik) **exercise**: Exercises that make a muscle stronger by contracting or tightening the muscle and holding that tightness for a brief period. Isometric exercises do not involve making the muscle lift or stretch, so they can be done by people with limited movement.

Mental health care worker: This broad term can refer to a number of professionals trained in counseling and mental health—psychiatrist, psychologist, social worker, counselor, and case manager.

Multiple sclerosis (skle-ro'-sis): Demyelination occurring in patches throughout the white matter of the central nervous system, sometimes extending into the gray matter.

Psychiatrist (si-ki'-a-trist): A medical doctor trained in the diagnosis, treatment, and prevention of mental illness.

Psychologist (si-kol'-o-gest): A person trained to understand mental processes and behaviors.

Spasm (spaz'-em): A sudden, uncontrolled tightening or contraction of a muscle or a group of muscles.

Spasticity (spa-stis'-e-ti): Spasms in the muscles that cause them to tighten or jerk around.

Source: The Rehabilitation Research and Training Center on Aging with SCI, a joint project of Craig Hospital and the Department of Rehabilitation Medicine at the University of Colorado Health Sciences Center. Funded by the National Institute on Disability and Rehabilitation Research.

Locating Your Fatigue Trouble Spots

Go through these three checklists for the medical, mental, physical, and daily living causes of fatigue. By looking at where you have the most check marks, you can get a better picture of which area or areas might be affecting your fatigue.

MEDICAL CAUSES

Changes in your physical health can cause fatigue. Which, if any, of the following statements apply to you?

- ☐ I have a fever.
- ☐ I have swollen lymph nodes.
- ☐ I have a sleep disorder.
- ☐ I have a sore throat.
- ☐ I often have headaches.
- ☐ I feel sick to my stomach.
- ☐ I have night sweats.
- ☐ I have joint pain.
- ☐ I feel dizzy.
- ☐ I have been outside where I could have gotten a tick bite.
- ☐ I have been told I have a serious illness such as cancer, diabetes, or high blood pressure.
- ☐ I am taking prescription drugs.

If you checked off one or more of these statements, your fatigue may be the result of something going on inside your body. For example, you may have a low-grade infection, or you may have gotten Lyme disease from a tick bite. Make an appointment with your doctor or clinic so you can find out if there's a physical reason why you're tired.

Changes in your mental health also can cause fatigue. Something going on in your life may be affecting how you feel about life, yourself, and others. Which, if any, of the following sentences apply to you?

- ☐ I am worried about myself or a member of my family.
- ☐ I have money problems.
- ☐ I often feel sad, depressed, or "blue."
- ☐ I love someone who has died or become ill.
- ☐ I have lost my friends.
- ☐ I have moved to a new home or job.
- ☐ I have lost my job.
- ☐ I have been fighting with my spouse, children, or friends.

continues

continued

☐ I feel angry.
☐ I have a new caregiver.

If you checked off one or more of these statements, your fatigue may be the result of changes or losses in your life. Dealing with these changes may be making you tired. Meet with a mental health professional so you can talk about your fatigue and what's going on in your life. You can call a counselor, social worker, psychologist, or psychiatrist or your local mental health clinic for help in seeing how changes in your life may be affecting your energy levels.

PHYSICAL CAUSES

Sometimes a lack of physical activity or stimulation can cause fatigue. Which, if any, of the following sentences apply to you?

☐ I often don't leave the house for many days.
☐ I'm alone for long periods of time.
☐ I rarely have visitors.
☐ My life is pretty much the same from day to day.
☐ I often feel bored.
☐ I have few or no hobbies.
☐ I sit or lie in one position for many hours.
☐ I exercise rarely or never.
☐ My day is mostly spent watching television.
☐ I rarely read or listen to music.
☐ I don't have a pet.

If you checked off one or more of these statements, your fatigue may be the result of inactivity and boredom. A simple change in routine such as getting out of the house during the week or having people come for visits may reduce your boredom and your fatigue. Talk with your peers to see what they do during their days at home. You can also talk to a counselor, social worker, or someone at your independent living center to see if someone can help you get out more or increase your activities at home.

DAILY LIVING CAN CAUSE FATIGUE

Changes in your daily routine, problems getting around in your home or at your job site, or a different way of eating also can cause fatigue. Which, if any, of the following sentences apply to you?

continues

continued

☐ I am learning how to use assistive equipment.
☐ I find it hard to get around in my house or apartment.
☐ I have moved to a new house or apartment.
☐ I get less sleep than I once did.
☐ I get less exercise than before.
☐ I eat more or less than usual.
☐ I eat a lot of "junk" food.
☐ I use alcohol or other nonprescribed drugs.
☐ I use my arms and shoulders more during the day.
☐ I have started some new activities.
☐ I have made some new friends.

If you checked off one or more of these statements, your fatigue may come from changes in your daily life. You may be tired because you're still getting used to a new activity or routine. These changes also may affect your sleeping and eating patterns or may cause you to travel more in your wheelchair or on your crutches. Meet with a physical therapist to discuss how assistive technology, exercises, or new ways of completing your tasks of daily living might reduce your fatigue.

Notes:

Source: The Rehabilitation Research and Training Center on Aging with SCI, a joint project of Craig Hospital and the Department of Rehabilitation Medicine at the University of Colorado Health Sciences Center. Funded by the National Institute on Disability and Rehabilitation Research.

ALCOHOL AND SUBSTANCE ABUSE

Facts about Alcohol

OVERVIEW

Alcohol, a drug, is a central nervous system depressant. It is easily made and is the mood-altering ingredient in wine, beer, and liquor. Since it contains calories, it is considered a food, but the calories in no way contribute to good nutrition. In fact, even moderate drinkers may need to reduce their drinking to maintain ideal weight.

A 12-ounce bottle of beer contains approximately the same amount of alcohol as 5 ounces of wine or $1\frac{1}{2}$ ounces of 80 proof liquor.

PHYSICAL EFFECTS

Alcohol is absorbed in the blood stream and transmitted to virtually all parts of the body. Several factors influence the effects of alcohol, including the amount of alcohol consumed; the rate at which it is consumed; the presence of food in the stomach during consumption; and the individual's weight, mood, and previous experience with the drug.

With moderate drinking, a person may experience flushing; dizziness; dulling of senses; and impairment of coordination, reflexes, memory, and judgment. Taken in larger quantities, alcohol may produce staggering, slurred speech, double vision, dulling of senses, sudden mood changes, and unconsciousness. Taken in larger quantities over a long period of time, death may occur due to depression of the parts of the brain that control breathing and heart rate. Alcohol can be very damaging when used in large amounts or over a long period of time. It can cause damage to the liver, heart, and pancreas. It may lead to malnutrition, stomach irritation, lowered resistance to disease, and irreversible brain or nervous system damage. Drinkers who also smoke are more at risk for developing certain cancers.

WHO SHOULD NOT DRINK ALCOHOL

Pregnant women, young people, alcoholics, those taking contraindicative medications, and those engaged in dangerous recreational activities should not drink alcohol.

All people should limit their intake of alcohol if they are going to drive, operate other machinery, or—especially—use firearms.

DEPENDENCE

Increased tolerance to alcohol may lead to physical dependence. At that point, alcohol becomes part of a person's normal physical functioning. Physical dependence is characterized by the presence of withdrawal symptoms when use is discontinued suddenly.

Source: U.S. Department of Health and Human Services, Public Health Service, National Institute on Alcohol Abuse and Alcoholism, National Clearinghouse for Alcohol Information, Rockville, Maryland.

Definition of Alcoholism

Alcoholism is often a progressive and fatal chronic disease that has specific symptoms. Indications of alcoholism include inability to control drinking, preoccupation with drinking, continued use of alcohol in spite of negative consequences, and denial.

- **Progressive:** gets worse over time
- **Fatal:** leads to death
- **Chronic:** lasts for longer than six months
- **Disease:** a disabling illness with specific symptoms
- **Inability to control drinking:** unable to limit the amount of alcohol consumed and/or the frequency of drinking occasions
- **Preoccupation with drinking:** spending a lot of time thinking about drinking and its outcomes
- **Negative consequences:** problems such as poor physical health, poor judgment, emotional difficulty, and unwanted behavior created as a result of drinking
- **Denial:** inability to be aware of problems resulting from drinking alcohol

Notes:

Source: Department of Psychiatric Nursing, The Ohio State University Hospitals, © 1993.

Are You a Problem Drinker?

How can we spot early signs of potential problems? The United States Department of Health and Human Service's National Institute on Alcohol Abuse and Alcoholism suggests that honest answers to the following questions may provide clues. Check off those questions that apply to you. If you answer "yes" to as few as one-fourth of these (seven questions), you may have a problem with alcohol.

- [ ] 1. Do you drink to feel better about yourself?
- [ ] 2. Do you turn to alcohol when you have troubles?
- [ ] 3. Do you make excuses for the reasons you drink?
- [ ] 4. Do you feel guilty after drinking?
- [ ] 5. Do you drink to help you fall asleep?
- [ ] 6. Do you often have diarrhea, indigestion, or nausea due to drinking?
- [ ] 7. Have you had other problems related to your drinking?
- [ ] 8. Have you ever fallen down or burned yourself while you were drinking?
- [ ] 9. Do you feel worried, anxious, or depressed most of the time?
- [ ] 10. Do you find yourself not realizing you are repeating things while drinking?
- [ ] 11. Have you ever been unable to remember what happened while you were drinking?
- [ ] 12. Have you ever missed work or put off work because of your drinking?
- [ ] 13. Have you put yourself or others in danger by driving after drinking?
- [ ] 14. Have you had financial or legal problems in which drinking was involved?
- [ ] 15. Do you drink alone?
- [ ] 16. Do you drink less with others than you do when alone?
- [ ] 17. Do you feel isolated and alone?
- [ ] 18. Do you often feel the need to telephone people when you are drinking?
- [ ] 19. Have you changed friends to be around people who drink like you do?
- [ ] 20. Do you hide your drinking from your spouse or children?
- [ ] 21. Have others told you that they think you drink too much?
- [ ] 22. Is either parent or your spouse or housemate a heavy drinker?
- [ ] 23. Do you think you drink too much?
- [ ] 24. Do you plan activities around being able to drink?
- [ ] 25. Do you find yourself thinking of drinking in-between times?
- [ ] 26. Have you failed in promises to yourself to cut down on your drinking?
- [ ] 27. Are there times when you don't drink because you're afraid you'll lose control of yourself?
- [ ] 28. Do you drink and use other drugs?

Source: *For Women Who Drink*. USDHHS Publication No. ADM 82-1176, 1982, U.S. Department of Health and Human Service's National Institute on Alcohol Abuse and Alcoholism.

What Can I Do about My Drinking?

OVERVIEW*

Until recently, many people believed that the troubled drinker had to "hit bottom"—be totally defeated by alcoholism—before he or she could be treated successfully. This is a myth. Alcoholism can usually be arrested at any point: in fact, the earlier help is sought, the better the chances for recovery. But whether your drinking problem is in its early stages or you are severely addicted to alcohol, you can find the kind of help you need. The most important criterion for successful treatment is a real commitment to overcoming your dependency on alcohol.

Nevertheless, it is often difficult to make the decision to seek help. Most of us have grown up with the notion that an alcoholic person is somehow "weak" or "immoral." Although these false stereotypes are gradually fading, many people still think there is something shameful about acknowledging a drinking problem. In dealing with these feelings, it is important to recognize that you are suffering from an illness.

A good start toward getting help is to talk to someone you trust about your alcohol problem. The person you confide in can be anyone with whom you feel comfortable and secure: a family member, a friend, a coworker, a physician, a member of the clergy, or a counselor. Many recovered alcoholics say that the turning point in their illness occurred when they were able to face another person and say: "Yes, I am in trouble with alcohol." They knew, at that point, that they had accepted the fact of their illness and were ready to seek outside help in dealing with it.

Once you have acknowledged your drinking problem, you have already taken an important step toward recovery. Your next step is to find out what kind of help is available in your area and begin a program of treatment that best meets your particular needs.

HOW TO FIND HELP**

Your Local Community

In most communities, there are numerous local resources that can either provide you with information about treatment resources or direct you to actual treatment services. The following are some examples.

Physicians (including psychiatrists) are often the first ones to diagnose an alcohol problem. Some physicians may even be able to assist in the care of alcoholic patients and their families as part of their private practice. If your physician is not experienced in the treatment of alcoholism, request help in seeking a referral to alcoholism treatment resources that are most appropriate for you.

Information and referral programs are frequently available in local communities and can offer information on a wide range of subjects. Specialized alcoholism information and referral programs

continues

continued

also exist in some communities. Consult the telephone directory under "information and referral" or "alcoholism."

Private alcoholism treatment facilities exist in many communities. These facilities offer a variety of alcoholism treatment services and can be contacted directly for information about costs and services provided by their specially trained staff. These centers are usually listed in your telephone directory under "alcoholism" or "alcoholism treatment."

Hospitals are sources of information about alcoholism treatment and also provide a variety of alcoholism treatment services. Community and private hospitals, Veterans Administration hospitals and facilities, and Indian Health Service hospitals are important resources in the treatment of alcohol-related medical problems.

Your **local county health department and social services department** are sources of information about community facilities, including those providing alcoholism services. These public health and social service agencies are found in the telephone directory under local government listings.

Many localities operate **community mental health centers**. Alcoholism treatment is part of the continuum of health care and social services provided by the centers. Community mental health centers are also excellent sources of information about other treatment sources nearby. The centers are usually listed under "mental health" in the telephone directory.

A **family service agency** in your community is an important source for referral information and may itself offer a variety of services—including treatment or referral for the alcoholic and his or her family. Check the telephone listings or contact the community council or United Way in your area.

Your **clergyman or spiritual counselor** can be a source of information and referral regarding alcoholism treatment. Clergy and religious leaders may also be skilled and experienced counselors. Many religious organizations sponsor or operate treatment facilities.

Your **employer** may have joined thousands of other organizations and businesses in establishing an employee assistance program. These programs employ professionals trained in providing you with information and, if necessary, referral for treatment.

Your State and National Resources

If you have had difficulty identifying a satisfactory community resource for treating alcohol problems or if there is not an appropriate service in your area, you may wish to contact the following state and national resources for more information. (In addition, there are many local affiliates of these organizations in your community.)

Each state has a **department of alcoholism services**, a government agency that is responsible for alcohol-related programs, resources, and initiatives offered throughout the state. States vary widely in the title of their alcoholism agencies and in their organizational affiliation within state government structures. In some instances, the alcohol and drug abuse agencies are combined. To locate your state alcoholism agency, look in your telephone directory under "state government"

continues

continued

listings. Or contact the National Association of State Alcohol and Drug Abuse Directors, 444 N. Capitol Street, NW, Suite 642, Washington, DC 20001. Or call (202) 783-6868.

National Clearinghouse for Alcohol and Drug Information (NCADI) is an information service of the Office for Substance Abuse Prevention (OSAP). The Clearinghouse staff can answer your questions about prevention, intervention, and treatment of alcohol and other drug problems. Information is disseminated free to the public. Write to NCADI, PO Box 2345, Rockville, MD 20847-2345. Or call (301) 468-2600 and ask for an information specialist.

National Council on Alcoholism (NCA) is a nonprofit national voluntary health agency with several hundred local affiliates that are well acquainted with the problems of alcoholics and are dedicated to helping them. Information about alcoholism and treatment opportunities is available through local affiliates. In some instances, counseling of alcoholics and their families may be provided through the local unit as well. Look for the listing of your local NCA affiliate in the telephone directory. If you are having difficulty locating a unit near you, write to NCA at 12 West 21st Street, Seventh Floor, New York, NY 10010. Or call (212) 206-6770.

Alcoholics Anonymous (AA) is a voluntary fellowship open to anyone who wants to achieve and maintain sobriety and is an important adjunct to many treatment programs. The fellowship was founded in 1935 by two individuals in an effort to help others who suffer from the disease of alcoholism. AA is the oldest of the organizations designed to help alcoholics help themselves. It is estimated that there are more than 1 million members in local chapters worldwide. For further information, look under "Alcoholics Anonymous" in your telephone directory. The Alcoholics Anonymous General Service Office can help in locating a nearby affiliate. Write to them at PO Box 459, Grand Central Station, New York, NY 10163. Or call (212) 870-3400.

Al-Anon is an organization for spouses and other relatives and friends of alcoholics. The Al-Anon groups help families and friends cope with the problems that arise from another's drinking and help foster understanding of the alcoholic through sharing experiences. Local groups are listed in your telephone directory under "Al-Anon Family Groups." Al-Anon Family Group Headquarters can assist you in finding a nearby affiliate. Write to Al-Anon Family Group Headquarters at PO Box 862, Mid Town Station, New York, NY 10018. Or call (212) 302-7240.

Alateen, a part of Al-Anon, is for young people whose lives have been affected by the alcoholism of a family member or close friend. Members of Alateen fellowships help each other by sharing their experiences and their strength. Alateen is listed in some telephone directories, or information may be obtained by contacting local Al-Anon groups. If you are having trouble locating an Alateen affiliate near you, contact Al-Anon Family Group Headquarters at the previously listed address and telephone number.

Women for Sobriety, Inc., is a national organization with local units that address the specific needs of women with alcohol-related problems. The program is used by many women in combination with other alcoholism treatment programs or as an alternative to other programs. Consult your telephone listings for a local unit or write to Women for Sobriety, Inc., PO Box 618, Quakertown, PA 18951 for assistance and more information. Or call (215) 536-8026.

[*]Source: U.S. Department of Health and Human Services, Public Health Service, National Institute on Alcohol Abuse and Alcoholism, National Clearinghouse for Alcohol Information, Rockville, Maryland.
[**]Source: National Clearinghouse for Alcohol and Drug Information, Rockville, Maryland.

Alcoholics Anonymous: Basic Information

Much has been written about Alcoholics Anonymous (AA), and many substance abuse treatment centers routinely refer all of their clients to this self-help group. Other popular 12-step groups, such as Al-Anon, Alateen, Adult Children of Alcoholics (ACOA), Narcotics Anonymous (NA), and Emotions Anonymous (EA), are modeled after the successful AA program, which has been described as the most effective treatment for alcoholism.

Alcoholics Anonymous was founded in Akron, Ohio, in 1935, and the "Big Book," entitled *Alcoholics Anonymous*, was published in 1939. The AA program stresses abstinence from alcohol (and any other mind-altering substance). Abstinence is the primary and basic goal for members of AA, but the individual members have their own goals as well. "Sobriety" is seen as a state of being very different from being "dry," and it takes longer to achieve. Many AA members report that sobriety is a way of life in which a person not only doesn't drink, but also returns as an active participant in life. For this reason, the framework of AA is based on 12 steps and 12 traditions. AA members do not view sobriety as a passive process, but rather an active attempt to work toward a contented and productive life free from substances.

Anonymity is another key component of AA. For its members, the promise of public anonymity makes the program a safe outlet from exposure to neighbors, bosses, and others. Although sports superstars and actors have made alcoholism seem almost fashionable, there is still a stigma attached to alcoholism. Additionally, many substance abusers enter AA with feelings of guilt, low self-esteem, and shame. Confidentiality gives newcomers a chance to observe the program without fear of exposure. As a member of AA becomes comfortable with the program and begins to gain sobriety, he or she often recognizes other benefits from remaining anonymous, including the therapeutic value of being just one of many alcoholics.

For persons with disabilities, AA or other 12-step groups are an often-needed means of cost-free, ongoing support. In recent years, the AA General Service Office and area committees have taken a special interest in making AA accessible to all members, including persons with disabilities. Among the AA Conference–approved literature is a new pamphlet, entitled "Twelve Steps Illustrated." This pamphlet contains not only the actual AA Steps, but also applicable illustrations and simplified interpretations of each Step. It also is becoming more common for area AA committees to publish listings of local meetings that include identifiers that allow persons with disabilities to locate wheelchair-accessible and sign language–interpreted meetings.

Other efforts for making AA materials accessible to persons with disabilities have been very successful. The AA "Big Book" and other AA Conference–approved literature is available in large print and Braille. These materials are also available on tape, and at least one chapter of the "Big Book" is available in American Sign Language on videocassette. With the ongoing success of these materials, it is likely that additional accessible materials will be developed as well.

There are many different types of AA meetings that allow for the special needs and/or interests of various individuals. Meetings can be either open (for AA members, anyone interested in finding out more about AA, family members, and friends) or closed (for persons who profess to have problems with alcohol). Additionally, the meetings can take on a variety of formats. Some meetings

continues

continued

are called speaker meetings or "leads" where one or more persons share their experiences with alcohol, what happened to instigate change, and what being sober has been like for them. Discussion meetings, on the other hand, allow more persons to actively participate. Generally, one alcoholic facilitates the meeting, and a topic about a problem with alcohol, one of the 12 steps, or another issue relating to sobriety is discussed. In addition to the types of meetings already mentioned, there are specialized meetings geared toward specific AA members. For example, there are men's, women's, young people's, gays', deaf persons', and physicians' meetings, which still focus on recovery from alcoholism by working the 12 steps. Efforts have been made in several communities to develop disability-specific AA meetings. Some of these meetings are affiliated with treatment centers specializing in substance abuse and disability. Others are independent of sponsoring agencies.

Many members of AA relate to the "program" and the 12 steps as a new way of life, and the search for sobriety as an active process. Most AA members do more than just attend meetings. They may spend time talking to other members and find a sponsor, as the program suggests. Generally a sponsor is an AA member with a longer period of sobriety who can assist the newcomer in becoming involved in the AA program. Finding the right sponsor may be very difficult for new AA members, especially if the new member has a disability. Beginners' meetings and assistance from professionals can be helpful. Persons going through traditional treatment centers often can meet AA members who volunteer with the center. Persons receiving other types of assistance may need additional help in finding appropriate, accessible meetings in their communities.

A variety of materials published by AA are available at meetings, treatment centers, the AA General Service Office in New York, and local AA offices. For additional information about AA or their Conference-approved literature, call the Alcoholics Anonymous phone number listed in the phone book or contact the General Service Office of AA, PO Box 459, Grand Central Station, New York, NY 10163.

Source: J.A. Ford and D. Moore, *Substance Abuse Resources and Disability Issues Training Manual for Professionals*, School of Medicine, Wright State University, Dayton, Ohio, © 1992.

Symptoms of Substance Abuse by Adolescents with Spinal Cord Injury

Some of the symptoms included in this list may be a normal part of adolescence and developing independence; however, the number and severity of symptoms should be considered when there is a concern about substance abuse. If adolescents with spinal cord injury are exhibiting several of these symptoms, a substance abuse assessment should be conducted by a professional trained in both substance abuse and adolescents with SCI. Any time a parent of or professional working with an adolescent with SCI suspects alcohol or other drug use, the problem areas must be explored and addressed.

SOCIAL

- Changing several friends or changing peer groups
- Suddenly popular with friends who are older and unknown to family
- Becoming involved with peers when formerly isolated from peers
- More frequent phone calls
- Social activities occurring more often, sometimes at odd hours
- Engaging in thrill-seeking behaviors evidenced by law breaking, promiscuity, and other dangerous physical situations

FAMILY

- Using SCI as a means for isolation from family members (hiding in room, locking bedroom door) and avoiding family activities
- Exhibiting negative attitude toward rules and parents
- Failing to follow through on promises
- Sneaking out of the house
- Blaming SCI for negative behaviors
- Becoming manipulative
- Lying

SCHOOL

- Lacking motivation and lower grades
- Sleeping in class
- Skipping class or school
- Blaming SCI for poor performance in school or negative behaviors
- Dropping out of school activities
- Becoming disrespectful of teachers, administrators, and rules

continues

continued

- Frequently needing discipline
- Suspended or expelled

PHYSICAL

- Smelling of alcohol, marijuana, or stale smoke
- Frequent minor illnesses (headaches, nausea, slight tremors, flu-like symptoms, vomiting, sluggishness)
- Neglects taking prescribed medications or takes more medications than usual
- Memory lapses
- Weight changes or unusual eating patterns (types of foods, amounts, time of day)
- Frequent use of eyedrops for bloodshot eyes
- Change in normal sleep patterns (more or less than usual, frequent naps)
- Injuries occurring more often
- Frequent infections or infections that don't heal
- More frequent complaints of pain or illness

LEGAL

- Shoplifting or stealing from family members
- Unruly behaviors like skipping school and not following family rules
- Charges for public intoxication, DWI, vandalism, breaking and entering, underage use (or these incidents occur but no charge is made)
- Involved in car accidents or near misses
- Selling drugs

EMOTIONAL

- Impaired judgment (putting self in dangerous situations)
- Talking about or attempting suicide
- Violent or threatening (verbally or physically)
- Lethargic or apathetic
- Mood swings
- Blaming SCI for all that goes wrong
- Burned out
- Operating at an inappropriate maturity level

OTHER

- Poor management of money
- Spending large sums of money and asking for money

continues

continued

- Having drug paraphernalia in bedroom or school locker
- Reading drug-oriented magazines
- Wearing drug-oriented clothing and accessories
- Using drug slang, talking about drugs

It is important to remember that exploring independence, becoming self-involved, and focusing on peer groups are normal parts of adolescence. Some adolescents will exhibit one or more of these symptoms, which may not be related to the use of alcohol or other drugs. However, if you suspect substance abuse in an adolescent with a spinal cord injury, it is better to explore these symptoms further.

Notes:

Source: J.A. Ford and D. Moore, *Substance Abuse Resources and Disability Issues Training Manual for Professionals*, School of Medicine, Wright State University, Dayton, Ohio, © 1992.

Substance Abuse Symptoms Checklist

1. **Frequent intoxication:**
   - ☐ Does the person report being or appear to be frequently high or intoxicated?
   - ☐ Do recreational activities center around drinking or other drug use, including getting, using, and recovering from use?
2. **Atypical social settings:**
   - ☐ Does the immediate peer group of the individual suggest that substance abuse may be encouraged?
   - ☐ Is the person socially isolated from others and is substance abuse occurring alone?
   - ☐ Is the person reluctant to attend social events where chemicals won't be available?
3. **Intentional heavy use:**
   - ☐ Does the person use "social drugs" with prescribed medications?
   - ☐ Does the person use more than is safe in light of medications or compromised tolerance?
   - ☐ Does the person have an elevated tolerance as evidenced by the use of large quantities of alcohol or other drugs without appearing intoxicated?
4. **Symptomatic drinking:**
   - ☐ Are there predictable patterns of use that are well known to others?
   - ☐ Is there a reliance on chemicals to cope with stress?
   - ☐ Has the person made lifestyle changes yet the drug use has stayed the same or increased (e.g., changed friends or moved to another area)?
5. **Psychological dependence:**
   - ☐ Does the person rely on drugs as a means of coping with negative emotions?
   - ☐ Does the person believe that pain can't be coped with without medication?
   - ☐ Does the person obviously feel guilty about some aspect of the person's use of alcohol or other drugs?
6. **Health problems:**
   - ☐ Are there medical conditions that decrease tolerance or increase the risk of substance abuse problems?
   - ☐ Are there recurring bladder infections, chronic infections, bed sores, seizures, or other medical situations that are aggravated by repeated alcohol or other drug use?
   - ☐ Did the spinal cord injury occur when the individual was under the influence, even if it is denied by the person?
7. **Job problems:**
   - ☐ Is the person underemployed or unemployed?
   - ☐ Has the person missed work or gone to work late due to use of alcohol or other drugs?
   - ☐ Does the person blame the spinal cord injury for work-related problems?
8. **Problems with significant others:**
   - ☐ Has a family member or friend expressed concern about the person's use?
   - ☐ Have important relationships been lost or impaired due to chemical use?

continues

continued

9. **Problems with law or authority:**
   - ☐ Has the person been in trouble with authorities or arrested for any alcohol- or drug-related offenses?
   - ☐ Have there been instances when the person could have been arrested but wasn't?
   - ☐ Does the person seem angry at "the system" and at authority figures in general?
10. **Financial problems:**
    - ☐ Is the person's spending money easily accounted for?
    - ☐ Does the person frequently miss making payments when they are due?
11. **Belligerence:**
    - ☐ Does the person appear angry or defensive but doesn't know why?
    - ☐ Is the person defensive or angry when confronted about chemical use?
12. **Isolation:**
    - ☐ Does increasing isolation suggest heavier substance abuse?
    - ☐ Is the person giving up or changing social and family activities in order to use?
13. **"Handicapism":**
    - ☐ Does the person focus on the spinal cord injury to the exclusion of other aspects of life?
    - ☐ Does the person blame the spinal cord injury for what goes wrong?

Exhibiting one of these symptoms is not necessarily indicative of substance abuse; however, several or more of these symptoms in combination may suggest that issues related to substance abuse should be explored at greater length. If a consumer exhibits several of the above symptoms, it might be advisable to consult with a substance abuse specialist.

Source: J.A. Ford and D. Moore, *Substance Abuse Resources and Disability Issues Training Manual for Professionals*, School of Medicine, Wright State University, Dayton, Ohio, © 1992.

Substance Abuse: Suggestions to Help You at Home

- Get rid of all drinking/drug use materials (wine, liquor, beer, pot, pills, rolling paper, and drug paraphernalia).
- Vary your daily routine:
  - Change the order in which you do things.
  - Drive different routes.
  - Do not sit in your favorite drinking chair.
  - Do something different after dinner, e.g., walk, read, talk to a friend.
  - Avoid people who drink/use (when possible).
  - Avoid routine TV shows.
- Get a good night's sleep each night.
- Shower or bathe in lukewarm water if you are jittery, nervous, irritable, feel panicky, or your skin itches.
- Begin an exercise program.
- Keep busy:
  - Read.
  - Go to a movie.
  - Visit a nondrinking/nonusing friend.
  - Go to an AA meeting.
  - Revive a hobby.
  - Fix something around the house.
  - Knit or sew.
- Develop new eating habits:
  - Use coffee or caffeine-related products (chocolate, aspirin), sugar, and desserts in moderation.
  - Take a multivitamin.
  - Eat three balanced meals a day.
- Make plans for your difficult times:
  - Know your supports.
  - Identify your needs and take care of yourself.
  - Do not wait for others to fix or rescue you.
- Practice saying the word *STOP*, either out loud or silently, when you have a thought about drinking or using.
- Do not pick up the first drink or drug.
- Use "One Day at a Time."
- The urge to drink will go away whether or not you drink.
- Tell your friends that you have stopped drinking.
- Whenever you feel tense or uncomfortable, take deep breaths.
- Understand what you really want in a situation.

continues

continued

- Be good to yourself. Give yourself daily rewards:
  - Treat yourself to a bubble bath.
  - Buy the hardback version of a book rather than the paperback.
  - Get the game or puzzle you've been wanting.
  - Go to an AA or NA meeting.
  - Have lunch or dinner with a nondrinking friend.

Notes:

Source: Department of Psychiatric Nursing, The Ohio State University Hospitals, © 1993.

ADAPTING TO SPINAL CORD INJURY

Examining Your Feelings Toward Disabilities

It's often said that one of the hardest things about coping with abrupt onset of disability is that you're suddenly thrust into it with all your able-bodied beliefs, attitudes, and misconceptions.

Do you know any people with disabilities? Are any friends or family members disabled? How about fellow employees or fellow students? If you have known someone well, you have probably discovered that the disability gradually seemed less important as the relationship grew. First impressions or initial attitudes are not always accurate, and they may change over time.

Many people have varying attitudes and impressions that show how they feel about people with disabilities. You may discover that you possess some of these beliefs as well, especially if your association with people with disabilities has been very limited or nonexistent. What are some common attitudes toward, or first impressions about, people with *obvious* physical disabilities? Here are some examples:

- Pity or sympathy for the individual, which often results in a condescending or patronizing attitude.
- Personal discomfort, anxiety, or fear of being around the individual with a disability. Therefore, such a person is actively avoided.
- Assumed cognitive/mental impairment because of physical disability.
- Assumed dependency because of physical disability.
- Assumed "second class" citizen status. Therefore, people with disabilities may not be included in many activities or functions of their communities, or they may not be treated with equal respect by others.
- Unearned praise of the individuals because they are "so brave" or "have coped so well."

However, your attitudes about yourself and the attitudes of others (family, friends, and even strangers) can change. But beliefs do not change overnight. This is a gradual process that occurs with new learning and behaving. You may find that you are a "student" in the rehabilitation facility and a "teacher" on the outside who helps others to reassess their attitudes about physical disability.

Source: Margaret Hammond, et al., eds., *Yes, You Can! A Guide to Self-Care for Persons with Spinal Cord Injury*, Paralyzed Veterans of America, Washington, DC, © 1989. Original body of text produced by the Seattle Veterans Affairs Medical Center.

"Normal" Feelings

It is important to keep in mind that the personal and psychological issues you face will, over time, be less focused on your injury and have more to do with everyday life. The following discussion of feelings applies to emotions of crisis (right after your injury) as well as emotions that may come and go throughout your life. It is normal for people to experience a wide range of feelings after a major crisis. Anger, sadness, frustration, irritation, confusion, and isolation are common. How *you* feel is probably different from how others may feel. However, some people like to know that others have similar feelings. This handout will discuss what you can do to help yourself in dealing with the emotional reactions you experience. Not all those emotions are going to be uncomfortable ones! The process of rehabilitation also involves humor, pride, hope, and a sense of accomplishment.

ANGER

If you find yourself snapping at others, yelling when things go wrong, or "boiling over" most of the time, know that *many* people experience anger. However, it may become difficult for you to work with others if that anger carries over into everything you do. A good test is to ask yourself: "Would I like to be treated the way I treat others?" If the answer is "No," ask yourself: "Who or what is getting in my way? Why am I angry?"

This kind of self-talk can help you step back from a problem, cool off, and develop a positive plan of action. Also, ask others to help you stay calm by talking about problems openly, rather than letting something build up to the boiling point and exploding in anger.

HUMOR

When was the last time you had a good, long, belly-shaking laugh? It seems that this type of "therapy" is often overlooked or discounted, especially when you are in the hospital. Recent medical writers have discussed the positive effect that laughing has upon both mental and physical health. Norman Cousins, author of *Anatomy of an Illness*, discusses how he has used joke books, funny movies, and other forms of humor to help improve his ability to combat illness. Certainly, laughing is no "cure," but it can help you deal with difficult problems, and it usually sets up a positive mood.

Some suggestions to help you find humor are the following:

- Spend more time with friends who make you laugh.
- Go to a bookstore and look at joke books or humorous notecards.
- Read newspaper comics or comic books.
- Watch a funny movie.
- Start a joke contest.

continues

continued

SADNESS

It is very common for someone to feel intense sadness after a major loss or significant change in health. This is similar to the grief you might feel when someone close to you has died. Some people express this sadness with tears, withdrawal, avoidance of the "usual routine," or talking about the sad feelings with a close friend. These are normal, common reactions. However, when these feelings seem to be overwhelming, persistent, or hopeless, you should consider getting help in dealing with your sadness. The main differences between *grief* and *significant depression* are that depression is often accompanied by hopelessness, a sense of "giving up," physical exhaustion, trouble sleeping, and a change in appetite. Try talking to someone close, thinking about something positive in your future, or maybe setting out to do something enjoyable (like listening to a concert, having a special dessert, or reading a good book). If you feel like "it's not worth trying," then talk with a member of your rehab team about those feelings. You can get some help.

PRIDE

How you feel about yourself is very important, especially in a rehabilitation setting. It influences how you look, talk, and act. Think of someone you know who is very proud and confident (not false pride). How does he or she look and act? When you feel good about yourself, other people will know because you care enough to groom well and present yourself nicely to others. This feeling starts when you tell yourself: "I am worthwhile as a person." Sure, you have faults, but you have some unique qualities as a person. You can learn to feel good about those qualities and that will begin to help you improve your sense of pride. A book called *A New Guide to Rational Living* by Albert Ellis and Robert Harper describes specific ways of improving and maintaining a positive sense of self-esteem and pride.

FRUSTRATION/CONFUSION

Having to try new ways of doing things can be both frustrating and confusing. First, try to identify the *source* of frustration. If you can identify a person, talk with that person about the problem as openly as you can. Clear communication helps! If talking about things makes you more upset, ask for a "third party" to help out or try to use some relaxation activities before you talk. Being calm and relaxed can help!

Sometimes you can identify why you are frustrated, but you can't figure out how to improve or change it. Ask for help! Another person can help you "brainstorm," which may lead to a solution, or you may find a way to stay relaxed in the face of some very frustrating situations.

Source: Margaret Hammond, et al., eds., *Yes, You Can! A Guide to Self-Care for Persons with Spinal Cord Injury*, Paralyzed Veterans of America, Washington, DC, © 1989. Original body of text produced by the Seattle Veterans Affairs Medical Center.

Learn to Let Others Know What You Need Without Being Rude

Many times, people feel upset, angry, and frustrated when they miss out on something they want. You can learn how to achieve certain things without hurting or stomping on others. This involves being assertive without being nasty or aggressive.

There will be times when you need to ask for assistance with something you cannot accomplish on your own, or you may need to let someone else know they are doing something that really bothers you. Also, recent research has shown that people with spinal cord injuries often need to take the extra step in making some nondisabled persons feel comfortable when talking to someone in a wheelchair. This often helps to set the stage for positive communication.

The following discussion will focus on three basic communication styles: assertion, aggression, and passivity.

The general style will be described, followed by descriptions of specific behaviors that are typical of each style. Notice that these are behaviors, not words. It is *how* you say something (body language, tone of voice, etc.) that is important, not necessarily the *words* you use.

ASSERTION

Assertion involves standing up for your own personal rights. Express your ideas and feelings directly and honestly, but take into account other people's feelings, too. This involves respect—respect for yourself *and* respect for other people. To do this requires that you communicate clearly and that you ask what others might think and feel. In other words, cooperation and fair play are essential to being assertive.

In assertive behavior, your body actions are consistent with the verbal messages and add support, strength, and emphasis to what is being said verbally. The voice is appropriately loud to the situation, eye contact is firm but not a stare-down, body gestures that denote strength are used, and the speech pattern is fluent—expressive, clear, and with emphasis on key words—without awkward pauses.

AGGRESSION

Aggression involves standing up for your personal rights, but in a way that ignores others' rights. This is not an honest way to communicate. It is almost always inappropriate and may create strong negative feelings, such as anger or disgust.

The usual goal of aggression is domination and winning, forcing the other person to lose. Winning is ensured by humiliating, degrading, belittling, or overpowering other people so that they become weaker and less able to express and defend their needs and rights. The basic message is: This is what I think—you're wrong for believing differently. This is what I want—what you want isn't important. This is what I feel—your feelings don't count.

continues

continued

In aggressive behavior, the nonverbal behaviors are ones that dominate or demean the other person. These include eye contact that tries to stare down and dominate the other person, a forceful voice that does not fit the situation, sarcastic or condescending tone of voice, and parental body gestures such as excessive finger pointing.

PASSIVITY

Passivity involves violating your own rights by failing to express honest feelings, thoughts, and beliefs. Expressing your thoughts and feelings in such an apologetic, self-defeating style may allow others to easily disregard you. The total message communicated is: I don't count—you can take advantage of me. My feelings don't matter—only yours do. My thoughts aren't important—yours are the only ones worth listening to. I'm nothing—you are superior.

Passivity is nonassertion and shows a lack of respect for your own needs. It also shows a subtle lack of respect for another person's ability to take disappointments or to shoulder some responsibility. The goal of nonassertion is to appease others and to avoid conflict at any cost.

In nonassertive behavior, the nonverbal behaviors include avoiding eye contact, hand wringing, clutching the other person, stepping back from the other person as an assertive remark is made, hunching the shoulders, covering the mouth with a hand, nervous gestures that distract the listener from what the speaker is saying, and wooden body posture. The voice tone may be singsong or overly soft. The speech pattern is hesitant and filled with pauses, and the throat may be cleared frequently. Facial gestures may include raising of the eyebrows, laughs, and winks when expressing anger.

In general, the nonassertive gestures are ones that convey weakness, anxiety, pleading, or a self "put-down." They reduce the impact of what is being said verbally, which is precisely why people who are scared of acting assertively use them. Their goal is to "soften" what they're saying so that the other person will not be offended.

Source: Margaret Hammond, et al., eds., *Yes, You Can! A Guide to Self-Care for Persons with Spinal Cord Injury*, Paralyzed Veterans of America, Washington, DC, © 1989. Original body of text produced by the Seattle Veterans Affairs Medical Center.

Family and Friends

When an acute spinal cord injury occurs, people who are close to you are likely to be as emotionally shaken up by your injury as you are. They may feel shock (numbness), disbelief, sadness, and anger as they see you move from surviving your injury through your rehabilitation process.

Their reactions may be quite familiar to you, or they may be very unexpected. You may or may not be able to understand the hows and whys of their reactions and actions. In any case, try to remember that this sudden change for you was just as unexpected and unwanted for them. Give yourself and them some time to adjust and think about all of these changes. Some tips on how to help both you and your family and friends during this time of transition follow:

- Try to talk about how all of you feel. By bringing it out into the open, no one has to guess how everyone else is taking it, especially *you*. They love you, and you love them, and that's not a bad place to start.
- Since your close friends and family may be afraid to bring up the subject for fear of causing you or them more pain, you may have to start the ball rolling. It will be hard, but it may be best in the long run. Timing is very important, however. Adapting is a healing process, so trust your gut instinct in dealing with certain issues. If either you or your close ones aren't ready to discuss something, let it go for a little while. There will come a time in the natural course of adaptation when you will both feel right about it.
- Try not to hide all of your feelings. You don't have to be strong for your family and friends. This only makes it harder for them to talk with you.
- Also, remember that your family and friends are part of society and may have the same misconceptions and attitudes about people with disabilities. When you're able to, try to talk to them about this. You need to teach them the truth. Soon enough, you'll find them educating their friends and families too!
- If your family members live close to a spinal cord injury center, they may want to attend a family support group. Check the bulletin board for day and time.
- Sometimes, family and friends go overboard trying to do just about everything for you. For some people with disabilities, this becomes a smothering experience. For others, this is merely what they always expect from their close ones. This type of behavior may be okay, or it may get tiring for both you and your family and friends.
- Figure out how and with what you'd like to have help. If your family and friends are doing too much, talk to them about it. Let them know how it makes you feel and why you'd prefer that they not do so much for you.

After living with spinal cord injury for a period of time, the feelings you have about your injury may be very different from those you experienced when you were first injured. You may be more comfortable with this change in your body and what you need to do to keep it healthy.

continues

continued

As you became more experienced in getting around town (either by car, van, or wheelchair), you may have gained a new sense of freedom as well. These challenges have helped you learn and adapt to this new way of life.

Adapting to life with a spinal cord injury is a unique experience. Each individual does it in his or her own way. Whatever way you have chosen is okay, as long as it keeps you healthy, both in mind and body.

Your family and friends have also adapted to your spinal cord injury. Many have come to realize that you are still the same person they've always loved except for some physical changes. Unfortunately, a few may not have been able to adjust to the new physical you, no matter how much they love you. Some people just can't. Relationships change in everybody's life, no matter if you're disabled or not! Being a person with a spinal cord injury is a challenging experience that offers a potential for growth.

Notes:

Source: Margaret Hammond, et al., eds., *Yes, You Can! A Guide to Self-Care for Persons with Spinal Cord Injury*, Paralyzed Veterans of America, Washington, DC, © 1989. Original body of text produced by the Seattle Veterans Affairs Medical Center.

Being a Parent

You can be a parent if you decide you can or want to be a parent. Many feelings and a great amount of thinking will contribute to that decision. Common feelings may be uncertainty about your ability to provide the physical care and financial support. Fear may arise about how a child will respond to you now that you are in a wheelchair. You may experience feelings of depression or discouragement that cause you to wonder about caring for another person. Or you may experience great joy and satisfaction as you realize your children need and respond to your caring and attention. You may be surprised how accepting and adaptable children are.

As you review your feelings and thinking, it is good to remember that bringing up children is a tough job and that every parent can feel uncertain at one time or another. Although your injury may change how you physically care for a child, it does not create insurmountable barriers. There are many adaptive tools, techniques, and even books that you can explore. Consult your rehabilitation team members for ideas.

When you are making changes because of a spinal cord injury, your children should be included in the process. If you are absent from the home due to a hospital stay, your children, of whatever age, need to have the absence explained at their level of understanding. You and your children need to know that a physical limitation need not change your relationship. Research has shown no difference in emotional and social development between children whose parents have a spinal cord injury and children of nondisabled parents.

It is also important to remember that your rights as a parent don't change after a spinal cord injury. Custody of your children or your right to seek adoption cannot be denied solely on the basis of your disability.

SPECIFIC THOUGHTS TO KEEP IN MIND

- Include your children in your rehabilitation program. Find out about visiting hours and passes out of the hospital with your family.
- Introduce your children and spouse to other parents with spinal cord injury. Have your children talk with their children.
- Include your children in family meetings in and out of the hospital.
- Continue the discussions with your children about your injury or related feelings after you leave the hospital. Seek out community counseling services that are recommended by your social worker or psychologist.
- You can also work closely with your rehab team members about parenting concerns.

DECIDING TO BECOME A PARENT

As a first step, you may wish to explore your physical capability to have children. Check with your doctors. You may wish to consult with your social worker or psychologist if you are thinking about becoming a parent. If you discover you are physically unable to have children, consider adoption or artificial insemination.

Source: Margaret Hammond, et al., eds., *Yes, You Can! A Guide to Self-Care for Persons with Spinal Cord Injury*, Paralyzed Veterans of America, Washington, DC, © 1989. Original body of text produced by the Seattle Veterans Affairs Medical Center.

Accepting New Help as the Years Go By

INDEPENDENCE

The world we live in and we ourselves place a very high value on physical independence. We're raised on the expectation that we will ultimately take care of ourselves. As toddlers, we learn to dress and feed ourselves, and as teens we learn to drive and to think for ourselves. Finally, as adults, we assume responsibility for our lives. Hallelujah, we've finally grown up.

Spinal Cord Injury

Then, somewhere in there spinal cord injury arrives and everything gets turned around. Many survivors have to hand back a large measure of control—to hospital staff, caregivers, parents, and even the government. Some fight a sense of being returned to childhood, and most have to deal with the concept of living on the edge—of being independent now, but only a breath, a fall, a skin sore away from losing a big hunk of that independence.

What if you injure one of your shoulders and can no longer do transfers? What if you lose the manual dexterity for bladder care or the range of motion for dressing, or maybe just the energy to keep up with household tasks?

Aging

Add aging to the mix. What then? Even those who aren't disabled eventually come to realize that as the years go by, the buffer that separates independence from dependence grows progressively thinner and thinner. If we live long enough, we all eventually become dependent, for a greater or lesser period of time.

With a spinal cord injury, that realization comes early. You don't have to add many years to your injury to become painfully aware that your independence is fragile, and that at some point, the only thing that will stand between you and an impossible living situation is the help of another person. Yet you fought a long, valiant battle to win your independence after injury, and you'll do anything to preserve it. Any compromise seems like fundamental failure. For most survivors, weaned on the holy grail of self-sufficiency, that's a terrible dilemma.

The dilemma doesn't go away. But it may not be so terrible, either.

THE FACTS

Like it or not, the need for help is as much a part of the spinal cord injury (SCI) picture as wheelchairs. About 40 percent to 45 percent of SCI survivors use some kind of personal assistance, and the percentage increases with age. The British Longitudinal SCI Aging Study of survivors injured 20 or more years found that 22 percent had an increase in the amount of assistance they needed, regardless of how much help they did or didn't need initially.

continues

continued

Why? One-fourth of this 22 percent blamed fatigue or weakness; another fourth blamed some other medical condition. Weight gain was another major cause. The areas they needed more help with tended to be with transfers if they had paraplegia and mobility in general if they had quadriplegia. Other problematic areas were dressing, toileting, homemaking, and eating.

THE MINDSET

So, given the weight society places on independence, how do you deal with the prospect of more dependence?

The key is mindset. Try thinking about what determines your self-worth and quality of life: do you have to be able to do everything yourself, or it is enough to know that you can get the job done? Realize that you alone are responsible for that determination.

Consider two people:

- Gary is a 20-year-old college student with quadriplegia. Each morning his alarm wakes him at 4:00 A.M. He then spends over three hours getting ready for his first class. He seldom has time for breakfast.
- Jon is another student with quadriplegia. He sleeps in until 7:00 A.M. when the personal care assistant he hired and trained arrives. Thirty minutes later he is up, washed, and dressed. His bed is made, and he is on his way to the cafeteria for breakfast.

To a large extent, Gary's self-esteem comes from his fiercely held physical independence. He likes knowing that no help is needed.

But Jon knows that, regardless of who does each task, he, Jon, has complete control. He also has the freedom to spend the time and energy he once used for self-care on activities that are more important to him.

The Source of Esteem

Self-esteem and accepting help may not be so incompatible after all. For most people, as they get older, knowing they have the control and the resources to get things done becomes progressively more important than doing everything themselves.

People learn to interact with their environment by consuming services, and think little of it. Most people are comfortable with not being able to replace the transmission in their cars; they can hire a mechanic for that. Most people don't raise their own food, haul water, or produce fuel to heat their houses either—they hire those things out and they don't lose too much sleep over it.

continues

continued

Setting Priorities

If personal care services are looked at in much the same way, perhaps you can hire out tasks—that early morning dressing routine, that tub transfer, or whatever it is that impedes getting on with the day—and spend your energy on your education, career, or serving your community instead.

The point is: hang on to the activities that really matter to you, and delegate or negotiate away the ones that don't. Consider the following examples:

- You have the skills to work but don't have enough energy to do your self-care as well. If your work is your first interest, and especially if it will generate money to pay a helper, where is the defeat in hiring a personal care attendant to get you ready for the job?
- The volunteer time you put in is the most gratifying thing you do, but you need someone to help with showering and dressing before you can get there. Doesn't it make sense, if you can afford it, to accept that help and the richness it enables you to experience?
- Perhaps you work for an independent living center. But you need a dresser, driver, gofer, and leg bag emptier. Your work is helping people, so why should you balk at accepting help yourself?
- You love sit-skiing and you're totally independent. But there's no skiing without some assistance on the hill. Can't you continue to be bullheaded about your independence at home, and lighten up for a weekend of fun?

INDEPENDENCE IS RELATIVE

Independence is a relative thing. How many individuals are truly independent of other people? Physically, psychologically, or financially—and in a host of other ways—people are all *inter*dependent. It's part of being human. And accepting help, of course, in no way prevents people from helping others.

From this perspective, a decision to use more help is not an admission of failure but an act of empowerment. In fact, accepting additional care may provide optimal independence. For many, taking responsibility and control over an appropriate level of physical assistance brings more freedom and flexibility than rigidly refusing all help.

Source: The Rehabilitation Research and Training Center on Aging with SCI, a joint project of Craig Hospital and the Department of Rehabilitation Medicine at the University of Colorado Health Sciences Center. Funded by the National Institute on Disability and Rehabilitation Research. For more information about the "SCI & Aging" publications, contact the RRTC at 800-5-REHAB-8.

THE CAREGIVER

Tips for the Long-Term Caregiver

Share your feelings. Ask about support groups at rehabilitation centers, local chapters of the National Spinal Cord Injury Association, Paralyzed Veterans of America, or at independent living programs. No luck? Consider starting your own group, using one of these organizations as a resource. Computer users can find dozens of disability interest groups exchanging ideas on-line; look into services like CompuServe, Prodigy, and America Online. One very successful support group was started by a few wives of disabled men. Besides providing mutual support, they devoted one of their twice-monthly meetings to a specific topic and invited a speaker, for example, someone to talk about financial planning for long-term care.

Improve your relationship. Research suggests that the better you feel about your relationship, the less stress you will have. Talk with the person you are caring for. Get counseling. If there is serious conflict, invite a third person—one you both know and trust—to mediate. The results can be gratifying; spouses with the highest morale generally attribute it to the continuing companionship and good relationship they have with their disabled partner.

Avoid isolation—invite people in. Have visitors. Make your family show up occasionally, even if only to bring in gossip and fast food once a month. Research shows that people who have frequent visitors report lower stress levels.

Get out of the house—alone. Go to a movie, get your hair done, go to church. Arrange things so the tasks you're most worried about—bowel care and skin management, perhaps—are done before you leave. Family, neighbors, or paid services can often cover for you, at least for a few hours.

Consider respite care. Look for local programs that can provide you with a more extended break. Try church organizations. Chances are you don't need to be a member of the particular denomination to use its services. Check out elder day care programs. Some of them can provide trained caregivers during the day, at either your place or theirs. Consider starting a care-swapping program in which several caregivers can hire an individual—perhaps a retired person—to work several afternoons a week. Then each can get out of the house one afternoon a week. Consider students majoring in health care and related professions. They are often required to do volunteer work. Why not with you and your spouse? The shock of having a stranger provide intimate care dissipates when the caregiver is no longer a stranger. Your spouse may even welcome the change.

Try to get your finances in order. No matter how little or how much you have, get some help sorting through insurance policies, retirement programs, Social Security, and other government entitlements to find out what there really is to draw on. Keep in mind that your entitlements and eligibility for specific benefits and programs change from year to year, so recheck periodically.

You may not be able to do anything about the disability, but you can do something about how it impacts your time, energy, and quality of life. Nowhere is it written that, simply because you provide care for someone with a disability, you may not have a life of your own.

Source: The Rehabilitation Research and Training Center on Aging with SCI, a joint project of Craig Hospital and the Department of Rehabilitation Medicine at the University of Colorado Health Sciences Center. Funded by the National Institute on Disability and Rehabilitation Research. For more information about the "SCI & Aging" publications, contact the RRTC at 800-5-REHAB-8. Reprinted in *Spinal Cord Injury Life*, National Spinal Cord Injury Association, Silver Spring, Maryland, © Winter 1995.

9
Pain Management

> Most materials in the *Spinal Cord Injury Patient Education Resource Manual* are intended for the health care professional to share with the patient. Materials that are intended solely for the professional are labeled "Exhibit" in the table of contents.

Definition and Treatment

    Pain and Spinal Cord Injury: Overview 313
    Dysesthetic Pain Syndrome 315
    Treatment of SCI Pain 316
    Practical Management Strategies for
        SCI Pain 319

Alternative Pain Management Strategies

    Psychological Methods for Relieving
        Pain 320

    Relaxation Techniques 322
    Sample Relaxation Exercises 324
    Muscle Relaxation Exercises 325
    Biofeedback 326
    Creating an Imagery Script 328
    Creating a Personal Music Tape 330
    Where to Go for Help with Pain
        Management 331

DEFINITION AND TREATMENT

Pain and Spinal Cord Injury: Overview

How can you feel pain in places where you are not supposed to feel anything? While it may seem confusing, it is true that some persons with spinal cord injury (SCI) feel pain in places where they would not feel it if touched or stuck with a pin.

You will most likely feel pain after your injury. This may be due to broken bones or sore joints and muscles resulting from the accident. Movement of muscles and joints after periods of nonuse can also cause pain. Sometimes the pain will not go away and becomes too severe to ignore.

There have been many studies on pain and SCI. It appears that severe pain that does not go away is a problem for about one in three persons with SCI. If you have severe pain, it can interfere with your ability to carry out your daily routine, which can greatly affect your quality of life. Your pain may depend on where and how you were injured. For example, SCI caused by a gunshot tends to result in more pain than SCI from other causes. Also, if your spinal cord is damaged low in the spinal column, you may have more pain than someone whose damage is higher. You might also notice that things like smoking, being tired, changes in weather, being emotionally upset, or bowel, bladder or skin problems seem to make your pain worse. Or, you may not notice any pattern to the ups and downs of your pain.

You may not have told anyone about your pain or the things that make it worse for fear others will think you are "crazy." If you feel pain following SCI this does not mean you are crazy. You need to find out from your doctor the source and type of pain you have and what can be done to reduce or eliminate it.

TYPES OF SPINAL CORD INJURY PAIN

There are two kinds of pain: acute pain and chronic pain. *Acute* pain begins suddenly and is usually caused by physical damage to the body or from disease. Acute pain is a danger signal; it means something is wrong and help is needed. When the problem is fixed or the body heals, the pain goes away. *Chronic* pain may start suddenly or build up slowly over time; sometimes a cause is known, sometimes not. But it does *not* go away as you would expect. Chronic pain, though usually not as dangerous as acute pain, should not be ignored. Chronic pain remains a difficult condition to treat in many persons with SCI.

Five types of chronic pain are commonly felt by those with SCI.

Central Pain

Central pain can cause the most problems for you. You feel pain where you are not supposed to feel anything or where your feeling is different. Central pain often begins weeks or months after SCI and can cause a "pins and needles" feeling, numbness, or a burning feeling throughout the area below your level of injury. The pain may be constant. At best, it is bothersome; at worst, it can be so severe that it limits your ability to fully function in life. Doctors believe central pain may

continues

continued

be caused by changes in the functioning of nerves following spinal cord injury. It is thought that the brain receives pain signals that it, and you, think are coming from one place (your legs, for example) but are really coming from somewhere else.

Root Pain

Root pain is usually felt at or below the level of injury. Root pain has a distinct pattern. It often begins days to weeks after injury and may worsen over time. You may feel brief waves of stabbing or sharp pain or a band of burning pain at the point where your normal feeling stops. You may find that a light touch worsens this pain.

Mechanical Pain

Mechanical pain can range from a sudden sharpness to dull and aching and is often worsened by physical activity. It is felt in areas where you have normal sensation. This pain has several causes, ranging from muscle overuse or damage, unstable bone fractures, infection, or deforming change in your bones and joints.

Syrinx Pain

Sometimes the spinal cord heals itself in such a way that a hollow, fluid-filled cavity called a syrinx is formed. Although rare, it results in pain that varies in severity and can occur either above or below the site of your injury. A syrinx can slowly increase in size and extend up or down the spinal cord. Syrinx pain develops months to years after injury and can result in gradual loss of organ function, feeling, or movement.

Referred Pain

Referred pain is unusual because it is felt in areas away from where the source of the problem is. The source of the problem can be your organs, muscles, or other tissues. Where you cannot feel pain you may see or feel increased muscle spasticity. For example, if you had a heart attack, the pain you might feel might be somewhere in your left arm and shoulder.

Source: J. Scott Richards, *Pain and Spinal Cord Injury*, American Association of Spinal Cord Injury Psychologists and Social Workers, Jackson Heights, New York.

Dysesthetic Pain Syndrome

Of all pain types, dysesthetic pain is probably the most persistent and resistant to treatment. It also is arguably the most common.

TYPICAL CHARACTERISTICS OF SCI DYSESTHETIC PAIN SYNDROME

1. **Quality**
   - Burning, tingling, shooting, stinging, stabbing, piercing, crushing, cutting, dragging
2. **Onset**
   - Two-thirds occur within one year of injury
3. **Timing**
   - Tends to decrease over time
4. **Location**
   - Diffuse, poorly localizing, asymmetric, patchy legs, perineum, back, abdomen, arms in persons with tetraplegia, hands and feet
   - Hyperalgesic border zone reactions
5. **Predisposing Factors**
   - Any SCI level
   - More common in:
     - cauda equina injuries
     - central cord syndrome
     - incomplete injuries
     - gunshot wounds
     - increasing age
     - increasing intelligence
     - increasing anxiety
     - adverse psychosocial situation
6. **Exacerbating Factors**
   - Any noxious stimuli:
     - smoking
     - bladder or bowel complications
     - pressure sore
     - spasticity
     - prolonged sitting/inactivity
     - fatigue
     - cold, damp weather
     - changes in weather

Source: Elliot J. Roth, "Pain in Spinal Cord Injury," *Spinal Cord Injury: Medical Management and Rehabilitation*, Gary M. Yarkony, ed., Aspen Publishers, Inc., © 1994.

Treatment of SCI Pain

Treatments for SCI pain vary, depending on the type of pain. Acute pain, such as syrinx and referred pain, often responds well to treatment. Treatment of a syrinx involves neurosurgery and the draining of fluid, through a tube called a shunt, from the syrinx into another area of the body where it can be eliminated. This procedure can eliminate pain caused by a syrinx. As for referred pain, once the cause is found and treated, the pain will stop. Pain caused by unstable fractures stops when the fracture heals or is surgically stabilized. Pain from sore or damaged muscles, stiff joints, or muscle spasms can be reduced by several techniques, including stretching, range of motion exercises, strengthening, heat or cold application, certain medications, and additional methods as well.

TREATMENT OF CHRONIC PAIN

Chronic pain, such as root and central pain, can be difficult to treat. A number of treatments are available, but no one method works absolutely every time. In addition, some of these methods have unwanted side effects. Others may work at first, then lose their effectiveness over time. Management of the more difficult types of SCI pain often requires a combination of treatment methods. It is advisable to try the safest treatments first and avoid treatments with greater medical risk. Often, successful treatment necessitates learning to *cope with*, rather than *curing*, the pain.

MEDICATIONS

A number of medications are available for SCI pain. All have shown some success, but again, none completely in every instance. Some of the side effects of these medications can be serious and therefore treatment must be closely watched by your doctor. These medications include antidepressants, anticonvulsants, neuroleptics, and narcotics.

- *Antidepressants* have proven helpful in alleviating SCI pain. They work not because they help with depression, but because they affect the pain pathways in the spinal cord. These medications also relieve sleep problems and therefore are often given at night.
- *Anticonvulsants* have also been used to treat central pain with some success. They are often used in combination with antidepressants.
- *Neuroleptics* are another group of medications that have been helpful.
- *Narcotics*, including methadone, are generally not helpful and not often used for long-term management of chronic SCI pain.
- *Alcohol* is not medication. You may believe alcohol reduces your pain, but it is not helpful and can lead to alcohol abuse and other serious problems. Don't let pain be an excuse to drink alcohol more than you should. Discuss alcohol use with your doctor.

continues

continued

ELECTRICAL STIMULATION

Transcutaneous electrical nerve stimulation, called "TENS," has, in some, provided relief from SCI pain. This technique involves placing electrodes on the surface of your skin and sending low levels of electrical current into your body. The electrical current results in decreased pain. Risks of this procedure are low, and therefore it often is tried before other, more invasive, treatments.

NERVE BLOCKS AND SURGERY

Injections of certain drugs have been used to reduce chronic SCI pain. These methods generally have not proven helpful. Neurosurgical procedures are another group of options available that can, in some, reduce pain. These may involve cutting or destroying parts of the spinal cord or nerve roots thought to be the source of pain. One such procedure showing limited success is the dorsal root entry zone, also known as "DREZ." This method, however, has substantial risks, such as loss of bowel, bladder, sexual, or other functions. Surgery of this nature is a last resort and meant for extreme cases, since it is not reversible.

OTHER APPROACHES

While medical/surgical procedures for managing chronic pain are important, psychological approaches to coping with pain are just as important. A major difference is that medical/surgical procedures are basically passive: You allow professionals to do something to you to reduce your pain. With psychological approaches, much of the benefit will come from your being an active participant.

Distraction is one of the best methods for coping with chronic pain. Keeping yourself busy in enjoyable and meaningful activities, whether recreation, work, or volunteer activities, is most important. If you are inactive or bored and have nothing to look forward to when you wake up in the morning, you will find yourself increasingly focused on your pain.

Depression can accompany pain, as well as result from everyday living problems or coping with a spinal cord injury. Depression can magnify the pain experience and result in social isolation. Depression is best treated through counseling, either with professionals or peer counselors. When it becomes severe, it may require medication or other approaches. Successful treatment of depression can improve your ability to cope with chronic pain.

Stress can magnify pain. Managing stress more effectively can be learned through counseling, either individually or in groups. Psychologists can teach you stress and muscle tension reduction techniques through the use of muscle and mental relaxation training, biofeedback, and hypnosis. How you think about your pain may affect your way of coping with it. If you believe it is a sign that something is terribly wrong with your body, you may avoid certain activities or rely on medications. This can change your entire lifestyle. To decrease your concern over your pain so you may safely participate in as many activities as possible, it is important to consult your doctor to find out the type and cause of your pain and what you can and cannot do. Unnecessarily limiting yourself will

continues

continued

only make things worse. Family counseling may also prove helpful at times. Pain is an invisible disability; family members may not understand, at times be overprotective, or resent the use of medications, etc. Education and counseling can be helpful to you and your family members if your pain is becoming a family concern.

LONG-TERM SPINAL CORD INJURY AND PAIN

With advances in medicine and technology, people with SCI are living longer than ever before. However, your body was not designed to be used in many of the ways that you are now using it. For example, pushing a wheelchair, transferring, or brace walking overstresses the arms and shoulders and can result in excessive "wear and tear" on joints, tendons, ligaments, and muscles. Pain of this nature may begin after years of overuse. Do not assume these problems cannot be treated and must be suffered through. They can often be helped by a combination of medical and/or surgical techniques and changes in equipment.

Notes:

Source: J. Scott Richards, *Pain and Spinal Cord Injury*, American Association of Spinal Cord Injury Psychologists and Social Workers, Jackson Heights, New York.

Practical Management Strategies for SCI Pain

1. **Prevention and Treatment of Complications**
   - Pressure sores
   - Bowel and bladder dysfunction
   - Infection
   - Temperature extremes
   - Spasticity
   - Emotional distress
   - Prolonged immobilization/deconditioning
   - Contractures

2. **Health Promotion**
   - Smoking cessation
   - Maintain nutrition and hydration
   - Spine fracture management
   - Passive range of motion exercises
   - Proper positioning
   - Activity and exercise

3. **Psychological Interventions**
   - Reassurance, psychologic support
   - Relaxation training; hypnosis
   - Biofeedback

4. **Physical Modalities**
   - Exercise
   - Massage
   - Hydrotherapy
   - Ultrasound, short wave diathermy
   - Acupuncture
   - Biofeedback

5. **Medications**
   - Mild analgesics
   - Nonsteroidal anti-inflammatory agents
   - Narcotics
   - Tricyclic and other antidepressants
   - Anticonvulsants
   - Phenothiazines
   - Clonidine, mexiletine, other newer drugs

6. **Neurolytic Injections**

7. **Electrical Stimulation**
   - Transcutaneous electrical nerve stimulation
   - Epidural dorsal column stimulation
   - Deep brain electrical stimulation

8. **Neurosurgical Procedures**
   - Laminectomy
   - Sympathectomy
   - Cordotomy
   - Myelotomy
   - Selective posterior rhizotomy
   - Dorsal root entry zone lesion

Source: Elliot J. Roth, "Practical Pain Management Strategies," *Spinal Cord Injury: Medical Management and Rehabilitation*, Gary M. Yarkony, ed., Aspen Publishers, Inc., © 1994.

ALTERNATIVE PAIN MANAGEMENT STRATEGIES

Psychological Methods for Relieving Pain

Psychological treatment for pain can range from psychoanalysis and other forms of psychotherapy to relaxation training, meditation, hypnosis, biofeedback, or behavior modification. The philosophy common to all these varied approaches is the belief that people can do something on their own to control their pain. That something may mean changing attitudes, feelings, or behaviors associated with pain, or understanding how unconscious forces and past events have contributed to the present painful predicament.

PSYCHOTHERAPY

Freud was celebrated for demonstrating that for some individuals physical pain symbolizes real or imagined emotional hurts. He also noted that some individuals develop pain or paralysis as a form of self-punishment for what they consider to be past sins or bad behavior. Sometimes, too, pain may be a way of punishing others. This doesn't mean that the pain is any less real; it does mean that some people with pain may benefit from psychoanalysis or individual or group psychotherapy to gain insights into the meaning of their pain.

RELAXATION AND MEDITATION THERAPIES

These forms of training enable people to relax tense muscles, reduce anxiety, and alter their mental state. Both physical and mental tension can make any pain worse, and in conditions such as headache or back pain, tension may be at the root of the problem. Meditation, which aims at producing a state of relaxed but alert awareness, is sometimes combined with therapies that encourage people to think of pain as something remote and apart from them. The methods promote a sense of detachment so that the person thinks of the pain as confined to a particular body part over which he or she has marvelous control.

HYPNOSIS

No longer considered magic, hypnosis is a technique in which an individual's susceptibility to suggestion is heightened. Normal volunteers who prove to be excellent subjects for hypnosis often report a marked reduction or obliteration of experimentally induced pain, such as that produced by a mild electric shock. The hypnotic state does not lower the volunteer's heart rate, respiration, or other autonomic responses. These physical reactions show the expected increases normally associated with painful stimulation.

The role of hypnosis in treating people with chronic pain is uncertain. Some studies have shown that 15 to 20 percent of hypnotizable people with moderate to severe pain can achieve total relief

continues

continued

with hypnosis. Other studies report that hypnosis reduces anxiety and depression. By lowering the burden of emotional suffering, pain may become more bearable.

BIOFEEDBACK

Some individuals can learn voluntary control over certain body activities if they are provided with information about how the system is working—how fast their heart is beating, how tense their head or neck muscles are, how cold their hands are. The information is usually supplied through visual or auditory cues that code the body activity in some obvious way—a louder sound meaning an increase in muscle tension, for example. How people use this "biofeedback" to learn control is not understood, but some masters of the art report that imagery helps: They may think of a warm tropical beach, for example, when they want to raise the temperature of their hands. Biofeedback may be a logical approach in pain conditions that involve tense muscles, like tension headache or low back pain. But results are mixed.

BEHAVIOR MODIFICATION

This psychological technique (sometimes called operant conditioning) is aimed at changing habits, behaviors, and attitudes that can develop in people with chronic pain. Some people become dependent, anxious, and homebound—if not bedridden. For some, too, chronic pain may be a welcome friend, relieving them of the boredom of a dull job or the burden of family responsibilities. These psychological rewards—sometimes combined with financial gains from compensation payments or insurance—work against improvements in the person's condition and can encourage increased drug dependency, repeated surgery, and multiple doctor and clinic visits.

There is no question that the person feels pain. The hope of behavior modification is that pain relief can be obtained from a program aimed at changing the individual's lifestyle. The program begins with a complete assessment of the painful condition and a thorough explanation of how the program works. It is essential to enlist the full cooperation of both the person and family members. The treatment is aimed at reducing pain medication and increasing mobility and independence through a graduated program of exercise, diet, and other activities. The person is rewarded for positive efforts with praise and attention. Rewards are withheld when the person retreats into negative attitudes or demanding and dependent behavior.

Source: "Chronic Pain: Hope Through Research," U.S. Department of Health and Human Services, Public Health Service, National Institutes of Health, Office of Scientific and Health Reports, National Institute of Neurological Disorders and Stroke, 1989.

Relaxation Techniques

QUIET BREATHING TECHNIQUE

1. Assume a comfortable sitting position.
2. Take a deep, slow breath.
3. As you exhale, envision all your tensions and anxieties flowing outward with each breath.
4. Repeat as needed.

PROGRESSIVE RELAXATION

1. Assume a comfortable sitting position.
2. Close your eyes and breathe slowly.
3. Continue slow breathing, feeling the tension leaving your body and becoming heavy.
4. Perform progressive relaxation of muscles, tightening muscles during inspiration and relaxing muscles during expiration.
5. Begin with muscles in feet and progress upward through the body muscles.

GUIDED IMAGERY

1. Assume a comfortable sitting position.
2. Use your imagination to experience a pleasant place or event.
3. Using all your senses, smell the pleasant smells, feel the warmth or softness, taste something pleasant, see the pleasant surroundings, and hear the pleasant sounds.

AUTOGENIC TRAINING

1. Assume a comfortable sitting position.
2. Take several slow, deep breaths.
3. Have someone say these phrases in a slow, monotonous tone three times; then you say them silently and begin to relax:

- My right arm is heavy and warm.
- My left arm is heavy and warm.
- My forehead is cool, and my face is relaxed.
- My neck and shoulders are warm and heavy.
- My breathing is slow and steady.
- My heartbeat is slow and steady.
- My entire body is warm and relaxed.

continues

continued

THOUGHT-STOPPING TECHNIQUE

1. Identify a few very pleasant experiences.
2. Whenever an unpleasant thought enters your mind, say, "Stop."
3. Begin thinking about a pleasant experience.
4. As this process is repeated, it will become habit-forming.

MASSAGE

1. Use warm lotion with massage to relax muscles.
2. Use a light, gliding stroke to relax muscles.
3. Use strong, circular movements to loosen tight muscles and to improve circulation.
4. Use a kneading-type motion to relax tight muscles.

Notes:

Source: Donna Meyers, *Client Teaching Guides for Home Health Care*, Aspen Publishers, Inc., © 1989.

Sample Relaxation Exercises

EXERCISE 1

- Let all your muscles go loose and heavy. Just settle back quietly and comfortably. Wrinkle up your forehead now . . . wrinkle and smooth it out. Picture the entire forehead and scalp becoming smoother as the relaxation increases. . . . Now frown and crease your brows and study the tension. . . . Let go of the tension again. Smooth out the forehead once more. . . .
- Now, close your eyes tighter and tighter. Feel the tension . . . and relax your eyes. Keep your eyes closed, gently, comfortably, and notice the relaxation. . . .
- Now clench your jaws, bite your teeth together. Study the tension throughout the jaws. . . . Relax your jaws now. Let your lips part slightly. . . . Appreciate the relaxation. . . .
- Now, press your tongue hard against the roof of your mouth. Look for the tension. . . . All right, press your lips together tighter and tighter. . . . Relax the lips.
- Note the contrast between tension and relaxation. . . . Feel the relaxation all over your face . . . all over your forehead and scalp . . . eyes, jaws, lips, tongue . . . and your neck muscles.

EXERCISE 2

- Press your head back as far as it can go and feel the tension in the neck. . . . Roll it to the right, and feel the tension shift. . . . Now roll it to the left. Straighten your head and bring it forward and press your chin against your chest. . . . Let your head return to a comfortable position, and study the relaxation. . . . Let the relaxation develop. . . .
- Shrug your shoulders right up. Hold the tension. . . . Drop your shoulders and feel the relaxation in your neck and shoulders. . . . Shrug your shoulders again and move them around. Bring your shoulders up . . . and forward . . . and back. Feel the tension in your shoulders and in your upper back. . . . Drop your shoulders once more and relax.
- Let the relaxation spread deep into the shoulders . . . right into your back muscles. . . . Relax your neck and throat and jaws and other facial areas as the pure relaxation takes over and grows deeper . . . deeper . . . ever deeper.

Source: Seymour Diamond, "Pharmaceutical Management of Headaches in the Elderly Patient," *Topics in Geriatric Rehabilitation*, Vol. 5:4, Aspen Publishers, Inc., © 1990.

Muscle Relaxation Exercises

Relaxation is very important in obtaining good breathing control. Once the feeling of muscular tightness is recognized, it will be easy to appreciate the contrast of muscular relaxation. Remember to:

- Practice daily.
- Perform these exercises in a quiet, comfortably warm room.
- Avoid pain.
- Perform all exercises slowly and smoothly.
- Breathe naturally throughout all exercises.

SHOULDER SHRUGGING

Sit in a chair and let your arms hang loosely by your side. Shrug your shoulders and tighten the muscles as much as possible. Hold the position until the muscles of the neck and shoulders feel tight. Hold for a count of five. Release the tension and let the shoulders drop. Repeat three times.

HEAD CIRCLES

Sitting in a chair, let your arms hang loosely, with shoulders relaxed and drooped. Roll your head slowly and loosely from side to side. Reverse direction of the head circle. Repeat three times to each side.

SHOULDER ROLLING

While sitting comfortably, roll a shoulder slowly, clockwise, then counterclockwise. Repeat three times for each side and then three times rolling both shoulders together clockwise, then counterclockwise.

ARM AND FIST TIGHTENING

While sitting comfortably, clinch the right fist tightly and bend the elbow. Hold for a count of five. Release the fist and contraction of the arm, and allow the arm to straighten slowly. Repeat three times.

ARMS OVERHEAD WITH CHEST TIGHTENING

Lying on your back with arms resting at both sides, slowly raise extended arms overhead until palms of your hands meet. Slowly press palms together until you feel a contraction of your chest muscles. Hold for a count of five. Gradually release the pressure at the hands and return arms to your side. Repeat three times.

Source: Carolyn J. Humphrey, *Home Care Nursing Handbook*, ed 2, Aspen Publishers, Inc., © 1994.

Biofeedback

INTRODUCTION

When a person experiences acute pain where actual tissue damage is occurring, the body's automatic and protective reaction is to tense up and restrict movement of the painful area. This is a helpful reaction that serves to promote survival. However, in chronic pain there is often no ongoing tissue damage, so the body's natural reaction to tense up leads to chronically tense muscles that can actually become a major reason for the pain to continue. In addition, most people experience increased stress and worry with a chronic pain problem. This adds to tension levels affecting muscles, joints, and connective tissues. The nervous system also is more active under stress and can have increased sensitivity to pain. Because these physical signs of tension can greatly increase pain, tension reduction methods such as biofeedback are common treatments in pain centers.

Biofeedback helps people learn to better recognize and control physical tension that aggravates their pain. Biofeedback has also been found helpful in treating anxiety, high blood pressure, Raynaud's disease, insomnia, teeth grinding, and irritable bowel syndrome.

WHAT IS BIOFEEDBACK?

Biofeedback is a way of providing auditory and visual feedback on certain biological functions (hence the name biofeedback). When people get feedback on what is going on in their bodies, they can learn how to better control their physiology. For chronic pain patients, biofeedback is most commonly directed at general tension levels and also specific muscles that are problematically tense and overreactive. The biofeedback instruments provide immediate auditory or visual information on whether specific muscles are becoming more or less tense, which helps people learn how to relax them more deeply. Biofeedback in the pain management center is also directed at temperature and perspiration changes that reflect general tension levels.

The biofeedback treatments involve attaching electrical leads only to the surface of skin. No needles are involved and the procedure does not cause discomfort. In fact, most people find biofeedback treatments a relaxing and enjoyable experience.

Most people stay relatively unaware of the many biological changes occurring in their bodies. Increases in muscle tension levels can easily go unnoticed until pain is realized. Many people stay chronically tense, so their pain seems unrelated to fluctuations in stress levels. With the aid of the biofeedback instruments, patients learn to recognize problematic physiological changes and how to reverse them before they set off an episode of increased pain. Thus, biofeedback helps patients feel and be in greater control of their physiology, instead of feeling helpless to decrease chronic pain and pain flare-ups. This increased sense of control is a key factor underlying all behavioral strategies for pain management.

continues

continued

HOW IS IT DONE?

The first biofeedback appointment is for evaluation. This consists of measuring levels of physiology, such as muscle tension, during various tasks. If abnormalities are detected, then it is more likely that a patient will benefit from biofeedback treatment.

There are three stages of biofeedback treatment. First, patients learn to adjust their physiology (i.e., muscle tension) to a normal range while receiving auditory or visual feedback. Second, a patient learns to maintain this more normal physiology without receiving biofeedback from the instruments. This is verified in the office and then the patient learns to maintain this control while practicing at home. Third, a patient learns to maintain this control and functioning in a range nearer to normal while undergoing common daily activities.

Patients usually do not begin to experience benefit from biofeedback therapy until they are well into the first stage, which usually requires several appointments. Treatments are typically provided once per week until the first two stages of treatment are completed. Thereafter, patients are seen once or twice per month.

Research has shown that most individuals derive maximum benefit from about 10 treatments. Further treatments produce diminishing returns. However, for some individuals and some disorders, the maximum benefit is achieved only after dozens of treatments. This is particularly true with seizure disorders and neuromuscular rehabilitation.

Patients may also report additional improvements in the months following completion of treatment as they continue to practice the skills. For patients with chronic disorders, home practice at a frequency of at least three times per week is needed to maintain the benefits. Studies have shown that benefits persist for at least 10 years following treatment if the patient continues to practice at home.

CONCLUSION

Biofeedback is not magic nor a cure-all for pain disorders. For biofeedback to be successful, regular practice of the exercises by the patient is required. As with any single approach for chronic pain, it does not work for everyone. It does, however, provide one step, or piece of the puzzle, toward managing pain for many patients. Biofeedback is most beneficial for chronic pain when it is combined with other treatment approaches, such as physical therapy, self-hypnosis, counseling, TENS, medication, patient education, and pain management groups.

Source: Robert W. Lutz, The Medical Center at the University of California, San Francisco, California, © 1990. Published with permission of the Regents of the University of California.

Creating an Imagery Script

Imagery helps access and control both acute and chronic psychophysiologic pain. The following exercise can be done in 10 to 20 minutes.

PAIN IMAGERY SCRIPT

- Close your eyes and let yourself relax. . . . Begin to describe the pain in silence to yourself. Be present with the pain. . . . Know that the pain may be either physical sensations . . . or worries and fears. Let your pain take on a shape . . . any shape that comes to your mind. Become aware of the dimensions of the pain. . . . What is the height of your pain? . . . the width of the pain? . . . and the depth of the pain? Where in the body is it located? . . . Give it color . . . a shape . . . feel the texture. Does it make any sound?
- And now, with your eyes still closed, . . . let your hands come together with palms turned upward as if forming a cup. Put your pain object in your hands.
- Let yourself decide what you would like to do with the pain. There is no right way to finish the experience . . . just accept what feels right to you. You can throw the pain away . . . or place it back where you found it . . . or move it somewhere else. Let yourself become aware . . . of how pain can be changed. . . . By your focusing with intention, the pain changes.

It is not unusual for the pain to go completely away or at least lessen after this exercise. You can learn to manipulate the pain so that it is not the controlling factor of your life. The exercise is also effective with severe pain. After taking pain medication, use the imagery process to relax.

SPECIAL/SAFE PLACE IMAGERY SCRIPTS

Identify a special place that is a safe retreat. This is an easy place for novices to start. It takes 10 to 20 minutes. Several different approaches can be useful.

- Let your imagination choose a place that is safe and comfortable . . . a place where you can retreat at any time. This is a healthy technique for you to learn . . . this place will help you survive your daily stressors. This safe and special place is very important, particularly while you are in the hospital [if applicable]. . . . Any time that there are interruptions, just let yourself go to this place in your mind.
- Form a clear image of a pleasant outdoor scene, using all of your senses. Smell . . . smell the fragrance of flowers or the breeze. Feel . . . feel the texture of the surface under your feet. Hear . . . hear all the sounds in nature, birds singing, wind blowing. See . . . see all the different sights around as you let yourself turn in a slow circle to get a full view of this special space. [Include taste, if appropriate.]

continues

continued

- Let a beam of light, such as the rays of the sun, shine on you for comfort and healing. Allow yourself to experience the warmth and relaxation.
- Form an image of a meadow. Imagine that you are in the meadow. . . . The meadow is full of beautiful grass and flowers. In the meadow, see yourself sitting by a stream . . . watching the water . . . flowing by . . . slowly and gently.
- Imagine a mountain scene. See yourself walking on a path toward the mountain. You hear the sound of your shoes on the path . . . smell the pine trees and feel the cool breeze as you approach your campsite. You have now reached the foothills of the mountain. You are now higher up the mountain . . . resting in your campsite. Look around at the beauty of this place.
- Imagine yourself in a bamboo forest. . . . You are walking in a large bamboo forest. The bamboo is very tall. . . . You lean against a strong cluster of bamboo . . . hear the swaying . . . and hear the rustling of the bamboo leaves, gently moving in the wind.
- Look into the sky of your mind . . . see the fluffy clouds. A cloud gently comes your way, . . . and the cloud surrounds your body. You climb up on the cloud and lie down. Feel yourself begin to float off gently in a gentle breeze.

RED BALL OF PAIN IMAGERY SCRIPT

To decrease psychophysiologic pain, you can learn to use distraction. This kind of imagery is good for both acute and chronic pain, as well as for the discomfort or pain of procedures. It takes 10 to 20 minutes.

- Scan your body . . . gather any pains, aches, or other symptoms up into a ball. Begin to change its size . . . allow it to get bigger . . . just imagine how big you can make it. Now make it smaller. . . . See how small you can make it. . . . Is it possible to make it the size of a grain of sand? Now allow it to move slowly out of your body, moving further away each time you exhale. . . . Notice the experience with each exhale . . . as the pain moves away.
- Try changing the size of the ball several times in both directions. This serves as a distraction and shows how to manipulate the pain experience rather than being trapped or overwhelmed by the pain. It provides a tremendous sense of control as well as pain relief.

Source: Barbara Montgomery Dossey, "Imagery: Awakening the Inner Healer," *Holistic Nursing: A Handbook for Practice*, ed 2, Barbara Montgomery Dossey et al., eds., Aspen Publishers, Inc., © 1995.

Creating a Personal Music Tape

Individuals can create their own tapes to match their moods and musical preference. If their mood is tense or angry and a quiet outcome is desired, they may start out with a short selection (three minutes or less) of music that resonates with the mood and then add selections that increasingly move to a relaxed state.

Before creating a personal tape, an individual should spend some time experimenting with music—trying a variety of musical selections and learning what happens when listening to specific selections. "Experimental listening" involves listening to various types of music at different times of the day and week. For example, spend 20 minutes listening to each type of music and then systematically evaluate your response to the selection, according to the following procedure:

1. Set aside 20 minutes of relaxation time.
2. Find a comfortable position.
3. Find a quiet place where you will not be interrupted.
4. Check your pulse rate.
5. Observe your breathing pattern (fast, slow, normal).
6. Assess your muscular tension (pain, muscle tightness, shoulder stiffness, jaw and neck tension). Are you loose, limp, sleepy?
7. Evaluate your mood state (angry, happy, sad).
8. Listen to the music for 20 minutes. Let your body respond to the music as it wishes: loosen muscles, lie down, dance, clap, hum.
9. Following the session, assess your breathing pattern.
10. Assess your muscular tension. (Are you more relaxed? more stimulated? tighter? tenser? calmer?)
11. Evaluate your mood state.
12. Record the name of the music selection and your before-and-after responses in a music notebook for use when developing your own therapeutic tapes.
13. On a separate page in your notebook, recall and write down the many ways that music has empowered your life psychologically, physically, and spiritually. Include your most dramatic, intimate, and emotional memories associated with music. You will begin to realize the importance of sound in your life and recognize its healing potential.

Based on your response, create your own relaxation music tape of 20 to 30 minutes in length. The more regularly you use the tape, the more effective it will become. Music therapy may be incorporated into daily living activities, such as taking a "music bath" after a morning shower as a means of balancing the body and mind for the events of the day.

Source: Cathie E. Guzzetta, "Music Therapy: Hearing the Melody of the Soul," *Holistic Nursing: A Handbook for Practice*, ed 2, Barbara Montgomery Dossey et al., eds., Aspen Publishers, Inc., © 1995.

Where to Go for Help with Pain Management

- Seek out a large rehabilitation center affiliated with a university hospital or other primary care hospital.
- Choose a doctor experienced in SCI management who is knowledgeable about pain.
- Choose a doctor who works with other health care professionals as part of a multispecialty team and can provide referrals, including to psychosocial professionals experienced in pain.
- Choose a doctor with access to several professional resources.
- Choose only those treating professionals whom you can communicate with and trust.
- Your responsibilities include:
  —being flexible and cooperative
  —working jointly with health care professionals to find solutions to managing your pain
  —following treatment instructions
  —taking an active role in treatment

If you cannot find help:

- Call your state Society of Physical Medicine and Rehabilitation and ask them to help you locate a physician experienced in treating SCI pain. If you cannot find this number, contact the American Academy of Physical Medicine and Rehabilitation (312) 464-9700 in Chicago and ask for the phone number of your state society.
- Contact the nearest comprehensive pain center for an evaluation. Your doctor can help you locate such a center near you.

Notes:

Source: J. Scott Richards, *Pain and Spinal Cord Injury*, American Association of Spinal Cord Injury Psychologists and Social Workers, Jackson Heights, New York.

10
Medications

> Most materials in the *Spinal Cord Injury Patient Education Resource Manual* are intended for the health care professional to share with the patient. Materials that are intended solely for the professional are labeled "Exhibit" in the table of contents.

General Instructions

Medications: Overview	335
Tips for Taking Medications Safely	338
Medication Instruction Sheet (Form)	339
Daily Medication Schedule (Form)	340

Medications for Spinal Cord Injuries

Bladder Medications	341
Bowel Medications	344
Pain Medications	347
Spasticity Medications	348
Miscellaneous Medications	349

GENERAL INSTRUCTIONS

Medications: Overview

WHAT IS THE PURPOSE OF MEDICATIONS?

Medications are taken to help your body adjust to the changes that have occurred since your spinal cord was injured. To give you the best possible care, your doctor must be told your *complete medical and surgical history*:

- Tell the doctor what over-the-counter and prescribed medications you are taking right now.
- Describe any allergies to medications you might have.
- **Always notify your doctor if you are pregnant.** Medications you take will affect your baby, too.

HOW DO MEDICATIONS WORK?

Medications contain chemicals that interact with your body:

- They replace chemicals that may be low in your body.
- They help body systems that aren't working right.
- They maintain the chemical balance throughout your body.

Drugs also interact with each other. One drug can stop another from working properly or can make another drug have a greater effect than is needed.

- Your doctor **always** needs to know **all** the medications you are taking to be sure they work well together.
- Check with your doctor about drinking beer, wine, or liquor, because alcohol affects the way many drugs work.
- Take the medications your doctor has ordered exactly as they are prescribed. Always check with him or her if you feel you need to increase or decrease the dose.

When you return to your clinic, you and your doctor will work together to wean you off any medications you no longer need for your health.

KNOW YOUR MEDICATIONS

Medications come in different forms. They vary in size, shape, or color and have distinct markings on them. They may be in the form of tablets, capsules, ointments, or liquids.

- Know the **names** of your medications.
- Know what they **look like**. (Remember: Generic medications may look different.)

continues

continued

- Know the **dosages** and **times** they should be taken.
- Know **why** you are taking them.
- Know any **side effects** they might cause.

You alone are responsible for all this information so that you can be independent in caring for yourself. If someone else is giving medicine to you, *personally verify each medication* before you take it.

Use a chart to help you keep a record of your medications. You and your nurse should fill this out before your hospital discharge. In the future, if your doctor orders a new medication, take the time to find out its name and purpose and add it to your chart. With these details in one place, you can now be sure your medications are taken as directed.

SIDE EFFECTS

Most medications can cause side effects in your body. These usually are not a problem because they can be controlled by regulating the amount of drug you take and when you take it. *Notify your doctor if you notice any discomfort from your medicines.*

DRUG ALLERGIES

An unpredictable side effect can cause an allergic or anaphylactic (*ANN-ah-fill-ACK-tick*) reaction. Some reactions occur immediately and some are delayed several days. Know what to look for and what to do:

- The most common symptom is a skin reaction such as itching or rash.
- Call your doctor **right away**.
- If you have difficulty breathing or any other **severe** reaction to any medicine, **CALL THE AMBULANCE** immediately and go to the emergency department.

HOW DO YOU KNOW WHEN TO TAKE YOUR MEDICATION?

Medication is usually scheduled for two, three, or four times each day. The schedule will be written on the prescription bottle or on the envelope containing your pills. Most medications are spaced at least four hours apart. Taking them more often is unwise, but feel free to ask your doctor how best to fit medications into your personal daily schedule. Learn how long you should continue the medication. Be prepared to renew your medication *long* before your supply runs out.

continues

continued

GUIDELINES TO SUCCESS IN TAKING YOUR MEDICATION

- If refrigeration is required, keep the medicine in the refrigerator. This will avoid spoilage or loss of potency.
- If directions say to mix a medication with water or juice, do so. This will provide faster absorption.
- Do not give your medications to friends or relatives. Your medications are specifically prescribed for you. They may be dangerous for another person.
- Keep medications out of reach of children.
- If you have any questions about your medication, contact your doctor, nurse, or spinal cord clinic.

Notes:

Source: *Spinal Cord Injury Manual*, Kessler Institute for Rehabilitation, West Orange, New Jersey.

Tips for Taking Medications Safely

To use medications safely, you will need to:

- Understand why the medicine is being taken, for example:
  - to control blood pressure
  - for an infection
  - for pain
- Know how much (the dose), how often, and when it is to be taken.
- Know when to stop taking the medication. Always take the whole prescription, unless the doctor says otherwise.
- Tell the doctor about any problems (negative side effects) that may happen when taking a medicine, for example:
  - feeling dizzy
  - trouble with voiding
  - constipation
  - feeling tired
  - sexuality changes/concerns
  - bleeding or bruising
  - rash
- Ask the doctor if there are any foods or medications that should be avoided when taking a medicine.
- When adding a new medication, ask the doctor if it is possible to stop taking another medication. **Never** stop taking a medication without talking to the doctor first.

Have a "brown-bag session" with the doctor. A brown-bag session is when all medications—including "over-the-counter medications"—are put in a bag and taken to a doctor visit. (Over-the-counter medications are those bought without a doctor's prescription, for example, Tylenol.) A brown-bag session gives the doctor a clear picture of what you are taking. This session is a chance to ask questions and discuss side effects and/or concerns.

Source: Kelly B. Wascher, ed., *Patient Education and Discharge Planning Manual for Rehabilitation*, St. Joseph Rehabilitation Hospital and Outpatient Center, Aspen Publishers, Inc., © 1995.

Medication Instruction Sheet

NAME OF MEDICATION

DOSE

PURPOSE

SIDE EFFECTS

SPECIAL INSTRUCTIONS

NAME
DATE

Source: Kelly B. Wascher, ed., *Patient Education and Discharge Planning Manual for Rehabilitation*, St. Joseph Rehabilitation Hospital and Outpatient Center, Aspen Publishers, Inc., © 1995.

Daily Medication Schedule

TIME	MEDICATIONS

Source: Kelly B. Wascher, ed., *Patient Education and Discharge Planning Manual for Rehabilitation*, St. Joseph Rehabilitation Hospital and Outpatient Center, Aspen Publishers, Inc., © 1995.

MEDICATIONS FOR SPINAL CORD INJURIES

Bladder Medications

DITROPAN

- **Why is it prescribed?**
  —To relax the bladder and help it to hold more urine
- **How should you take this medicine?**
  —Follow instructions given by your doctor.
- **What are side effects to look for?**
  —Drowsiness, dizziness, or blurred vision—drive with caution.
  —Dry mouth—suck on hard candy.
  —Diarrhea—call your doctor.
- **What should you know about this medicine?**
  —May cause overheating, fever, or heat stroke due to decreased sweating.
  —Be careful when in the sun or a hot room.

EPHEDRINE

- **Why is it prescribed?**
  —To relieve bladder spasms and prevent leaking
- **How should you take this medicine?**
  —Follow instructions given by your doctor.
- **What are side effects to look for?**
  —Drowsiness, dizziness, or blurred vision—drive with caution.
  —Dry mouth—suck on hard candy.
- **What should you know about this medicine?**
  —If side effects continue, call your doctor.

HYTRIN

- **Why is it prescribed?**
  —To relax the sphincter
  —To help control dysreflexia
- **How should you take this medicine?**
  —Take medicine at bedtime.
- **What are side effects to look for?**
  —Dizziness and fainting
- **What should you know about this medicine?**
  —Do not drive a car until the effect of the medicine is known.
  —Call the doctor if dizziness persists.

continues

continued

MINIPRESS

- **Why is it prescribed?**
  —To relax the sphincter
  —To help control dysreflexia
- **How should you take this medicine?**
  —Follow instructions given by your doctor.
- **What are side effects to look for?**
  —Dizziness due to lowered blood pressure
- **What should you know about this medicine?**
  —If side effects continue, call your doctor.

PROBANTHINE

- **Why is it prescribed?**
  —To reduce bladder spasms
  —To increase bladder volume
  —To help control sweating
- **How should you take this medicine?**
  —Do not take antacids at the same time that you take this medicine.
  —Space apart 1 to 2 hours.
- **What are side effects to look for?**
  —Dizziness, nervousness, drowsiness, blurred vision, nausea, constipation, difficulty in breathing—call your doctor.
  —Dry mouth—suck on hard candy.
- **What should you know about this medicine?**
  —May cause overheating, fever, and heat stroke due to decreased sweating. Be careful when in the sun or a hot room.

SUDAFED

- **Why is it prescribed?**
  —To help prevent bladder leakage
- **How should you take this medicine?**
  —Take medicine in the morning.
- **What are side effects to look for?**
  —Dry mouth, nervousness
- **What should you know about this medicine?**
  —If medicine keeps you awake, call the doctor.
  —Notify your doctor if you have high blood pressure.

continues

continued

TOFRANIL

- **Why is it prescribed?**
  —To help prevent bladder leakage
- **How should you take this medicine?**
  —Take with a meal or snack to prevent stomach upset.
- **What are side effects to look for?**
  —Drowsiness, dizziness, or blurred vision—drive with caution.
  —Confusion, fainting, sore throat, skin rash—call your doctor.
- **What should you know about this medicine?**
  —Avoid alcohol.
  —Wear sunscreen—this medicine may make you burn more easily.

URECHOLINE

- **Why is it prescribed?**
  —To help the bladder wall muscle contract to push out urine
- **How should you take this medicine?**
  —Follow instructions given by your doctor.
- **What are side effects to look for?**
  —Dizziness due to lowered blood pressure
  —Sweating
  —Changes in bowel function
- **What should you know about this medicine?**
  —Take with food or milk to decrease stomach upset.
  —Call your doctor if side effects continue.

URISPAS

- **Why is it prescribed?**
  —To help prevent bladder leakage
- **How should you take this medicine?**
  —Follow instructions given by your doctor.
- **What are side effects to look for?**
  —Drowsiness, dizziness, or blurred vision—drive with caution.
  —Nausea, vomiting—call your doctor.
- **What should you know about this medicine?**
  —If side effects continue, call your doctor.

Source: Adapted from Donna Schachtel, et al., *Key to Independence Personal Care Manual*, Shepherd Spinal Center, Atlanta, Georgia, © 1989. To order a complete version of the manual, contact the Shepherd Center at 404-350-7361, and *Spinal Cord Injury Manual*, Kessler Institute for Rehabilitation, West Orange, New Jersey.

Bowel Medications

ANESTHETIC CREAMS

Nupercainal Ointment
Anusol Cream

- **Why is it prescribed?**
  - To prevent dysreflexia
  - To decrease feeling of discomfort or pain
- **What should you know about this medicine?**
  - It should be put into rectum 5 to 10 minutes before giving suppository, doing digital stimulation, or manual removal.

BULK FORMERS

Citrucel
Metamucil
Fiber Cookies

- **Why are they prescribed?**
  - To soften and increase size of stool
- **What should you know about this medicine?**
  - It will cause constipation if you do not drink enough fluids.

ENEMA

Fleet's enema

- **Why is it prescribed?**
  - To increase movement of the bowel
- **What should you know about this medicine?**
  - It should only be used if you are very constipated, and as prescribed by your doctor.
  - It should not be used all the time, as it decreases bowel elasticity.

"MINI" ENEMA

Theravac Enema
Fleet's Bisacodyl

- **Why is it prescribed?**
  - To start movement of the bowel
  - To soften and lubricate stool

continues

continued

- **What should you know about this medicine?**
  - It may be used to start a bowel program.
  - It often costs more than suppositories.

PERISTALTIC STIMULATORS

Pericolace
Doxidan
Dialose-plus

- **Why are they prescribed?**
  - To start movement of the bowel
- **What should you know about this medicine?**
  - If stool becomes too soft or loose, decrease the number of pills taken in a day or stop the medication (per your doctor's instructions).
  - Drink plenty of fluids.

STOOL SOFTENERS

Colace
Surfak
Dialose
Ducosate Sodium

- **Why are they prescribed?**
  - To soften stool, allowing for easier movement through the bowel
- **What should you know about this medicine?**
  - Drink plenty of fluids.
  - If stool becomes too soft, decrease number of stool softener pills taken in a day or stop pills for a short period, restarting pills when stool is firm (per your doctor's instructions).
  - It prevents, but does not treat, constipation.

HEMORRHOIDAL SUPPOSITORIES

Anusol Suppositories

- **Why are they prescribed?**
  - To decrease swelling of hemorrhoids
- **What should you know about this medicine?**
  - It should be taken $\frac{1}{2}$ to 1 hour before bowel program to lessen discomfort and/or bleeding, as prescribed by your doctor.

continues

continued

SUPPOSITORIES

Dulcolax (firm, cone-shaped)
Glycerine (soft, pencil-shaped)

- **Why are they prescribed?**
  —To irritate the lining of the rectum to start bowel movement
- **What should you know about this medicine?**
  —It is used to START bowel program. You may stop using suppositories as the bowel is trained (per your doctor's instructions).
  —Be sure suppository is placed against bowel wall, or it will not work.
  —Be sure to remove any stool in the rectum before inserting suppository.
  —Glycerine is often less costly and less irritating.
  —Dulcolax may cause cramping.

Notes:

Source: Adapted from Kelly B. Wascher, ed., *Patient Education and Discharge Planning Manual for Rehabilitation*, St. Joseph Rehabilitation Hospital and Outpatient Center, Aspen Publishers, Inc., © 1995, and *Spinal Cord Injury Manual*, Kessler Institute for Rehabilitation, West Orange, New Jersey.

Pain Medications

ELAVIL

Same as Norpramin

NORPRAMIN

- **Why is it prescribed?**
  - To treat neurogenic pain
  - In high doses, to treat depression
- **What should you know about this medicine?**
  - Avoid alcohol.
  - This drug can cause drowsiness.

TEGRETOL

- **Why is it prescribed?**
  - To control neurogenic pain
  - To control seizures
- **What should you know about this medicine?**
  - Must have routine blood work done, because Tegretol can cause anemia in some people.
  - This drug can cause dizziness or drowsiness.

Notes:

Source: *Spinal Cord Injury Manual*, Kessler Institute for Rehabilitation, West Orange, New Jersey.

Spasticity Medications

BACLOFEN (Lioresal)

- **Why is it prescribed?**
  - To relax skeletal muscle to decrease spasticity
  - To relax the external sphincter to allow the passage of urine when the bladder contracts
- **What should you know about this medicine?**
  - It must **not** be discontinued abruptly; dosage must be decreased gradually down to zero. (If, for some reason, you suddenly cannot take it by mouth, intravenous (IV) Valium will be used to wean you slowly.)
  - If discontinued abruptly, this drug can cause hallucinations, increased spasticity, abdominal cramping, and tiredness.
  - Avoid drinking alcohol.

CLONIDINE (Catapres)

- **Why is it prescribed?**
  - To lower high blood pressure
  - To reduce spasticity
- **What should you know about this medicine?**
  - With prolonged use, get routine eye exams.
  - Can cause increased constipation (in which case, your bowel medication will be adjusted to help relieve this effect).
  - This drug can cause lowered blood pressure.

DANTRIUM

- **Why is it prescribed?**
  - To relax skeletal muscle to reduce spasticity due to injury to the spinal cord or brain
- **What should you know about this medicine?**
  - This drug can cause muscle weakness or liver damage (blood level tests must be done to check the health of the liver).
  - Avoid alcohol or over-the-counter medications.

DIAZEPAM (Valium)

- **Why is it prescribed?**
  - to relax skeletal muscle to reduce spasticity
  - To decrease anxiety
- **What should you know about this medicine?**
  - This drug can cause addiction, tiredness, or decrease in alertness.
  - Avoid alcohol.

Source: *Spinal Cord Injury Manual*, Kessler Institute for Rehabilitation, West Orange, New Jersey.

Miscellaneous Medications

COUMADIN

- **Why is it prescribed?**
  — To thin the blood and prevent clots that lead to deep vein thrombosis and pulmonary embolis
- **What should you know about this medicine?**
  — Take on an empty stomach at the same time each day.
  — Use a soft toothbrush, as gums may bleed.
  — Report any sign of bleeding to your doctor.
  — This drug can cause bruising to occur easily.

CIMETIDINE (Tagamet) AND RANITIDINE (Zantac)

- **Why is it prescribed?**
  — To prevent or treat stomach ulcers by lowering the secretion of acid in the stomach

DIDRONEL

- **Why is it prescribed?**
  — To prevent calcium from being added to areas of excess bone growth (heterotopic ossification)

INVERSINE

- **Why is it prescribed?**
  — To treat severe sweating that comes with spinal cord injury
  — To treat moderate to severe high blood pressure
- **What should you know about this medicine?**
  — This drug can cause lowered blood pressure.

ANTIBIOTICS

- **Why are they prescribed?**
  — To kill bacteria that cause infections
- **What should you know about this medicine?**
  — Take only by doctor's orders.
  — Take **ALL** that is prescribed even if the signs and symptoms are no longer present. This is to destroy **ALL** the bacteria involved.
  — Wounds and urine will be tested once in a while to make sure that the correct antibiotic has been used to treat the infection.

Source: *Spinal Cord Injury Manual*, Kessler Institute for Rehabilitation, West Orange, New Jersey.

11

Independent Living Strategies

> Most materials in the *Spinal Cord Injury Patient Education Resource Manual* are intended for the health care professional to share with the patient. Materials that are intended solely for the professional are labeled "Exhibit" in the table of contents.

Personal Attendants

What Are Personal Assistance Services?	353
My Needs Inventory	354
Assessing My Lifestyle	355
The Job Description	357
Job Description Worksheet (Form)	358
Options for Finding Personal Assistants	359
Sample Employment Application (Form)	361
Interviewing: Overview	363
Questions to Think about When You Interview an Attendant	364
Request for Reference Information (Form)	366
Reference Information Waiver	367
Agreement Between Employer and Attendant (Form)	368
Guidelines for Attendant Training (Form)	369
Emergency Backup Attendant Care	370
Communicating with Your Attendant	373
Who Pays for Personal Assistance?	376

Travel

Travel after a Spinal Cord Injury	377
Tips for Hassle-Free Flying	379

The Americans with Disabilities Act

Understanding the ADA	381

PERSONAL ATTENDANTS*

What Are Personal Assistance Services?

When you incur a severe disability, such as a spinal cord injury, you must come to terms with many issues. You may need to rely on others to accomplish the basic tasks of daily living. Independent living is encouraged, but what does this mean? Many people with new injuries expect that they will be able to do everything for themselves. However, because of physical limitations you may be unable to do certain tasks. Does the fact that you will have to rely on others to meet some of your needs mean that you have failed at independent living? Not at all. Many people with no spinal cord injury rely on others to fulfill needs. Thus, independence should be seen as being able to control what is done, how it is done, who does it, and when. The use of personal assistants to meet your needs in no way takes away from your independence.

Various types of services are available:

- *personal services*—including assistance with bathing, personal hygiene, bowel and bladder care, dressing, grooming, transferring, feeding, and giving medications
- *household services*—including assistance with meal preparation, shopping, cleaning, and laundry
- *communication services*—including assistance with reading and writing
- *mobility services*—including escort and driving

A personal assistant is there to provide physical assistance with tasks you are unable to do on your own. You make the decisions and the assistant provides his or her physical ability.

*Note: Because the terms *attendant* and *assistant* are often used interchangeably in the field of SCI, both are incorporated into this chapter.

Source: Melvyn R. Tanzman, *Living Independently with Personal Assistance*, American Association of Spinal Cord Injury Psychologists and Social Workers, Jackson Heights, New York.

My Needs Inventory

Communicating your needs clearly is very important when working with an attendant. To communicate clearly, you must be specific and make sure your needs are as well defined and as detailed as possible. The following worksheet will help you to be very specific about the different aspects of attendant care that you need.

PERSONAL CARE NEEDS

Bathing:	Type of bath (shower, bed bath, set-up)? How often? What time of day? How long does it take?
Dressing:	Complete help? Partial help? Special considerations? How long does it take?
Oral hygiene:	How often?
Bowel care:	Type of bowel program? If any, how often? Time of day? How long does it take?
Bladder care:	Type of bladder program, if any? How often? Times of day? How long does it take?
Toileting:	Bedpan? Commode, toilet?
Transferring:	Type of transfer? When needed? Special considerations?
Eating:	Other than meal preparation, any special help? Special diet?
Medication:	Type? How often needed? Who administers? Attendants may or may not be able to assist with this.
Exercises:	Type? How often? How long does it take?

HOMEMAKING NEEDS

Laundry:	How often? Where done?
Housecleaning:	How often? How many rooms? Specific chores?
Meal preparation:	Times of meals? Who will plan?
Grocery shopping:	How often? Where? Who will go?

OTHER NEEDS

Job or school:	Schedule of work or classes? Help needed?
Social needs:	Activities? Help needed?
Finances:	Help with banking, checking, or correspondence?
Transportation needs:	Special equipment needs, equipment maintenance?

Source: Sara Roberts and Nancy Sydow, *Consumer's Guide to Attendant Care*, Access to Independence, Inc., © 1984.

Assessing My Lifestyle

This worksheet is especially for use by people who need a live-in attendant, but some aspects of it are also relevant to those who have come-in attendants. Because you will be working so closely with an attendant, it is important that you have not only a clear understanding of your needs, but also an awareness of your own personal habits and skills. Completing this worksheet may also help you discover areas in which you may need to gain more knowledge. For example, if you have never had to be responsible for housekeeping, you may need to learn what kinds of household products are needed and how they are used because it's possible that your attendant may need direction from you in this area. This worksheet also can help you decide what information about your personal habits you feel is important to communicate to your attendant.

FOOD AND EATING ARRANGEMENTS

- What kind of foods do I usually eat?
  - Likes?
  - Dislikes?
- Am I good at supervising someone who cooks?
- Where do I shop for groceries?
- Do I eat at regular times or when I feel like it?
- How do I feel about eating with my attendant?
- How do I feel about giving cooking instructions to my attendant?

HOUSEKEEPING

- What do I know about housekeeping and laundry?
- Do I like things very neat, or am I not particular?
- How do I feel about giving cleaning instructions?
- Would I like a definite schedule for cleaning and laundry—for example, vacuum on Monday, scrub floors on Tuesday, etc.—or would I prefer to be more flexible?

PERSONAL CARE

- How often do I need to bathe?
- How often do I need a shampoo?
- Is my personal appearance important to me?

PERSONAL HABITS, ETC.

- Do I smoke?
- Do I drink alcohol?
- Do I take drugs or smoke pot?

continues

continued

- Do I like to sleep late in the morning or get up early?
- What time do I usually go to bed at night?
- Do I go out to visit friends and to participate in other social activities?
- Will I want to entertain friends and family in my apartment?
- Would it be troublesome to me if my roommate wanted to have a friend stay overnight?
- Do I usually like activities well planned, or do I like them to be spontaneous?
- What do I like to do for entertainment?
- Do I like to listen to music?
  - What kind?
  - What volume?
- Do I like a quiet atmosphere?
- Do I like to watch TV?
- What hobbies do I have?
- Do I consider myself a flexible person? Example?
- How do I react if I have to change my plans at the last minute?
- Describe my personality:
- Is there a spiritual aspect to my life that is important?
- In general, could it be said that I take responsibility for my own life?

Notes:

Source: Sara Roberts and Nancy Sydow, *Consumer's Guide to Attendant Care*, Access to Independence, Inc., © 1984.

The Job Description

Before you begin the advertising and interview process, you must know the kind of help you need. You should list your needs, such as dressing, using the bathroom, and washing, as well as cleaning and washing the car, mowing the lawn, or defrosting the freezer. Include all your needs and what you expect from the personal assistant. This list will be part of the job description. A complete job description includes these six sections:

1. **Job Title:** The title "personal assistant" is used most. Other titles may be personal care attendant, companion, homemaker, or driver.
2. **Summary of Work:** This is a brief description of the type of services you need. For example, "John Jones needs assistance preparing for work in the morning, driving to and from work, and preparing for bed."
3. **Qualifications for a Personal Assistant:** When you interview the person for your job, these are some qualifications you may want to consider:
   - a certificate, training, and/or experience
   - dependability
   - respect for you and your property
   - cleanliness
   - drug and alcohol free
   - physical strength
   - ability to follow directions

   You may want to list other qualifications that suit your needs, such as nonsmoker, animal lover, etc.
4. **Duties:** This is where you will include the complete list of your needs.
5. **Schedule:** You should list the hours you want your assistant to work. Also, set up a system to make changes in the schedule. For example, you might want to make sure that you and your assistant give two weeks' notice (except in emergencies) to request a schedule change.
6. **Salary:** You have three choices: list a set salary, list a salary range (e.g., $5–$7/hr.), or state that the salary will be based on qualifications and experience.

This job description will help you in many ways. It is an informal contract that lists what you expect. If both you and your assistant keep this contract, there will be fewer problems. As your needs change, you can change the job description with your personal assistant.

Source: Melvyn R. Tanzman, *Living Independently with Personal Assistance*, American Association of Spinal Cord Injury Psychologists and Social Workers, Jackson Heights, New York.

Job Description Worksheet

BATHING: _____

_____

DRESSING: _____

_____

HELPING TO BATHROOM: _____

_____

BLADDER CARE: _____

BOWEL CARE: _____

TYPE OF TRANSFER: _____

EXERCISES: _____

PREPARATION OF MEALS: _____

_____

HOUSEKEEPING: _____

LAUNDRY: _____

GROCERY SHOPPING: _____

CORRESPONDENCE, FINANCES: _____

OTHER NEEDS—SCHOOL, SOCIAL, JOB, OCCASIONAL ASSISTANCE TO ACHIEVE A SKILL TO INCREASE INDEPENDENCE: _____

_____

TRANSPORTATION: _____

TIME OFF: _____

_____

Source: Sara Roberts and Nancy Sydow, *Consumer's Guide to Attendant Care*, Access to Independence, Inc., © 1984.

Options for Finding Personal Assistants

When you are ready to use personal assistance services, your first task, after learning what kind of help you need and for how many hours, is to find assistants. The use of hired personal assistants, rather than nurses or family members, will afford you the most control. Nurses have been trained to perform tasks in a set manner and may be unwilling to take directions from you. They may also feel that household tasks are not their professional job. Family members may tend to take control and resist your input. They may do "for you" instead of doing "with you." A hired assistant must take directions from you or be fired. You can choose to hire through an agency, or you can advertise and hire on your own. You must choose the method you prefer.

HOME HEALTH AGENCIES

Your local Yellow Pages will probably have listings for home health agencies. These agencies often provide personal assistants, as well as nurses. There are many good reasons to use an agency. First, they can provide an assistant within several days of your request. Second, they can provide backup assistance on an emergency basis. Third, agencies are a good choice if you are unsure about training and directing your own assistant. You will also not have to handle the financial details.

However, there are bad points to using an agency. You will be giving up much of the direct control over your assistant. The agency nurse will train and manage your assistant. Thus, the nurse will be in charge of what the assistant does and does not do. You may be seen as a patient, rather than an employer. Another bad point of using an agency is the high cost. You can expect that the cost will be twice that of hiring an assistant on your own.

Some states may have employment agencies for health personnel. These agencies are often less costly because you and the personal assistant agree on the salary. You may have to pay a one-time fee to the employment agency. Employment agencies do not train personal assistants, but they should make sure that they are qualified.

HIRING PERSONAL ASSISTANTS ON YOUR OWN

If you decide that you want to hire on your own, there are many issues to think about:

- How many hours of help do you need?
- Do you need a person who lives nearby or has his or her own transportation?
- Do you need a driver?
- Do you want a male or a female personal assistant?
- Do you need personal care, homemaking, or both?
- Can you offer room and board in exchange for personal assistance?
- How much can you pay?

After thinking about these points you may want to try a "word of mouth" approach. For example, you can speak with friends, neighbors, and professionals. Consider the following resources:

continues

continued

- college job placement offices
- local bulletin boards in supermarkets, libraries, churches, and other public places
- hospital and nursing home bulletin boards
- local newspapers
- local independent living centers for the disabled
- state unemployment offices
- county or local offices for the disabled

If this does not work, you may consider placing an advertisement. It is important to keep the advertisement short and to the point. For example:

> PERSONAL ASSISTANT for individual with a disability. $__/hr in the northeast part of town. Six hours of assistance needed daily, 7–10 A.M. and 6–9 P.M. Assistance with personal needs, homemaking, and driving (license required). Male or female OK. Needed immediately. Call John at 546-6758.

or

> FREE ROOM AND BOARD and $__ per week in exchange for personal assistance to disabled professional. Quiet neighborhood, near transportation. Must be able to work 2–3 hours in the morning and 1–2 hours at night, to assist with personal needs and light housekeeping. Own bedroom and use of common kitchen and bath. Female preferred. Apply immediately. Call Susan at 695-4782.

Remember, the more you publicize the job, the more responses you will receive and the better your chance of finding the right assistant to match your needs.

Source: Melvyn R. Tanzman, *Living Independently with Personal Assistance*, American Association of Spinal Cord Injury Psychologists and Social Workers, Jackson Heights, New York.

Sample Employment Application

Name:_____ Date:_____ Phone:_____
Address:_____ ZIP:_____
      street   city   state
How long have you lived here?_____
Sex:_____ Age:_____ Birthdate:_____
In case of emergency, notify:_____
_____
Experience in attendant work/nursing/companionship/aide? _____
How long?_____ If so, where: _____
Date available:_____
Hours willing to work: Full-time_____ Part-time_____ Come-in _____
                   Live-in_____ Mornings_____ Afternoons _____
                   Evenings_____ Weekends_____ Overnight_____
How many hours per week?_____
Permanent_____ Temporary _____
Are you willing and able to do emergency attendant work? _____
If you are a student, what is your class schedule?
  Monday_____ Thursday_____
  Tuesday_____ Friday_____
  Wednesday _____
What is your means of transportation?_____ Valid driver's license? _____
Have you been convicted of a felony or misdemeanor or other offense within the past three years?_____If so, please explain:_____
_____

Are there any jobs that you would **not** want to do, (for example, drive, work for opposite sex, duties listed in job description, etc.)? _____
Who referred you?_____ Salary acceptable:_____
Restrictions on location of employment: _____
COMMENTS: _____
_____

continues

continued

Please list MOST RECENT employer FIRST.

Employer: _____

Address: _____ ZIP: _____

Work you did: _____

Dates of work: From _____ to _____

Reason for leaving: _____

Supervisor: _____ Phone: _____

Employer: _____

Address: _____ ZIP: _____

Work you did: _____

Dates of work: From _____ to _____

Reason for leaving: _____

Supervisor: _____ Phone: _____

Employer: _____

Address: _____ ZIP: _____

Work you did: _____

Dates of work: From _____ to _____

Reason for leaving: _____

Supervisor: _____ Phone: _____

PLEASE indicate which supervisors you want to use as references (you MUST indicate at least **two**.)

Additional references (use, if needed):

(include name, address, phone number, and relationship)

1. _____
   _____ ZIP: _____
   Phone: _____ Relationship: _____

2. _____
   _____ ZIP: _____
   Phone: _____ Relationship: _____

I understand that the information provided will be used in pursuit of employment.

Signed: _____ Date: _____

Source: Sara Roberts and Nancy Sydow, *Consumer's Guide to Attendant Care*, Access to Independence. Inc., © 1984.

Interviewing: Overview

The interview process should have two steps: a short telephone interview to see who might be good for the job and a face-to-face interview to make your final choice.

THE TELEPHONE INTERVIEW

This is an important tool that can help you save time and energy by ruling out those not suited to your needs. When a person calls in response to your advertisement, give the key information: the schedule you will need, the salary you are able to pay, and a list of your needs. Ask other questions as needed.

If you decide to interview the person, ask the applicant to bring the following:

- proof of citizenship (birth certificate, passport, voter's registration card)
- proof of address (driver's license, utility bill)
- Social Security number
- two references

THE FACE-TO-FACE INTERVIEW

Keep a record of each person, including name, address, phone number, good points, bad points, and your overall view. This list can be helpful in the future. When the person arrives, begin the interview in a friendly manner.

Get to know the person. Discuss the person's work experience: Did he or she enjoy the work; did he or she get along with other people; how long did he or she remain on each job? Length of time on each job is helpful for showing dependability. Discuss his or her personal history, such as social problems, health problems, driving record, and any criminal convictions.

During the interview, you should also do the following:

- Let the person know you. Talk about your disability and your needs. What are your personal likes and dislikes? What is your lifestyle? What are your goals? Such an open discussion can be useful, as it will help you and the person decide whether you can work together.
- Describe the job in detail. This is a time to share the job description with the person and to go over it together.
- Ask the person's thoughts about these duties. Are there any tasks he or she could not or would not do? Why does he or she want this job?
- Review the person's transportation needs. How close does he or she live to you? How would the person arrive if his or her main transportation failed?
- Ask for references.
- End by describing your hiring process. Tell how and when you will make your choice. Ask the person for any questions.

Source: Melvyn R. Tanzman, *Living Independently with Personal Assistance*, American Association of Spinal Cord Injury Psychologists and Social Workers, Jackson Heights, New York.

Questions to Think about When You Interview an Attendant

During the interview, keep in mind the qualities that you like in other people. This person does not have to become your best friend, but should be someone you can like and respect. The following questions may help you discover if your lifestyles are compatible, but don't limit yourself to these.

FOOD AND EATING ARRANGEMENTS

- What kind of food do you usually eat?
  - Likes?
  - Dislikes?
- Are you a good cook?
- Where do you shop for groceries?
- Do you eat at regular times or when you feel like it?
- How do you feel about eating together?
- How do you feel about taking cooking instructions from me?
- If you like different foods than I do, will you be willing to prepare my meals and yours?

TRANSPORTATION

- Can you drive?
- Do you have a valid driver's license?
- How do you feel about accompanying me on errands?

HOUSEKEEPING

- Have you had experience with housekeeping and laundry?
- Do you like things very neat, or are you not particular?
- How do you feel about taking cleaning instructions from me?
- Do you like a definite schedule for cleaning and laundry—for example, vacuum on Monday, scrub floors on Tuesday, etc.—or do you prefer to be more flexible?

PERSONAL CARE

- Do you think it would bother you to help me with toileting, catheter irrigations, or suppositories, if necessary?
- Will you be able to bathe me?
- Is there any aspect of personal care with which you feel uncomfortable?

continues

continued

PERSONAL HABITS, ETC.

- Do you smoke?
- Do you drink alcohol?
- Do you take drugs or smoke pot?
- Do you like to sleep late in the morning or get up early?
- What time do you usually go to bed at night?
- Are you a light sleeper?
- Do you go out to see your friends?
- Will you expect to entertain your friends in my apartment?
  —All the time?
  —Some of the time?
  —Never?
- Might you ever want a friend to stay overnight?
- Do you usually like activities well planned, or do you like to do things on the spur of the moment?
- What do you like to do for entertainment?
- Do you like to listen to music?
  —What kind?
  —At what volume?
- Do you like quiet surroundings?
- Do you like to watch TV?
- What hobbies do you have?
- Do you consider yourself a flexible person? What examples can you give?
- How do you react if you have to change your plans at the last minute?
- Describe your personality:
- What do you personally expect to give to this job?
- Are you on any medications?
- Do you have any emotional problems that might interfere with your work?

Source: Sara Roberts and Nancy Sydow, *Consumer's Guide to Attendant Care*, Access to Independence, Inc., © 1984.

Request for Reference Information

To Whom It May Concern:

A personal care attendant is someone who helps a physically disabled person with daily living activities such as personal care (e.g., bathing, dressing, toileting, and transferring), meal preparation, housekeeping, laundry, grocery shopping, and errands. I am currently interviewing people for a position as an attendant.

Enclosed is a reference waiver form signed by the applicant. _____ has applied for a _____ attendant position. Please furnish me with the following information as soon as possible:

Place of Employment: _____

Dates of Work: _____

Reason for Leaving: _____

_____

Is there any reason why this person might not be suited for this kind of work? _____

_____

Dependability:	Excellent	Good	Fair*	Poor*
Honesty:	Excellent	Good	Fair*	Poor*
Relating well to others:	Excellent	Good	Fair	Poor

*Please explain if **Fair*** or **Poor*** are marked: _____

_____

Personality: _____

_____

Comments: _____

_____

Signature of person filling out form: _____

(References will be kept confidential.)

Thank you for your cooperation.

Sincerely,

Source: Sara Roberts and Nancy Sydow, *Consumer's Guide to Attendant Care*, Access to Independence, Inc., © 1984.

Reference Information Waiver

I, _____, have applied for an attendant care position. In order that they may better evaluate my qualifications, I wish that they may be fully advised of my record with you.

I hereby respectfully request that you furnish the necessary information, and I authorize its release without penalty or liability due to an invasion of privacy or civil rights.

_____
Signature of Applicant

_____
Witness

_____
Date

Source: Sara Roberts and Nancy Sydow, *Consumer's Guide to Attendant Care*, Access to Independence, Inc., © 1984.

Agreement Between Employer and Attendant

(Cross out items that are not applicable.)

1. Following are the hours the attendant will work:

   Monday_____   Friday_____
   Tuesday _____   Saturday_____
   Wednesday_____   Sunday_____
   Thursday_____

2. The attendant will have the following time off:

   _____
   _____

3. Salary includes room, board, utilities, phone, and $_____per week and/or $_____ per _____ to be paid _____.
4. When leaving, the attendant will give the approximate time of return and, if possible, leave a phone number where he or she can be reached. Also, when the attendant will be late in returning, he or she will call to let the employer know.
5. Any nonlocal telephone calls will be paid for by the person who made the call.
6. The attendant will carry out the duties and responsibilities listed in the job description.
7. When an **unscheduled** backup is needed, money to pay the backup will be deducted from the regular attendant's salary.
8. Both parties to this agreement will respect each other's individuality and treat each other accordingly. Both will attempt to be flexible and work at solving problems as they arise.
9. At least two weeks' notice will be given by either party regarding termination of this agreement.
10. Other agreements:

_____   _____
Employer   Date   Personal Care Attendant   Date

Source: Sara Roberts and Nancy Sydow, *Consumer's Guide to Attendant Care*, Access to Independence, Inc., © 1984.

Guidelines for Attendant Training

Now that you have interviewed attendants and selected one to work for you, you will be focusing on training. Of course, what you teach that person to do depends on what you need and will vary from person to person.

Begin by explaining your disability in as much detail as you are comfortable with.
_____
_____

Explain any technical words that you use; be as descriptive as you can.
_____
_____

Be sure to emphasize anything relating to safety or emergencies.
_____
_____

When giving instructions involving a procedure such as transferring, include **each step** as you go. Describe why it's important to you that something be done a certain way.
_____
_____

Don't take for granted that the attendant knows what you mean. Ask for feedback.
_____
_____

Be patient. Your attendant probably will not get everything right the first time or second.
_____
_____

Try to be aware of your attendant's feelings as you train. Put yourself in his or her shoes.
_____
_____

Use others to help train, for example, a previous attendant, nursing home staff, visiting nurse service, family member, etc.
_____
_____

Source: Sara Roberts and Nancy Sydow, *Consumer's Guide to Attendant Care*, Access to Independence, Inc., © 1984.

Emergency Backup Attendant Care

What do you do when you suddenly find yourself without an attendant? This can be one of the more frightening, disconcerting, unnerving, anxiety-producing situations anyone can face. There are steps you can take to **prevent** it.

Many circumstances can lead to being without attendant care. An attendant may suddenly become ill and not be able to work; you and your attendant may not be getting along and he or she quits the job without notice; you feel your own personal safety is in jeopardy because of the attendant's behavior so you fire him or her without notice.

PLANNING AHEAD IS THE ANSWER

An attendant is unlikely to be healthy and able to work 365 days per year. Therefore, it is **essential** that you have an available list of people to call in an emergency.

In the case of poor relations between you and your attendant, these problems don't occur overnight. Many things can be done to prevent the kind of blowup that results in an attendant suddenly quitting or being fired. Angry outbursts, rudeness, and behaving in an inconsiderate manner on either side only serve to escalate a situation to a crisis. These situations in particular can be and are avoidable. If you find yourself in this kind of situation often, it is probably advisable to seek training and counseling in attendant management.

WHAT CAN YOU DO?

To prepare for the time when, for any reason, you find yourself without an attendant, you can take certain steps:

- Take the time **now** to review what your **essential** personal care needs are. It is important to be flexible in a time of crisis. Remember: you may have to modify your personal care schedule, get along with less care than usual, and/or skip nonessential activities in order to get basic needs met. Preparing a brief description of your essential needs will help you be more specific when you approach people to serve as backups.
- Develop a list of people who can be available as emergency backup attendants for you. People you could ask include family and friends; former attendants; people you go to school with, volunteer with, or know from church or social organizations; or other working attendants you know. When you ask if they are willing to help in an emergency situation, find out under what general circumstances or at which times they'd be available. Keep this information handy.
- Develop a short, descriptive letter to recruit other emergency backup attendants. It can be sent to many places where people may be looking for extra work, such as your local Job Service, technical school, college or university, residents in your apartment building or neighborhood, your local grocery store, church bulletin, etc.

continues

continued

- If the people you recruit to be emergency backups are people you don't know, give them a job description and information about hours and salary and interview them as you would any attendant. Add their names, phone numbers, and hours they can work to the backup list you've made.
- Set aside money each month, since it is easier to find an emergency attendant if you can offer a little higher salary than usual. Often those who agree to help in an emergency have to disrupt their own schedule to some degree in order to help. They may have to travel across town at their own expense for two or three hours' work. Offering more than your usual rate may help in your search for backup care.
- Every six months or so, update your emergency backup list. A brief phone call to check if the people are still interested and if they have any changes in the times they are available can save you a lot of frustration when you need to find someone on short notice. (This step is particularly important if any of your backups are students, because their schedules will change each semester.)

WHEN YOU NEED TO FIND A BACKUP

These are a few things to keep in mind when you actually need an emergency attendant:

1. Begin the process as quickly as possible. Even a few hours' lead time may give your potential backup person an edge in being able to rearrange his or her schedule to meet your request.
2. Take a few moments to collect your thoughts before you begin calling people on your list. Make sure you know the answers to the following questions:
   —What kind(s) of assistance am I requesting that they do?
   —When do I need them, and for what period of time?
   —How much can I pay?
3. When you do call someone about doing emergency backup for you, be as specific as possible. Include information that answers the questions in item 2 above. Provide the specifics to help the person make a decision more quickly, and there will be less likelihood of misunderstandings later.

EMERGENCY BACKUP ATTENDANT LIST

The sample format below is just one you could use. "Restrictions" could range from only wanting to do certain tasks to the amount of lead time the person may need.

continues

continued

Name/Address	Phone #	Hours/Weekdays/ Weekends Available	Restrictions?
Example:			
John Doe 123 Main Street	555-1212	After 3:30 M–F; all day Sat & Sun	No heavy lifting

1. _____
2. _____
3. _____
4. _____
5. _____
6. _____

Source: Sara Roberts and Nancy Sydow, *Consumer's Guide to Attendant Care*, Access to Independence, Inc., © 1984.

Communicating with Your Attendant

This information sheet places a strong emphasis on communication. Learning good communication skills and using those skills are the keys to working effectively with an attendant.

GOOD WORK ENVIRONMENT

Attendant work is usually not well paid and offers few, if any, fringe benefits. Therefore, those who take this kind of job often do it because it has other rewards, such as personal satisfaction or a chance to work closely with other people. That makes the work environment a most important factor in keeping your attendant.

Good employers create a work environment that will bring out the best an attendant has to offer. You will want your attendant to have good morale, be happy and satisfied with his or her work, and therefore be a productive employee. Good communication between you and your attendant can help do this.

To create that good work environment:

- **Reward** attendants for the work they are doing. Besides paying them, it is important to praise them frequently, as well. Everyone wants to feel appreciated, needed, and important. For example, your attendant has transferred you very smoothly from your bed to your wheelchair. You might say, "That was a really smooth transfer. You do it very well, and I feel very safe." You have communicated your appreciation in a very concrete way and your attendant will know that he or she has performed this task well.
- When you must criticize something your attendant has or has not done, it is important to be open and honest and to criticize the action, not the person. For example, your attendant has returned an hour later than planned. He or she did not call to explain and you are angry. You might say, "You said you would be home an hour ago. I feel frustrated and angry when people are late. In the future, I would appreciate it if you would call me and let me know you'll be late." Don't say, "You idiot! You're always late! I don't know what I'm going to do with you." This will only make your attendant defensive and angry, and you won't resolve anything.
- Don't let small irritations build up until an angry explosion occurs. Anger vented in these explosions often is expressed in a hurtful and destructive way. If you feel irritated about something that is happening, talk about it as soon as possible. This may happen daily, especially if you have just begun to work together.
- Respect your attendants. They are human beings and should be treated accordingly. Use the Golden Rule and treat your employee as you would like to be treated. Be honest, fair, kind, respectful, and patient.
- Attendants have their own lives, too. Especially with people who live in, it is important to be sure to respect their privacy, leave them alone during their time off, and realize that unexpected events sometimes disrupt schedules. Although your attendant has responsibili-

continues

continued

ties to you, you should not attempt to control his or her life. Flexibility and compromise are important qualities for both of you.
- Ask your attendant how he or she feels about the work and about you as an employer. Set a regular time to share feelings about your relationship. And then, **both** of you be open to making changes in the routine, in attitude, or in anything else that can correct a problem. After all, you are not in a nursing home where routines are set—this is **your home**, where changes can and should be made.
- When things just don't work out even after repeated attempts, it is time to terminate the agreement. There are good and poor ways to do this, as well.
  - **Do** state your reasons clearly without attacking him or her personally.
  - **Do** give a period of notice, usually two weeks. This allows time for him or her to find a new job and/or a place to live and for you to find a replacement.
  - **Do not** withhold payment of wages even if you are not satisfied with his or her work. Just give notice and terminate the agreement.

To summarize, you—as the employer—have the opportunity to provide a positive work environment for your attendant. This in turn helps him or her to be happy, productive, and motivated to work for you. Good communication between the two of you is the key to this interdependent relationship. An attendant who is happy in his or her work will stay with you longer and do a better job, which will benefit both of you.

If you are interested in learning more about communication skills, check with your local social service organization, colleges, universities, or technical schools for classes in assertiveness, conflict management, or basic communication skills.

GIVING CRITICISM

- Give the criticism as soon as possible after the situation that you dislike occurs.
- Criticize only one incident at a time.
- Do not bring up things from the past. Stick to the present.
- Criticize the person's actions, not the person.
- Keep the criticism brief and to the point.

Use criticism as a tool for sharing information that will help your attendant do the job more effectively.

Follow these three steps for giving criticism:

1. Describe the situation or event that you disliked.
2. Tell what **your** feeling was when it happened.
3. State what would make it better next time. (Suggestion)

continues

continued

GIVING PRAISE

- Always be sincere. Don't say something you don't really mean.
- Give compliments often.

Follow these two steps for giving compliments:

1. Describe the situation or event that you liked.
2. Tell what your feeling was when it happened.

or

Say that you appreciated it.

or

Say "thank you."

Notes:

Source: Sara Roberts and Nancy Sydow, *Consumer's Guide to Attendant Care*, Access to Independence, Inc., © 1984.

Who Pays for Personal Assistance?

Personal assistance services are expensive and you must find a way to pay for these services. There is no single plan nationwide. Below are the major public and private resources that might pay for personal assistance.

PRIVATE RESOURCES

- **Health insurance:** Most insurance policies do not cover personal assistance. However, if you need skilled nursing or skilled therapy services, many health insurance plans may pay for a few hours of personal assistance.
- **Auto insurance:** In certain states, no-fault auto insurance may help pay for personal assistance if you are injured in an automotive accident.

PUBLIC RESOURCES

- **Medicare:** Over the years, Medicare has decreased the amount of home care it provides. The general rule is similar to private insurance. If you need skilled nursing or therapy, Medicare may pay for a few hours of a home health aide. In most cases, this will be under 30 hours of assistance each week.
- **Department of Veterans Affairs (DVA):** While the DVA does not directly provide personal assistants, there are two benefits that may assist you:
  - **Aid and attendance benefits:** The DVA will provide more income than your pension if you need assistance. If you were not injured while in the service, this amount is minimal and will not be enough to cover the cost of your care.
  - **Fee basis benefits:** If you are receiving a pension and have nursing needs, such as assistance with bowel and bladder care, the DVA will pay for services to meet these needs.
- **Vocational rehabilitation:** Your state office of vocational rehabilitation can provide some personal assistance if you are taking part in a vocational rehabilitation program. The state may provide assistance to prepare you for attending a training or education program, assistance while you are at the program, and assistance to return home. Once you are employed, services will end.
- **Crime victims compensation:** Some states provide compensation to victims of crimes. This could include cash and/or services, such as personal assistance.
- **Medicaid:** Some states include personal assistance as part of their Medicaid program. The amount of services varies from state to state. Medicaid will only accept clients who have a low income.
- **State-funded programs:** Some states may have personal assistance programs that are separate from Medicaid. You may be able to earn a salary above the poverty level and still receive these services.

These programs vary, so you should consult with an independent living center or social worker in your community to learn what is available. Generally, programs tend to be limited and may not provide you with all the assistance you need. In addition, some programs have long waiting lists.

Source: Melvyn R. Tanzman, *Living Independently with Personal Assistance*, American Association of Spinal Cord Injury Psychologists and Social Workers, Jackson Heights, New York.

TRAVEL

Travel after a Spinal Cord Injury

INTRODUCTION

Arranging travel is a fairly straightforward process for nondisabled individuals. Most people contact a travel agency, choose a destination, and hope that their baggage and the sun follow them.

For the traveler with a spinal cord injury (SCI), or other disability, there is much more to consider when planning a trip. Anxiety about air travel, the accessibility of accommodations and transportation, and attitudinal barriers can be extra "baggage" for the novice traveler with SCI. With proper planning, these issues can be minimized, and often avoided.

The purpose of this factsheet is to assist people with SCI to travel with greater ease and comfort. It provides useful travel tips, an overview of applicable laws, and a listing of up-to-date resources.

LOOK FOR AN EXPERIENCED TRAVEL AGENCY

Call or visit a few travel agencies. Ask if they have actual experience with coordinating travel for persons with SCI or other disabilities. An experienced agency will have readily available, fully researched sources on accessible accommodations. On-site visits of travel destinations should be conducted by either agency personnel or reliable area contacts to provide accurate accessibility information. Determining accessibility by telephone is risky unless performed by an individual who specializes in site evaluation. A reputable agency will ask about such specifics as door width, bathroom design, ramping, etc.

If the agency does not have experience coordinating travel for persons with SCI or other disabilities, ask if they would be willing to do the necessary research to successfully plan the trip. If so, how would they go about determining accessibility of the destination and any in-between ground transportation? Do they know airline procedure for requesting passenger assistance or proper storage of a power wheelchair?

An unexperienced agency may deliver acceptable results, but it takes much more time and effort on the traveler's part. The individual must be well versed in his or her personal requirements and able to articulate those needs. Of course, the travel agency must be capable of understanding those needs and following through with accessibility confirmation.

BE AWARE OF APPLICABLE LAWS AND RIGHTS

It is useful to spend some time becoming educated about how the Americans with Disabilities Act (ADA) and the Air Carriers Access Act (ACAA) affect the traveler with an SCI.

The ADA, passed in 1990, gives civil rights protections to individuals with disabilities. It guarantees equal opportunity in employment, transportation, public accommodations, telecommunications, and state and local government. For travelers with SCI, this means travel-related services such as lodging, dining, entertainment, bus and rail stations, cruise-ship terminals, and airports are impacted and should be more accessible as the industry comes into compliance.

continues

continued

The ACAA, passed in 1986, guarantees that people with disabilities receive consistent and nondiscriminatory treatment when traveling by air. An experienced travel agency will provide SCI travelers with a copy of the ACAA. It is recommended that travelers with SCI bring a copy of the ACAA whenever flying. Having a copy on hand can help both the passenger with an SCI and airline personnel clarify any misunderstanding about what is covered.

These laws have dramatically improved how individuals with SCI travel. However, travel industry suppliers need to be constantly educated about their obligations under these laws.

BE PREPARED

Seasoned travelers have organization down to a science, but most people need assistance in this area. Taking time to get organized before departure is time well spent:

- Make a list of "must bring" items such as medications, medical supplies, patch kits, etc. Keep these items in a carry-on bag to make certain they arrive with you. When packing, keep medication in its original container. This avoids questions at customs about the nature of the drugs the traveler is carrying.
- Write down important telephone numbers and store them in a carry-on bag.
- Power wheelchair users should consider using gel cell batteries whenever possible to avoid battery separation as may be required under Department of Transportation rules.
- Locate a medical supply/wheelchair repair company in close proximity to the destination. Airlines have limited financial responsibility for wheelchair damages; however, they may not know where or how to locate a repair company in a timely manner.
- Adaptive equipment, such as shower/commode chairs and lifts can be rented at many destinations.
- When making airline reservations, consider booking a nonstop or direct (one stop without getting off the aircraft) flight, although a connecting flight may be preferred to allow the passenger with SCI the opportunity to exit the aircraft.
- Travelers with SCI should be mindful of fluid intake prior to flying (wheelchair accessible aircraft lavatories are rare, see ACAA) but common sense should be exercised with regard to dehydration.
- Gate-check your wheelchair so you can use it up until boarding of the aircraft.

SUMMARY

In the not-too-distant past, travelers with SCI faced many obstacles. Architectural barriers and unenlightened attitudes prevented many people with disabilities from traveling with ease. The desire to travel was still alive, yet the potential for negative experiences made staying close to home the safest option.

Fortunately, laws such as the ADA and ACAA have dramatically improved travel options for individuals with SCI. Additionally, the travel industry is slowly recognizing that the disability community is a formidable market, with billions of dollars in expendable income. These factors mean that individuals with SCI and other disabilities can once again travel with confidence.

Courtesy of the National Spinal Cord Injury Association, 545 Concord Avenue, Suite 29, Cambridge, Massachusetts 02138. For more information, call (800) 962-9629 or (617) 441-8500.

Tips for Hassle-Free Flying

Flying on a commercial airline is an exciting, enjoyable experience, but it can be difficult if you do not make good arrangements. Keeping a few things in mind and knowing some tricks of the trade can make a big difference.

RESERVATIONS

- Make reservations early and ask for any special deals.
- Ask for the bulkhead seat in coach class, or buy a ticket for first class if you can afford it. Both have more knee room.
- Tell them you are in a wheelchair and will need assistance with transferring.
- Ask for flights that are nonstop.
- Have the tickets mailed to your home to save time and trouble.
- Pack an emergency kit (condoms, medicines, catheters, etc.) to carry with you on the plane to tide you over if your luggage gets lost or if you have a layover.
- If transfers must be made, plan enough time to switch airplanes.

ARRIVAL AT AIRPORT

- If possible, check all baggage at the outside ticket counter when you arrive.
- Be **sure** to have a tag put on your chair. Ask for your chair to be gate-checked.
- Check in early at the ticket counter.

BOARDING GATE

- Go to the bathroom before boarding. It may be a long time before you can go again.
- If you are taking a flight that lasts longer than five hours, ask your doctor if a Foley catheter can be inserted so that intermittent catheterization will not have to be done on the plane.
- Take a urinal with you on the plane.
- Your chair will not fit down the aisle on most planes. Ask for a boarding chair.
- Take any removable parts of your chair with you (armrests, backpack). Tape down any straps.
- It is difficult to transfer to the narrow boarding chair. **Ask for help and assume the flight attendant has never seen a disabled person before!**
- It is best to be lifted by two people. Be sure to tell them that you have little or no balance.
- Take your cushion with you and have a flight attendant put it in your seat.
- Most flight attendants' experience with wheelchairs involves elderly people who can walk. You must tell them that you are paralyzed. Be sure they strap you in the carryon chair before they let go of you. **Bring a strap or belt with you.**
- Be sure to remind them to load your chair!

ON THE PLANE

- You will be the first person on the plane.
- Be sure your cushion is in your seat. Your airplane seat cushion **can** be removed and replaced with your cushion.

continues

continued

- The outside arm on the plane seat usually does not lift up, so it is best to be lifted over it. Tell them to be sure that you clear the arm. A pillow or blanket can be placed on the armrest to protect your skin.
- Use the seat belt. If you have high-level tetraplegia, you may need someone to brace you on landing.
- Remember to do your weight shifts! Good methods to use are push-up, side to side, or leaning over your knees with a spotter to assist you.
- If you must empty your bladder, ask the flight attendant to provide privacy for you at the seat by using a sheet or blanket.

LANDING

- Ask the flight attendant to call ahead 20 minutes prior to landing for help in getting you off the plane.
- Ask the flight attendant to have your chair brought to the plane.
- You will be the last person off the plane. Tell the flight attendant that you cannot use an airport chair, or tell them your chair is gate-checked.
- Be sure to tell the people transferring you what to do. Remember, these are **not** the same people who put you on the plane.
- Do not forget your cushion.
- In case you must make a connecting flight, make sure they bring your chair to you to get to the next plane. This ensures that your chair is making the flight with you.

IN CASE YOU PLAN TO TRAVEL WITH AN ELECTRIC WHEELCHAIR

If you must transport an electric wheelchair on an airplane, there are some extra concerns you will need to find out about. First, check with the reservations office to see if the airline takes electric chairs on board. Most major airlines will take electric chairs at no cost if you follow special rules. If the airline does not take electric wheelchairs on board, be prepared to do the following:

- Tell the reservation agent about your chair.
- Disconnect the battery from the chair.
- Place the battery in a leakproof container, if it is a wet cell battery.
- Only **one** battery will be allowed on board the plane, so **do not** plan to bring an extra one.
- Check the wheelchair in at the ticket counter with your other baggage.
- Take all removable parts off of the wheelchair, such as footrests and armrests. Carry them on the plane with you or be sure to tag **all** the separate parts. Tape down sip and puff parts, arm straps, and anything that someone could grab and pull off by mistake.

Source: Donna Schachtel et al., *Key to Independence Personal Care Manual*, Shepherd Spinal Center, Atlanta, Georgia, © 1989. To order a complete version of the manual, contact the Shepherd Center at (404) 350-7361.

THE AMERICANS WITH DISABILITIES ACT

Understanding the ADA

In July 1990, the United States Congress passed the most important legislation ever to affect people with disabilities. The Americans with Disabilities Act (P.L. 101-336), or ADA, gives civil rights protections to people with disabilities and prohibits discrimination on the basis of disability.

For the purposes of this overview, a disability is a physical or mental impairment that substantially limits one or more of an individual's major life activities. Major life activities include functions such as caring for one's self, walking, performing manual tasks, breathing, speaking, hearing, seeing, learning, and working.

A disability can also mean a record of an impairment, or being regarded as having an impairment. A record of an impairment means that a person has a history of an impairment or has been misclassified as having an impairment. Examples include a person who has recovered from mental illness or cancer, or a person whose school records may have misclassified him or her as having a learning disability.

Being regarded as having an impairment means that a person is perceived or treated as having an impairment, even though the impairment itself does not substantially limit his or her major life activities. Examples include a person with controlled diabetes or high blood pressure, a person with physical disfigurements due to scarring, or a person who is rumored to have tuberculosis.

The ADA also prohibits discrimination against people without disabilities on the basis of their relationships or associations with people with disabilities. For example, an employer cannot refuse to hire someone who provides care for a spouse with a disability on the assumption that the caregiver will have a high absentee rate.

The ADA is divided into four major areas:

- Title I: Employment
- Title II: Public Services
- Title III: Public Accommodations and Commercial Facilities
- Title IV: Telecommunications

TITLE I: EMPLOYMENT

Private employers are prohibited from discriminating against qualified individuals with disabilities in job application procedures, hiring, termination, promotion, compensation, fringe benefits, job training, and other terms, conditions and privileges of employment. Beginning July 26, 1992, this applies to employers with 25 or more employees; as of July 26, 1994, the law applies to employers with 15 or more employees. Public service employers were required to comply as of January 26, 1992, regardless of the number of employees.

A qualified person with a disability is an individual who can meet the requirements of the position and perform the essential functions of the job, with or without reasonable accommodation.

continues

continued

Reasonable accommodation includes modifications in the work environment (including common areas such as lounges and cafeterias) and modifications in the way things are usually done. These changes are required to ensure that people with disabilities can enjoy equal employment opportunities. A person may also need reasonable accommodation during the job application process, to ensure access to testing facilities, or to take employment tests that relate directly to the job.

TITLE II: PUBLIC SERVICES

Title II of the ADA is divided into two subtitles.

Subtitle A

Subtitle A prohibits discrimination on the basis of disability by state and local government in the provision of services, programs, and activities, even when they are made available by contractors. This subtitle also covers communication with the public and the public's use of public facilities. All such programs must be administered in the most integrated setting possible.

Structural changes in existing public buildings may not be required as long as all services and programs are accessible. Public entities are also required to furnish auxiliary aids and services that provide communication to people with vision, hearing, and speech impairments. This communication must be as effective as the methods provided to people without disabilities.

In addition, emergency response services, such as 911 services, must provide direct access; a relay service is not adequate.

Subtitle B

Subtitle B prohibits discrimination on the basis of disability in the provision of accessible transportation services and transportation facilities. This includes rail and nonrail vehicles, such as minibuses, articulated buses, rapid rail, and light-rail cars, that are purchased by public entities, or private entities under contract with public entities. Transportation facilities include publicly operated depots and other stations, as well as airport passenger terminals.

TITLE III: PUBLIC ACCOMMODATIONS AND COMMERCIAL FACILITIES

Title III prohibits discrimination on the basis of disability by private entities in places of public accommodation, commercial facilities, and certain tests or courses related to professional or trade licensing or certification. According to Title III, businesses open to the general public must make their products and services available to all people, regardless of disability.

Places of public accommodation include restaurants, bars, or other establishments serving food or drink; movie theaters, auditoriums, and concert halls; hotels, inns, and motels; professional offices, e.g., accountants' or lawyers' offices; social service centers; retail sales or rental estab-

continues

continued

lishments; places of recreation; museums; and zoos. Commercial facilities include office buildings, factories, and warehouses.

No matter what the facility, all goods and services must be provided in an integrated manner. Facilities must provide auxiliary aids and services to customers or clients with vision, hearing, or speech impairments, to ensure effective communication. Structural barriers in existing facilities must be removed when removal does not require much difficulty or expense; building access is the first priority. New construction and alterations must be designed for accessibility.

TITLE IV: TELECOMMUNICATIONS

Title IV of the ADA ensures that people with hearing or speech impairments have equal access to universal telecommunications services. Common carriers must provide interstate and intrastate telecommunication relay services (TRS) throughout their respective service areas by July 26, 1993. The communication assistants who relay a conversation from voice to text and vice versa must be familiar with the cultures and languages of people with hearing and speech impairments. They must also be competent in the interpretation of typewritten American Sign Language (ASL).

Notes:

Courtesy of the STAR (System of Technology to Achieve Results) Program, Minnesota Advisory Council on Technology of People with Disabilities, St. Paul, Minnesota.

12

Home Modification and Assistive Technology

> Most materials in the *Spinal Cord Injury Patient Education Manual* are intended for the health care professional to share with the patient. Materials that are intended solely for the professional are labeled "Exhibit" in the table of contents.

Home Modification

Home Modifications for the Wheelchair
 User 387
General Home Construction Checklist 389
Helpful Bathroom Checklist 391
Helpful Kitchen Checklist 392
General Home Mechanical Checklist 393
Home Accessibility 395
How to Make a Wheelchair Ramp 397

Assistive Technology

Taking Care of Your Home 400
Preparing and Serving Food 403
Choosing and Adapting Clothing 408
Adapting Your Personal Care Routine 413
Reaching and Mobility Aids 416

Wheelchairs

Wheelchairs for People with Spinal
 Cord Injuries 420

Features to Consider When Purchasing
 a Wheelchair 424
Wheelchair Accessories Glossary 427
Important Information about Your
 Wheelchair Cushion 428
Wheelchair Information Sheet 430
Wheelchair Maintenance 431
Charging Guidelines for Power
 Wheelchairs: Lead Acid Batteries 432
Wheelchair Positioning 433
Basic Wheelchair Transfer
 Considerations 434
Wheelchair Safety: How to Handle and
 Push a Wheelchair 435
Switching to a Power Chair 440

Adaptive Driving

Adaptive Driving: The Basics 443
How to Select a Vehicle 446
Am I Ready for a Van? 448

HOME MODIFICATION

Home Modifications for the Wheelchair User

Before discharge from the hospital, a home visit by a rehabilitation professional may be done for possible home modifications (changes) and equipment needs.

OUTSIDE THE HOME

- Park close to the front door, if possible.
- If the wheelchair does not fit on the sidewalk, the sidewalk may need to be:
  —widened
  —repaired
- —cleared of bushes, trees, and weeds
- Reserve a parking space if living in an apartment.
- Make a ramp if there are steps to the front or back door (see How To Make a Ramp handout).

HALLS

- Clear hallways of unnecessary items.
- Fix doors:
  —Rehang doors to open into room instead of hall.
  —Remove doors completely, if possible.
- Remove or secure loose rugs that are in the way.

LIVING ROOM

- Rearrange furniture to clear a path.
- Raise or lower chairs, if needed.

DINING AREA

- Raise or lower the table so the wheelchair can fit under it.
- For safe transfers, use chairs that are the right height and shape (armless).

KITCHEN

- Keep commonly used foods and cooking items within easy reach. Use sliding shelves and wire racks on cupboard doors, shelves, or walls.
- Use hooks/magnetic strips for storing equipment.
- Add long handles to sink faucets and taps if needed.
- Remove door of cupboard under sink to allow easy reach.

continues

continued

BEDROOM

- To make transfers on/off the bed easier:
  - Move the bed.
  - Raise or lower the bed.
  - Use a firm mattress or a bedboard under the mattress.
  - You may need a hospital bed.
- Make sure storage areas are within easy reach.
- Replace closet doors with sliding doors or curtains.

BATHROOM

- Make sure the bath, toilet, and sink are usable from a wheelchair.
- Use a bath seat.
- Put grab bars in good positions for bath and toilet.
- Use a bath mat when sitting or transferring to prevent slipping.
- Put shower controls at sitting height, or use a hand-held shower over the bath.
- Remove the cupboard (cabinet) under the sink.
- Raise toilet seat.

Notes:

Source: Kelly B. Wascher, ed., *Patient Education and Discharge Planning Manual for Rehabilitation*, St. Joseph Rehabilitation Hospital and Outpatient Center, Aspen Publishers, Inc., © 1995.

General Home Construction Checklist

DOORWAYS AND DOORS

- ☐ Minimum clear width is 32 inches.
- ☐ Install fold-back hinges to widen a narrow doorway.
- ☐ Provide a five-foot space inside and outside the doorway.
- ☐ Doors should not open directly to the top of a staircase.
- ☐ Doors should open outward, especially in small rooms.
- ☐ Choose suitable doors for your individual needs. (Choose side hung, remote-controlled, sliding, folding.)
- ☐ Install kick-plates to protect door from wheelchair footrests.
- ☐ Provide mat wells for doormats to ensure level surfaces.
- ☐ Use easy-to-open door handles, pulls, and latches.
- ☐ Convert hard-to-grip round doorknobs to lever or push-type handles.
- ☐ Door handles should be placed at a height of at least three but no more than four feet.
- ☐ If locks are used, they should only require use of one hand.
- ☐ Avoid raised thresholds or upstanding door guides (used with sliding doors).
- ☐ Wooden thresholds may be beveled using weather stripping.

FLOORS, WALLS, WINDOWS, AND HALLWAYS

- ☐ Floors should have a hard surface (wood, vinyl, or tile).
- ☐ Carpet, if used, should be installed tight to the floor; avoid padding if possible.
- ☐ Tightly woven carpet is best; avoid loose weave or shag.
- ☐ Make sure floors are nonskid; avoid floor wax.
- ☐ For a tile floor, pick a pattern or dark color to hide wheelchair tire marks and other scuffing.
- ☐ Protect wall corners with clear plastic corner edging or metal plaster bead.
- ☐ Walls should be easy to clean and maintain.
- ☐ Use clear plastic shields to protect walls in hard-wear areas, such as above the sink.
- ☐ Windows should open outward and be easy to operate. Casement windows are the most difficult to use; horizontal sliding windows among the easiest.
- ☐ Cover radiators in front of windows to decrease risk of burns.
- ☐ Inaccessible windows may be remote controlled.
- ☐ Hallways should be four feet wide, wherever possible.
- ☐ Widen doors wherever narrow hallways must be used.
- ☐ Provide turning room at the ends of hallways, wherever possible.

continues

continued

BEDROOMS

- ☐ Ensure convenient access to bath and toilet rooms.
- ☐ Make sure light switch is in reach of bed.
- ☐ Provide room to move wheelchair around sides of bed.
- ☐ Bed should be level with height of wheelchair seat.
- ☐ Provide convenient storage within reach of bed for braces, clothing, etc. (Try a pullout storage system under the bed.)
- ☐ Bedroom furniture can be placed on wheels (casters) for easy movement.
- ☐ Make sure dresser drawers can be opened with only one hand.
- ☐ Use stops so that drawers can't be pulled all the way out accidentally.
- ☐ Use bedside tables with drawers for convenient storage and a place to put a clock, telephone, etc.

Notes:

Adapted from Robert Harold Jackson, *Spinal Cord Injury: Medical Management and Rehabilitation*, Gary M. Yarkony, ed., Aspen Publishers, Inc., © 1994.

Helpful Bathroom Checklist

Water Controls and Valves

- ☐ Single-handle control
- ☐ Lever or blade shape
- ☐ Shut-off valve easy to use
- ☐ Pressure balance and thermostatic control
- ☐ Insulated pipes
- ☐ 105°F delivery temperature

Counters and Sinks

- ☐ 27 inches deep
- ☐ Securely bracketed
- ☐ Within reach of toilet
- ☐ Knee space

Toilets

- ☐ Raised toilet 20 inches
- ☐ Raised toilet seat with cutout front and back
- ☐ Ample space for transfer
- ☐ Grab bars properly positioned
- ☐ Water level and rim $7\frac{3}{4}$ inches
- ☐ Easily used flushing device
- ☐ Toilet paper and sink within reach

Grab Bars

- ☐ Suitable height for individual ability
- ☐ Positioned in bath tub and shower

Medicine Cabinets and Storage

- ☐ Positioned for easy use
- ☐ Bottom edge 36 inches high
- ☐ Narrow shelves with single-row storage

Mirrors

- ☐ Bottom edge 36 inches high
- ☐ Full-length mirror

Bath Tubs

- ☐ Grab bars positioned for individual use and ability
- ☐ Bath seats or benches
- ☐ Lifts and hoists
- ☐ Bath mat or friction tape
- ☐ Shower wand
- ☐ Recessed shelf

Showers

- ☐ Roll-in
- ☐ Transfer with fixed bench
- ☐ Roll-in with removable bench
- ☐ Grab bars positioned for individual use and ability
- ☐ Adequate space for transfer
- ☐ Recessed shelf
- ☐ Shower wand
- ☐ Single-lever handle
- ☐ Thermostatic control valve

Towel Racks and Soap Dishes

- ☐ No more than 40 inches high
- ☐ Withstanding 250 pounds of pressure

Source: Robert Harold Jackson, *Spinal Cord Injury: Medical Management and Rehabilitation*, Gary M. Yarkony, ed., Aspen Publishers, Inc., © 1994.

Helpful Kitchen Checklist

Counters

☐ 30- to 33-inch height
☐ Pullout work counter, 30-inch height

Sinks

☐ 6 inches deep
☐ Rear drain
☐ Knee space under sink
☐ Spray attachment
☐ Insulated sink and pipes
☐ Temperature control hardware
☐ Mixing type faucet
☐ Shallow shelf over sink
☐ Garbage disposal

Refrigerators

☐ Side-by-side doors allow for most variation
☐ Standard one-door top freezer for ambulatory disabled
☐ Bottom freezer for person in wheelchair
☐ Self-defrosting

Ovens

☐ Side-hung or drop door
☐ Door strong enough to support food
☐ Cabinet space under oven
☐ Pullout board under oven
☐ Easily used, safe shelves

Cooktops

☐ No knee space under cooktop
☐ Burners in single row
☐ Burners flush to adjacent surface
☐ Range hood vent
☐ Controls in front
☐ Lip or drain along front edge

Cabinets and Shelves

☐ Easily used cabinet door pulls
☐ Cabinet space under counters and wall oven
☐ Full-height storage for variety of access
☐ High cabinet storage for those not in wheelchair
☐ High recessed base under cabinets to accommodate wheelchair footrests
☐ Narrow shelves for single-row storage

Miscellaneous

☐ Smooth, nonskid floor surface
☐ Open spaces for wheelchair passage
☐ Round table with pedestal base to allow for wheelchair
☐ Lighting under cabinets
☐ Bulb replacement within easy reach
☐ Strip plugs and accessible receptacles for small appliances
☐ Securely fixed drop ironing board with receptacle for iron
☐ Lap tray to help in carrying food and dishes
☐ Front-loading dishwasher, washing machine, and dryer

Source: Robert Harold Jackson, *Spinal Cord Injury: Medical Management and Rehabilitation*, Gary M. Yarkony, ed., Aspen Publishers, Inc., © 1994.

General Home Mechanical Checklist

LIGHT SWITCHES

- ☐ Position switches horizontal to door handle to locate them easily.
- ☐ Use two-way switches at staircases and hallways.
- ☐ Place light switches at a height from 3 feet to 3 feet and 3 inches. A wheelchair user's comfortable range of forward reach generally does not exceed four feet.
- ☐ Install rocker action switches for people with limited use of hands or fingers.
- ☐ Adapt existing switches with light switch extenders.
- ☐ There should not be more than two switches per plate.
- ☐ Place switches at points of entry to all rooms, staircases, and hallways.
- ☐ Use wireless remote control switches, cord switches, dimmer switches, timer switches, or pull chains for people with limited use of hands or fingers.

LIGHTING/ELECTRICAL OUTLETS

- ☐ Wall bracket lighting should be securely fastened to the wall and placed within easy reach.
- ☐ Use table lamps with wide bases for maximum stability.
- ☐ Use pull chains or pressure-sensitive push switches.
- ☐ Consider outside lighting for access paths and ramps.
- ☐ Place an electric tabletop strip console of switches and outlets alongside the bed to control lights, TV, etc., and in the kitchen to power appliances.
- ☐ Receptacles should be within easy reach (at a height between 18 and 24 inches) and unobstructed.

HEATING AND AIR CONDITIONING

- ☐ Place thermostat within easy reach.
- ☐ Consider space heating in heavily used bedrooms and bathrooms.
- ☐ Air conditioning is vital to those with breathing problems.
- ☐ Use ceiling fans to provide more heat, circulate air, and reduce expenses.

SHELVES AND COUNTERS

- ☐ A full wall of shelves provides the most convenient, easy-to-reach storage for wheelchair users and the able-bodied.
- ☐ Provide narrow shelves for single-row storage.
- ☐ Place writing surfaces 30 to 33 inches high.

continues

continued

SWIMMING POOLS

☐ Provide built-in stairs on the shallow end of the pool or in a corner and handrails for stability.
☐ Provide a rest area by building a recessed alcove into the concrete.
☐ Use overhead hoists, hydraulic lifts, and ramps for transfer.
☐ Provide a changing area with raised transfer mats.

SPECIAL CONSIDERATIONS

☐ Install a central vacuum system for convenient use throughout the house. The suction hose and attachments can be plugged into special outlets in each room.
☐ Install a large slot letterplate at the door with a letter basket inside at a height of 2 feet 4 inches to provide accessibility to outside mail delivery.
☐ Design an emergency evacuation plan in the event of a fire.

Notes:

Adapted from Robert Harold Jackson, *Spinal Cord Injury: Medical Management and Rehabilitation*, Gary M. Yarkony, ed., Aspen Publishers, Inc., © 1994.

Home Accessibility

INDIVIDUAL LIFTS AND HOISTS

Individual lifts and hoists are used to allow a person inconvenienced through disability to transfer from bed to wheelchair and to the bathtub, toilet, exercise mat, and back to the wheelchair. There are several types of these devices available, such as manual hydraulic, electrically powered, or portable. Some require assistance; others can be operated independently. These lifts provide accessibility inside the home for the individual and reduce or eliminate the need for attendant care. When attendant care is used, these devices will eliminate back strain and unnecessary exertion for the attendant.

MECHANICAL LIFTS

In remodeling homes where several stairs exist and space for ramps is not available, mechanical lifts may be the only solution to access for people with mobility limitations. There are both vertical and inclined platform lifts for wheelchairs. Vertical lifts are placed at the bottom of stairs, and the upper landing may need to be extended to meet them. Inclined platform lifts are mounted on walls or stairs or are post-mounted on tracks along the stairs. Both lifts can be installed with enclosing walls and electrically interlocked gates for safety. There should be enough space to propel the wheelchair directly onto the lift without the need for turning. Controls should be easy to use and conveniently located. Chair lifts have built-in seats for people with mobility limitations who can walk but cannot climb stairs. This type of lift does not serve wheelchair users well and therefore is of limited use.

ELEVATORS

Elevators often are used to provide access between floors. Some companies will manufacture residential type elevators with special car sizes to accommodate a wheelchair. They are constructed in a convenient location inside the home where a corner or closet area common to all floors exists. Local coding authorities should be consulted before design begins.

RAMPS

Ramps are the most reasonable means of access to and from a home. They can be installed to beautify the home by blending into an altered façade and accenting the grounds with flowers and shrubbery. It is important to go beyond standards of measure and into the imagination. The results will be a home that is accessed more easily by all family members and guests.

The ability of the person to navigate a ramp, as well as the ramp's location, convenience, style, and materials, should be considered before a ramp is built or purchased. Expanded metal provides traction but is a poor choice for some kinds of heeled shoes. Concrete ramps can be constructed with nonskid surfaces. Wood should be treated to resist rotting and should maintain space of no

continues

continued

more than $\frac{1}{2}$ inch to allow elements to pass through and to provide better grip. Carpeting should be avoided because it holds water and is more difficult to push on. People using crutches or canes often prefer stairs.

A manual wheelchair weighs from 25 to 65 pounds, and it can be tiring for some people to push themselves up a ramp, especially at the maximum slope of 1:12. On a long or steep ramp, there is the possibility of loss of control; the downward speed could cause friction burns on the hands. Level rest platforms are therefore necessary at 10-foot intervals for ascent and descent on a long ramp. Level platforms are also necessary to turn a wheelchair on a slope. Continuous hand rails should be installed on each side, extending beyond the slope at the top and bottom of a ramp. Ramps should have curbs on both sides so that a wheelchair cannot accidentally run off the ramp; curbs also are used to help brake a wheelchair in an emergency.

There should be at least 5 feet of straight clearance at the bottom of a ramp. Nonskid surfaces are essential. If possible, ramps should be protected from the elements. In any case, they should be kept free from ice and snow.

Notes:

Source: Robert Harold Jackson, *Spinal Cord Injury: Medical Management and Rehabilitation*, Gary M. Yarkony, ed., Aspen Publishers, Inc., © 1994.

How to Make a Wheelchair Ramp

Talk to a carpenter for building needs. Ask the therapist for additional information. (See drawings.)

RAMP GUIDELINES	
RAMP LENGTH	1 FOOT LONG FOR EACH 1 INCH OF HEIGHT For example, for two 7-in steps, a 14-ft ramp will be needed.
RAMP WIDTH	36 INCHES OR MORE The most common width is 42 to 48 in. A 48-in width is common because CDX 3/4-in plywood comes in sheets of 4 × 8 ft.
PLATFORM AT DOORWAYS	1. **IF door opens OUT:** 5-ft × 5-ft area is needed at the top of the ramp. This area should extend 1 ft on each side of the door. 2. **IF door opens IN:** 3-ft-deep × 5-ft-wide area is needed at the top of the ramp.
TURNS	Need 5-ft × 5-ft AREA to turn.
HAND RAILINGS	Attach a 32-IN-HIGH RAILING to the ramp. Use 2-in × 2-in, or 2-in × 4-in lumber, pipe, or commercial railing.
EDGES	Install edges at least 2-in high on both sides of the ramp. This prevents wheels from going over the edge.
SURFACES	Must have a nonslip surface. Any of the following will work: 1. Adhesive nonskid strips 2. Ribbed rubber matting 3. Textured roofing paper 4. Sand in paint 5. Sweep wet concrete

continues

continued

RAMP GUIDELINES

MATERIALS	Use: 1. Treated lumber 2. Concrete
BOTTOM OF RAMP	Need an area 6 ft long

Note: Portable ramps can be rented until a ramp is built.

HOW TO USE THE RAMP

MANUAL OR ELECTRIC WHEELCHAIR	**UP THE RAMP:** Face the wheelchair forward. **DOWN THE RAMP:** Face the wheelchair forward—or backward for steep ramps.

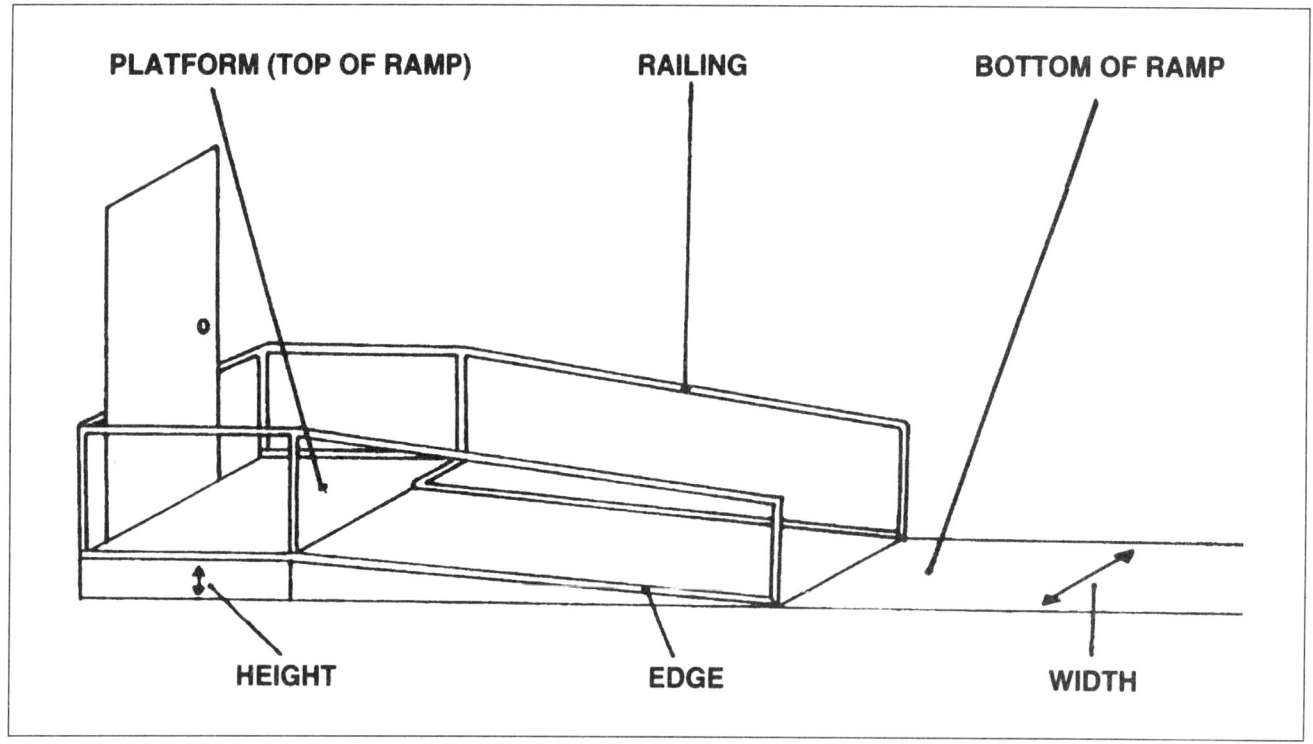

Straight ramp

continues

continued

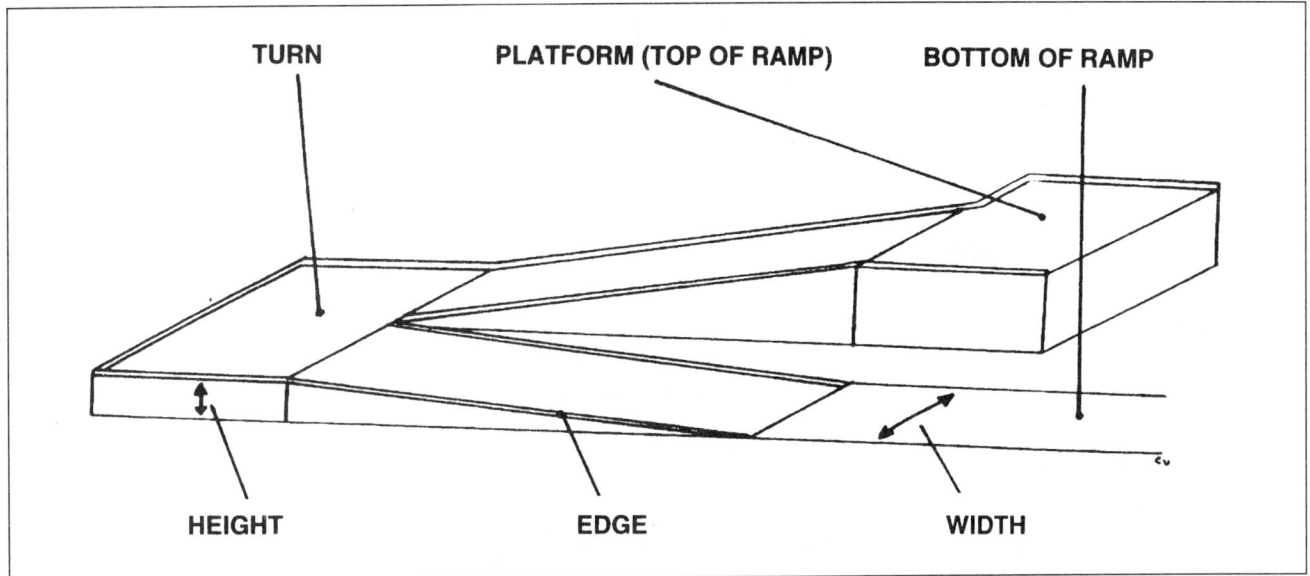

Ramp with a U-Turn

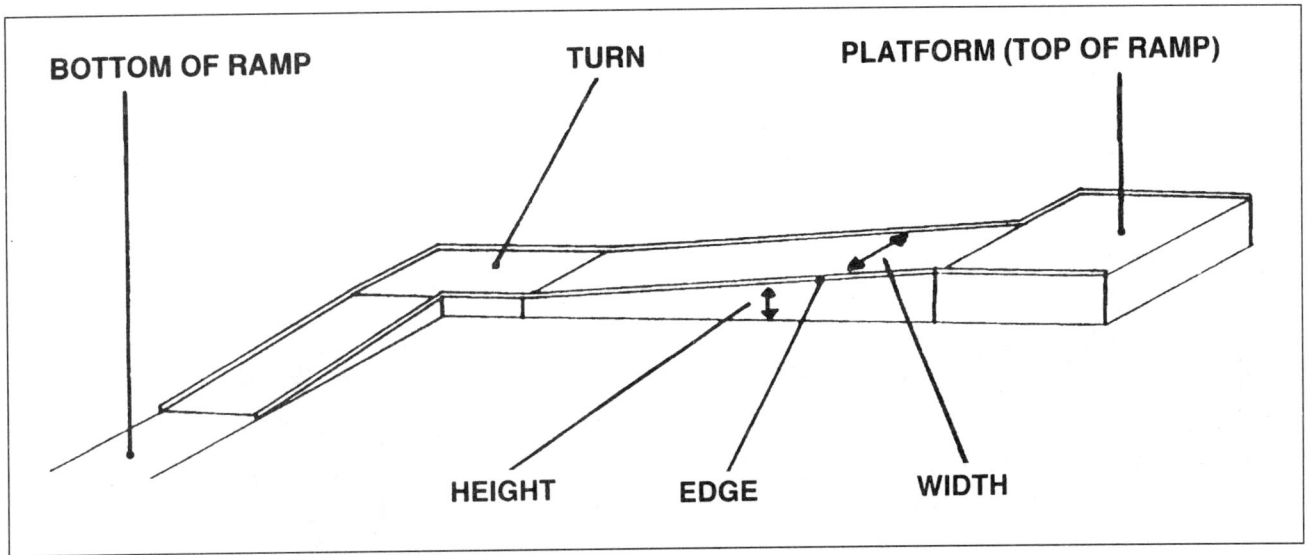

Ramp with a 90-Degree (Right-Angle) Turn

Source: Kelly B. Wascher, ed., *Patient Education and Discharge Planning Manual for Rehabilitation*, St. Joseph Rehabilitation Hospital and Outpatient Center, Aspen Publishers, Inc., © 1995.

ASSISTIVE TECHNOLOGY

Taking Care of Your Home

CLEANING

Floors

When purchasing a vacuum cleaner, think carefully about your upper body strength and don't buy a model that will be too heavy for you. As a rule, cannister types are lighter than uprights; attachments to clean upholstery, drapes, blinds, and corners also make them more versatile. On the other hand, uprights help with balance and support. A rotating brush on the power head, though more expensive, gets down into a carpet and picks up ground-in dirt. A drawback is that the heads move independently and can get away from you.

Electric brooms may be as useful as full-sized vacuum cleaners. They are lighter, less expensive, can be adapted for carpets or bare floors, and do not require vacuum cleaner bags. Practice emptying the dust compartment to make sure it is not more difficult than replacing a bag.

When buying a broom, look for one with a slanted edge and feathered bristles. Wide push-brooms can provide support while sweeping. Long-handled dustpans can be bought at some stores, or insert a broom handle in the hollow handle of a regular dust pan and then angle the pan so that it lies flat to the floor. You can also purchase attachable extra handles to give better leverage and reduce bending over when using long-handled tools.

Dust mops handily clean under beds and furniture and down steps. They also offer some help with balance and support. If you use a wheelchair, the handles of mops or brooms may be too long. Cut them off; you can then attach a bicycle-grip or D-grip handle to give yourself a better grip.

Dusting

Dust frequently; dust combines with airborne cooking grease to make a sticky film that requires scrubbing to remove. A reaching aid holding a soft cloth can reach awkward surfaces. A dusting mitt can be modified to fit over a foot, allowing you to dust along mop boards and under cabinet edges without bending over.

To save time and energy, make or buy an apron with plenty of large pockets to carry cleaning supplies, or attach a pocketed pouch

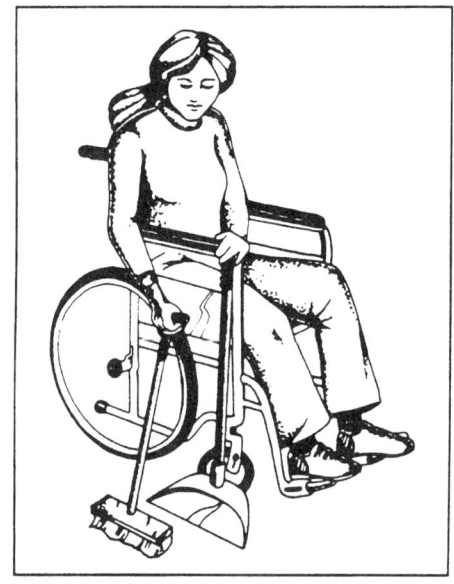

continues

continued

to your wheelchair. A small cart on casters can also be used to move cleaning supplies from place to place.

Windows

A lightweight, car-sized squeegee can be mounted on a broom handle. Use the sponge side with a warm water/vinegar solution to scrub windows and mirrors; then wipe clean and dry with the rubber blade.

STORAGE

Organization is the key to efficient, accessible storage. Most of the products referred to in this section are widely available at hardware and department stores. Be sure to take along accurate measurements and comparison shop to find the product that solves a storage problem the most effectively for the least money.

Accessible Storage

- From waist height to just above eye level is the most accessible.
- "Within reach" means six inches less than your arm's length, seated or standing; or, within reach of your reaching aid.
- Store heavy objects within easy reach so you can handle them safely.
- Store items close to where they will be used, to save motion.
- Some storage can be made movable for easier use, using roll-out shelves, hanging organizers on cupboard or closet doors, or storage carts on casters.

Kitchens

Make the most of already accessible space, as most kitchens have a lot of awkward or unusable space. Stacking shelves or bins come in plastic or metal in many sizes, designs, and prices. Roll-out shelves can make the back of a shelf as accessible as the front.

Under-shelf containers use wasted space; a Lazy Susan gives ready access to the back of a shelf. A blank wall becomes storage with a sheet of Pegboard and wire hooks.

Pull-out shelving allows access from both sides of an island counter. Corner cupboards can be better used by installing revolving or swinging shelves.

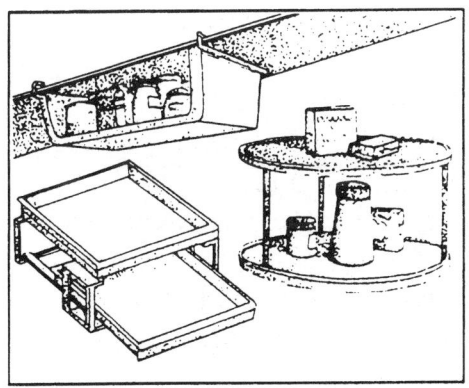

continues

continued

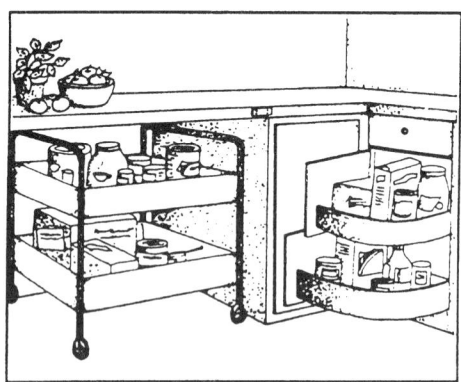

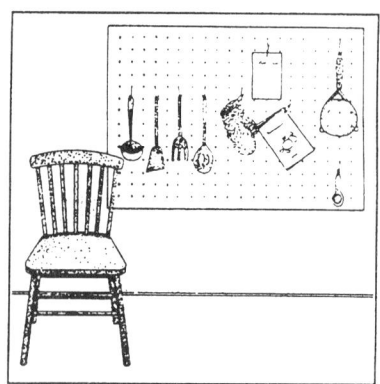

Bathrooms

Vertical towel bars, with rings to hang towels through, take up little space and are easily reached. Hanging racks, available in many bed and bath shops, can be very useful in the tub and shower. They can be attached to a wall, the side of the tub, or the shower fixture, and can hold shampoo, soap, brushes, etc. If you take baths instead of showers, a shelf across the tub can hold bathing items.

Closets

Stacking bins can create accessible storage at waist height on the floor of a closet; shelving units attached to the door can store cleaning, laundry, or kitchen supplies within easy reach. Full closet organizer "systems" are also available for $50 and up; look for a sturdy modular unit that allows you to set shelves at heights that you can reach easily. Lower the clothes bar if you use a wheelchair. Bifold doors will give easier access to the entire closet.

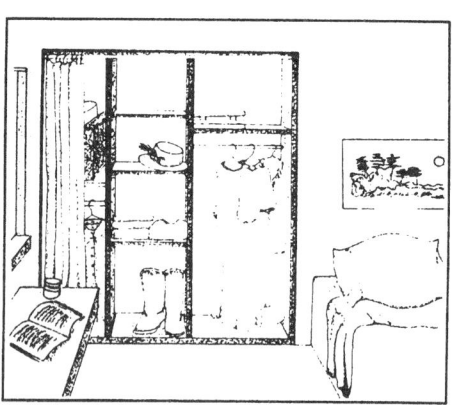

Source: "Around the House," produced by the Iowa Program for Assistive Technology, University Hospital School, Iowa City, Iowa. Reprinted with permission from the Status of Disabled Persons Secretariat, Department of Human Resources Development Canada. Copies of the brochure are available from IPAT. Additional information may be obtained from the Canadian Clearinghouse on Disability Issues, 25 Eddy Street, Suite 100, Hull, Quebec, Canada, K1A 0M5.

Preparing and Serving Food

FOOD PREPARATION

Cutting, Peeling, and Chopping

Cutting boards can be bought or made with stainless steel nails pointing up to hold meat, fruits, vegetables, cheese, etc., for one-handed cutting or peeling. Some have a raised angle for buttering bread. A peeler mounted on a clamp can be attached to a table top or a cutting board; the apple, carrot, or potato can be pushed or pulled across the blade with one hand. A hardwood chopping bowl comes with

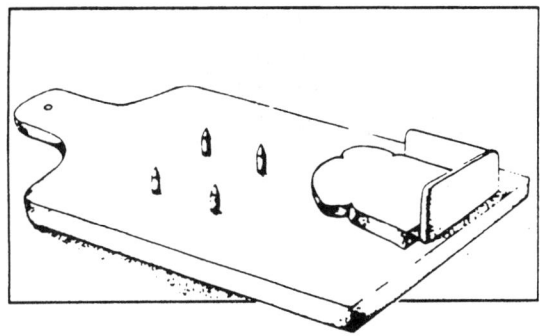

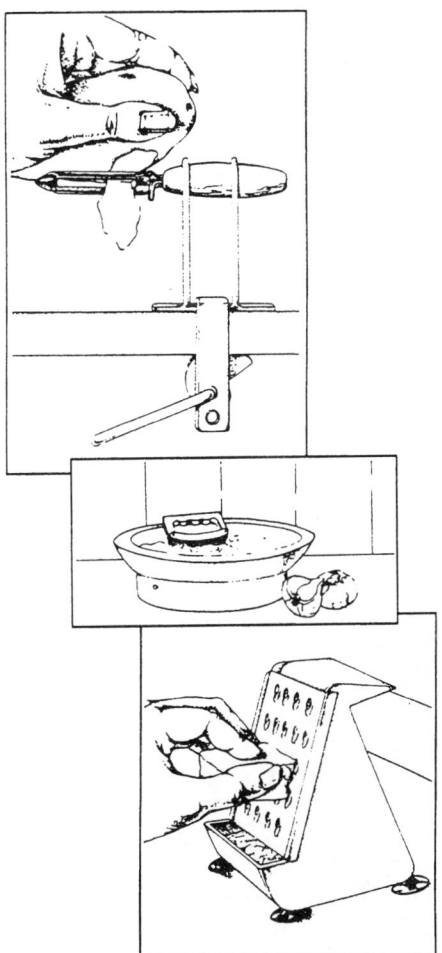

continues

continued

a five-bladed chopper and features a nontip plastic base, available at some medical/surgical supply stores. Also available is a grater with suction feet and a bin to hold grated food.

Opening and Closing Containers

An electric can opener can prevent a lot of frustration. Make sure the one you buy has nonslip rubber feet and a mechanism that can open any shape of can. Jar openers also come in many designs and are widely available. Boxes can be slit open with a knife and closed with a piece of masking tape or a rubber band. Plastic bags can be resealed with a rubber band or clothes pin by twisting the bag shut and tucking the twisted end under the rubber band.

Mixing and Beating

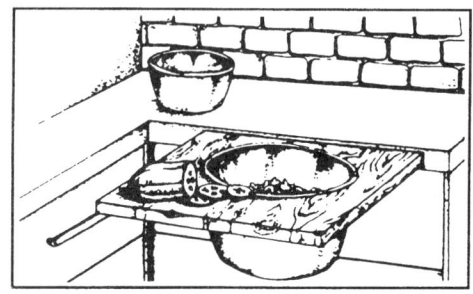

Bowls should be heavy enough to prevent sliding: a rubber ring on the base, a Dycem mat (from a medical/surgical supplier), or even a damp cloth can help. Bowls with handles are widely available. A hole cut in a piece of plywood or hardwood set over a drawer or sink will help steady a bowl while you use it, increasing your counter space at the same time. If the bowl is flush with the board's surface, you can easily push ingredients into the bowl as they are prepared.

Blenders, electric mixers, and food processors can be a big help; if you buy one, make sure the features are useful for your particular cooking needs, and that you can operate the controls.

Cooking

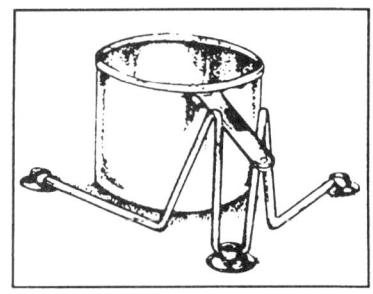

To hold a pot or pan steady while you stir, try a wire frame attached to the stove with suction cups, available from medical supply stores. You can also push the handle against the back of the stove or another pot to stabilize it. The lightest, easiest-to-manipulate pots are made from aluminum, stainless steel, and copper. These metals are also good conductors, so they heat and cool quickly. You will need to stir more frequently with lightweight pots.

Casserole dishes and oven-to-table ware of ceramic, porcelain, Corningware, and tempered glass come in all sizes and weights. They're heavy, but designed to look good on the table, which means less transferring of food from one container to another.

continues

continued

Handles and Knobs

Make sure the shape and size of handles and knobs are well-suited to the strength and flexibility of your grip. A long handle lets you brace against your wrist or arm, or use both hands, and also makes reaching a back burner easier. Handles on both sides of a pan distribute weight more evenly, but are sometimes smaller, and they require two hands and good coordination. A clip-on handle, available where camping supplies are sold, can function as an extra grip for a heavy or awkward pot.

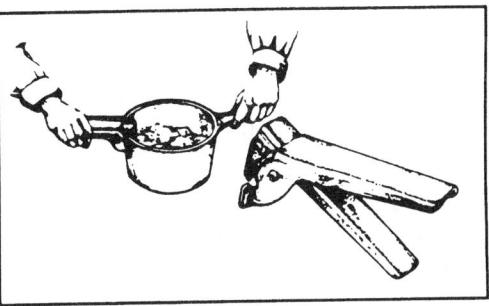

Lids should have a knob that won't slip out of your grip. You'll find replacement knobs at hardware stores. If you use a reaching aid, choose a knob that works well with your aid. Any part of a pot that you touch should be well insulated. Plastic and wood are the safest materials; solid and hollow-core metal handles will heat up eventually and could cause a burn.

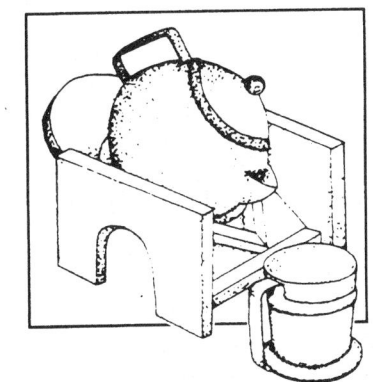

A tipping platform can make handling a teapot easier and safer.

For frying bacon and thinly sliced foods, place a cast aluminum fryer on top of the food, reflecting heat downward, so that it cooks without turning or stirring. A drainer/strainer that clamps over the pot is also a good idea. Oven mitts are essential when working with hot things; you can also use a reaching aid for some jobs. A commercial pizza shovel makes a good reacher to pull hot dishes out of the oven.

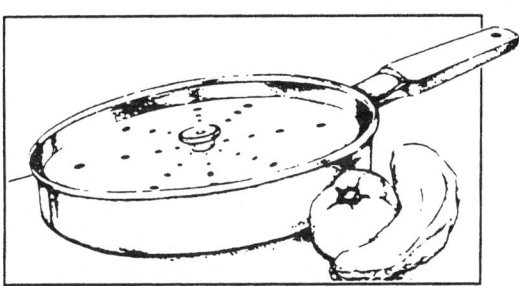

Place heatproof pads around the kitchen and use them as resting stops when carrying heavy, hot items over long distances. If you use a wheelchair, use a heatproof lapboard or wheelchair tray so that you can use both hands for traveling.

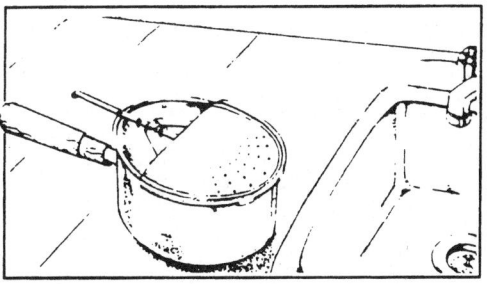

continues

continued

TABLE SETTING

Attractive table settings brighten mealtime and enhance the appreciation of good food. A variety of specially designed plates, dishes, cups, glasses, and silverware are described here; you may find other designs in catalogs from the manufacturers of independent living aids.

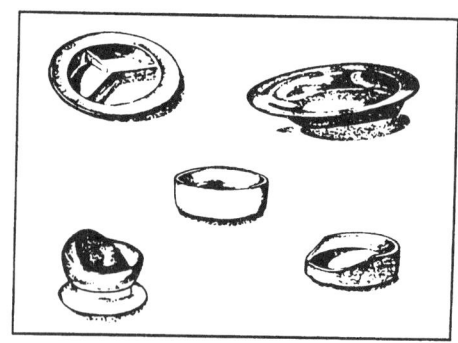

Several manufacturers have designed plates with a curved inner wall and a slightly raised outer rim to help guide food onto your fork or spoon. A heavier plate prevents slipping and retains heat longer. Other options include a nonslip scoop dish, which makes it even easier to push food onto your spoon; a partitioned plate; and dishes with high sides around all or part of the circumference. Available in ceramic or Melamine at medical/surgical supply stores.

A pedestal cup has been designed to make drinking easier for people with a weak grip. A lidded cup reduces spills and controls the flow of liquid. This design is particularly useful for people in bed.

Look for these features in a cup:

- easy-to-grip handle(s)
- insulation or large handles to prevent burns
- a wide base for good stability when empty or full
- break resistance
- easy-to-clean finish

Products are also available to adapt your own tableware: a plate guard in plastic or metal to help guide food onto your fork or spoon; nonslip matting (Dycem, available at medical supply stores) to keep plates from sliding around; handles or wide bases to add to glasses or mugs for better stability; angled or bendable straws that permit drinking from a regular glass while lying in bed.

Silverware

Specially designed knives, forks, and spoons described here can be found at medical supply stores and some "gourmet" kitchen shops. They have been designed to help you overcome the problems of weak grip, lack of flexibility, limited range of motion, and poor coordination.

A built-up handle makes it easier to grasp eating utensils. The simplest way to do this is to buy a length of Rubatoze at a medical supply store. This is foam-rubber tubing that comes with a variety of bore dimensions to fit a range of handle sizes. Or you can use a child's bicycle

continues

continued

handlegrip, as shown in the illustration. Several manufacturers make cutlery with square, round, oval, or built-up handles of varying lengths in light, standard, or heavy weights. Shop around to find which version is best for you. If you have trouble moving your wrist, fingers, or arm, try a fork or spoon with a swivel or self-leveling mechanism.

Extension spoons and forks to assist with limited range of motion can be set at any angle.

Also available are utensils designed to be attached to the palm rather than gripped by the fingers. The angle can be adjusted to compensate for lack of range of motion. Speaking of angles, you can buy "bent" or offset forks and spoons angled left or right in a variety of shapes. Knives come with straight or curved blades, either smooth or serrated, for easier cutting. A person with one hand can cut food easily by rocking a Nelson knife back and forth across the food. Another suggestion is to sharpen an ordinary pizza cutter and use it as a one-handed food cutter. Combination utensils are convenient if you don't use both hands, or if coordination is a problem. Known as "knoons," "knorks," and "sporks," they come in several different designs and weights, some with built-up handles.

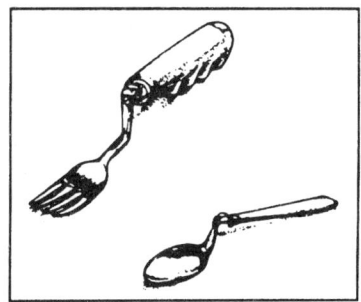

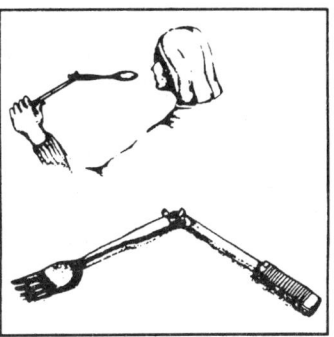

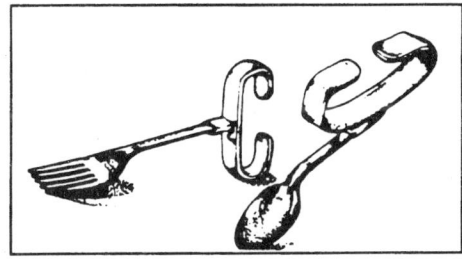

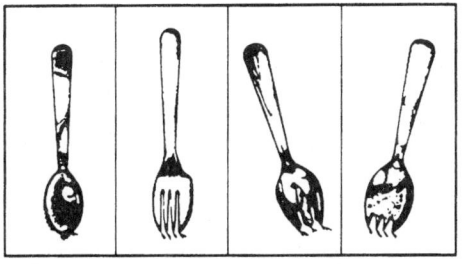

Source: "What's for Dinner?" produced by the Iowa Program for Assistive Technology, University Hospital School, Iowa City, Iowa. Reprinted with permission from the Status of Disabled Persons Secretariat, Department of Human Resources Development Canada. Copies of the brochure are available from IPAT. Additional information may be obtained from the Canadian Clearinghouse on Disability Issues, 25 Eddy Street, Suite 100, Hull, Quebec, Canada, K1A 0M5.

Choosing and Adapting Clothing

Everyone of us has fumbled with a button. But stiffness, pain, weakness, or paralysis can make dressing and undressing particularly difficult. This pamphlet provides information on types of clothing and simple adaptations, devices, and methods to make dressing and undressing easier.

CHOOSE ACCESSIBLE CLOTHING

Roomy, stretchy clothes with simple fastenings are your best bet. For ease and comfort, choose clothing with:

- side or front closings
- deep armholes or raglan sleeves
- pull-on, elasticized waists
- ample room to move freely
- "breathable," soft-surface fabrics

CLOTHING ADAPTATIONS

- Sew cuff buttons on with elastic thread; keep them buttoned all the time and simply slide your hand through.
- Remove buttons from the cuff or front of a blouse or shirt, and sew the button to the closed buttonhole borders. Sew Velcro on the two sides and press to close.
- Attach a ring or loop to the zipper tab so it's easier to catch with fingers or a dressing aid.
- Sew loops or tabs of ribbon or seam binding inside clothes to help in pulling them on or off.
- Adapt a brassiere by sewing up the back closure, cutting the front open and attaching Velcro strips or purchase a brassiere with a front closure.
- To keep a shirt or blouse tucked in, sew rubber strips to the inside of your skirt or slacks waistband. Be careful if no sensation is present.
- Slacks can be fitted with side zippers in the legs to ease in pulling them on and off. Zippers in the inside seam to the knee may accommodate a cast or brace.

Remember: Buttons require the most movement and coordination. Snaps or dome fasteners are easier. Zippers are faster and easier still, and simplest of all are Velcro strips.

SOME OTHER TIPS

Wheelchair-users should avoid long ties or scarves, full-length coats, wide pant legs, and floppy sleeves, which can catch in wheelspokes or pick up dirt from the tires.

Wrap-around skirts are particularly fast and easy to put on, and allow women in wheelchairs extra movement. Choose a shawl rather than a sweater for extra warmth.

continues

Jackets with side (not rear) vents are less likely to ride up. Pre-tied, clip-on ties are available in attractive patterns for a dressier look. Avoid using pants pockets. Keep your wallet in a breast pocket, secured with a strip of Velcro.

A customized apron of pockets designed for tools or items that you use most frequently may make work or hobby activities easier and more enjoyable.

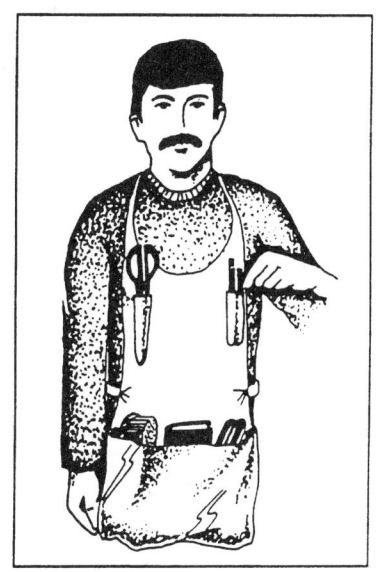

OUTERWEAR

Look for warm, waterproof designs that can bridge seasons, with the same design features—deep armholes or raglan sleeves, roominess—as indoor clothing.

A hooded poncho or cape is particularly suitable for protecting a wheelchair user from rain and cold, and can be purchased at camping supply stores. If you design your own, cut it just below waist level at the back and allow enough front length to drape over the knees. Taper the sides, so they won't bunch and catch

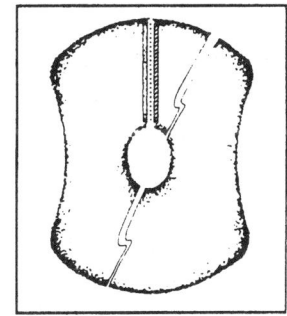

in the wheels. A zip-in insulated lining can make a rain cape into a cold-weather garment.

A hat is essential in winter since so much body heat escapes from an uncovered head. Elderly people may be especially susceptible to chilling. A well-designed winter hat covers the ears, is made of a natural fiber with good insulating properties, and is not tight. If gloves are difficult for you to wear, try mittens instead. They're warmer, much easier to get on and off, and come in a wide variety of colors and styles. A thumbless version is especially warm and easy to get on and off, and can be knitted by a friend.

continued

FOOTWEAR

Here are some ideas for accessible footwear:

- Both dressy and casual shoes are available in slip-on styles.
- Elastic shoelaces stay tied and simply stretch open when you put on or remove your shoes.
- Shoelace clips slide up and down the lace ends and lock into place.
- Many sport shoes and boots and a few dressier styles are available with Velcro tab fasteners. Try them out.
- A shoe button screws into the top lace hole on your shoe; once laces are tied, you just hook them over the button to fasten.

Inexpensive removable cleats attached to shoes or boots can improve your walking control on ice or snow. These can be purchased from a medical supply store.

DRESSING AIDS

When it comes to the actual process of dressing and undressing, dressing aids can make these activities easier.

A well-designed aid should be lightweight but sturdy, and will:

- help you reach your clothing and pull it toward you
- hold the garment so that you can put in your foot, arm, etc.
- pull the article on without straining your back, shoulders, or arms
- attach to and detach from clothing easily

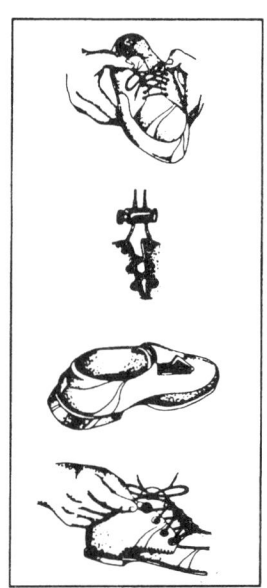

A very simple dressing aid can be made by attaching a clothes peg, hook, garter, or clamp to a piece of fabric tape, rope, or length of wood. The rope or tape can be tied into loops for easier handling; two aids can be used together to pull on slacks, pantyhose, or a skirt. An instant dressing aid can be improvised from a wire coat hanger: bend the triangular form into a long, thin handle; use the hook to reach, pull, or zip.

Sew small loops inside your clothes; catch them with the hook of your dressing aid to pull

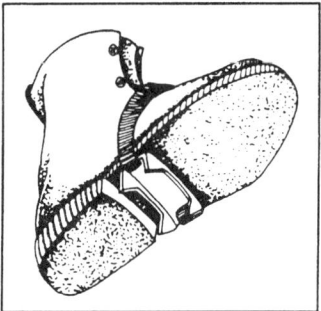

continues

continued

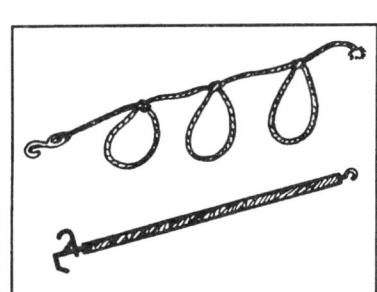 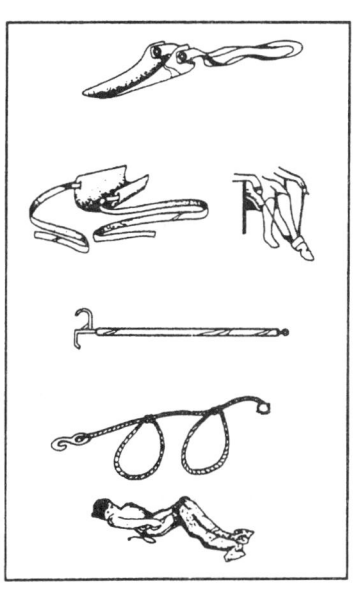 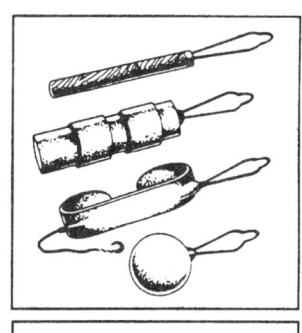 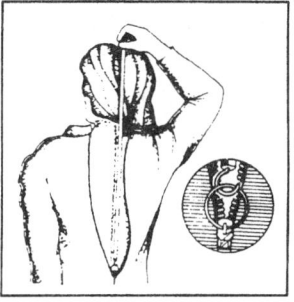

them toward you and to pull them on. Use belt loops on skirts or slacks, and buttonholes on shirts, blouses, and sweaters. If you own a reaching aid, you've probably already used it as a dressing aid. Most reachers have jaws or a projecting hook or lug for catching articles and retrieving them. You can find commercial dressing aids at most medical supply shops.

Once the garment is on, you'll need to fasten it. Buttons can be dealt with easily with a button hook, available in many sizes, with a variety of handles. Push the hook through the buttonhole, catch the button in the hook, and pull it through.

Attach a ring or loop to the zipper on slacks or jackets to make it easier to catch with your finger or the hook of a dressing stick. For back zippers, use a dressing stick if you can reach the zipper; otherwise attach a hook with a cord as shown in the illustration (before putting on the garment, if you can't reach behind), then grasp the cord or ring and pull the zipper.

SHOES AND BOOTS

A simple shoehorn can be your best friend when it comes to putting on shoes and boots, whether laced, buckled, or slip-on. Shop for a long-handled model to reduce bending and straining; check that the point where the horn joins the handle is sturdy, particularly if you use it for heavy shoes or boots. The handle can be

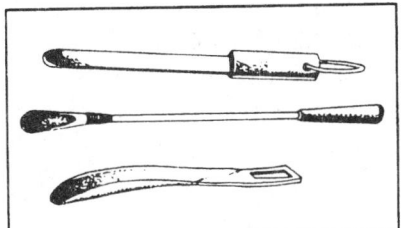

continues

continued

built up if you find it hard or painful to grip. Push your shoe up against the wall or a solid piece of furniture for stability when putting it on.

Removing shoes and boots can also be difficult, but a bootjack can be a great help. Place your heel between the prongs of the bootjack, and pull your foot out. A bootjack can be fastened to the floor in a convenient location or left free to be moved where needed. Or use the rung of a chair or stool to catch the heel when removing footwear.

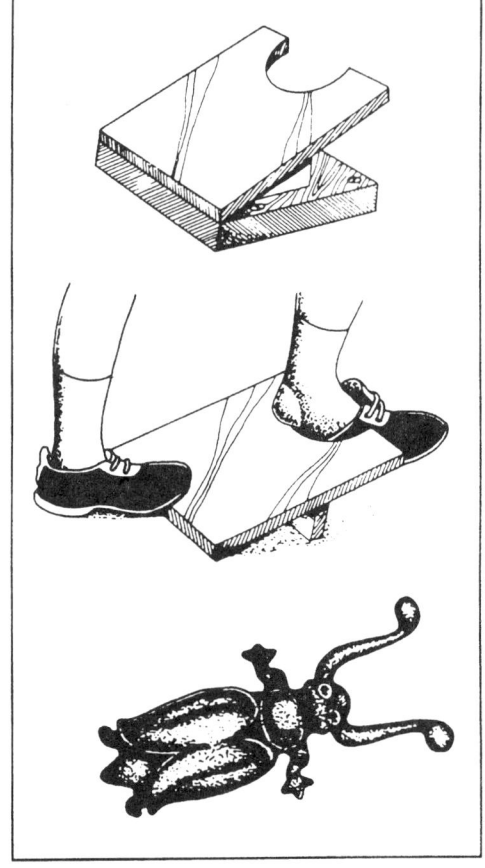

Source: "Zip It Up," produced by the Iowa Program for Assistive Technology, University Hospital School, Iowa City, Iowa. Reprinted with permission from the Status of Disabled Persons Secretariat, Department of Human Resources Development Canada. Copies of the brochure are available from IPAT. Additional information may be obtained from the Canadian Clearinghouse on Disability Issues, 25, Eddy Street, Suite 100, Hull, Quebec, Canada, K1A 0M5.

Adapting Your Personal Care Routine

GROOMING AIDS

Dental Care

You can build up your toothbrush handle for easier gripping by adding a ready-made, built-up handle, a child's bicycle handlegrip, or a palm or wrist cuff, as illustrated. Foam tubing called Rubazote, available from medical suppliers, has a hollow center in which to insert a handle. Extension handles, of the type used with eating utensils, can be helpful when you can't comfortably reach your mouth.

A denture brush can be attached to a sink or counter with a suction-cup device. Flossing may be easier if you use a floss holder, available at most drugstores; it also can be fitted with a built-up handle. "Pump" style toothpaste dispensers are easier for some people to manipulate. A twisting key is another possibility, and a third alternative is toothpowder, which you can simply dip a wet brush into.

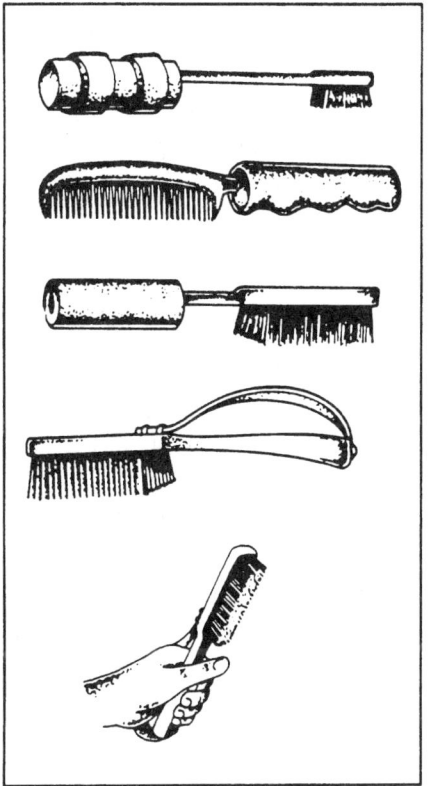

Hair Care

The handle adaptations illustrated here can be used to modify combs and brushes as well. Extension handles are particularly useful if arm or shoulder motion is limited, but your motions will lose some force due to loss of leverage. If you use a hair dryer, mount it on the wall to leave your hands free. The bracket should swivel so the dryer can blow in any direction. Hair washing is easiest in the shower. If you bathe in a tub, a hand sprayer is useful for rinsing. Pump dispensers or flip lids ease opening and closing shampoo and rinse bottles.

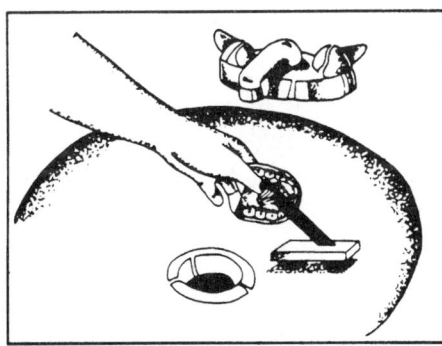

continues

Skin Care

A soap mitt eliminates fussing with slippery bars of soap and awkward facecloths. You can buy one inexpensively, or make a simple one yourself from a small amount of terrycloth.

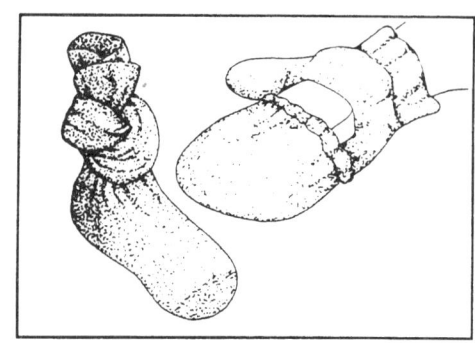

Shaving

Electric razors are easier to use and safer than blades. A bracket or clamp can be rigged to hold a razor firmly to a counter or wall while you move your face against it. A Velcro strap holder can help secure the razor in your hand.

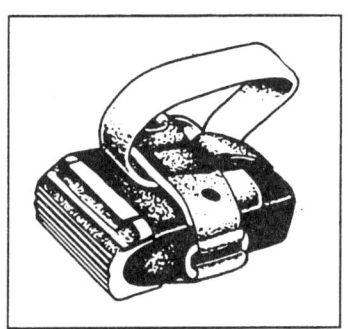

Nails

A nailbrush can be mounted on the edge of the counter or sink with suction cups. Attach a nail file or emery board to a piece of wood or tape it to the countertop to stabilize it for one-handed use. You can attach a nail clipper to a piece of plywood to give you better control, or increase the leverage by lengthening the handle as shown in the illustration. Larger clippers for trimming toe nails, available at most drug stores, may be easier to manipulate for fingernails, too.

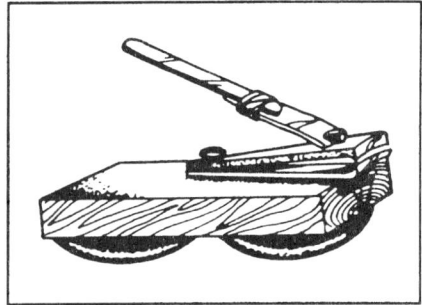

BATH AIDS

Safety is the first consideration. Safety treads or rubber mats on the bottom of tubs and showers are simple and inexpensive. Test and adjust water temperature before stepping into a bath or shower. Set water heaters below 120 degrees, and ask others not to run water elsewhere in the

continues

continued

house to prevent temperature fluctuations. For extra protection, pressure balancers to prevent surges of hot or cold water are available from plumbing supply stores.

Handrails that clamp to the side of the bathtub and gripping bars for tub and shower walls can be purchased from medical suppliers.

Organize items that you'll need before you get in the tub or shower. If you use a reaching aid, put it near the tub. A shelf across the tub keeps useful items near at hand and offers another surface to steady yourself against.

Bath brushes with long handles are useful for scrubbing various hard-to-reach places; handles can be built up or bent to improve your control.

Another way to scrub your back is to attach a piece of terrycloth, sponge, or loofah to a strip of sturdy fabric or plastic to pull from side to side. These scrubbers are available for sale at medical supply stores, but you could easily make your own.

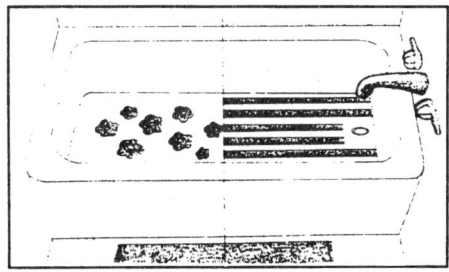

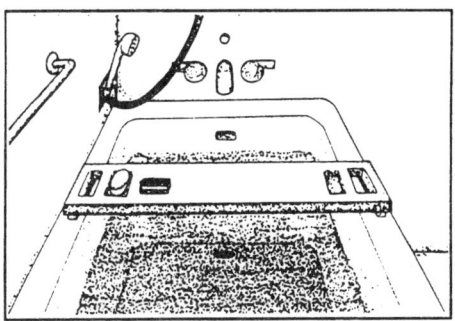

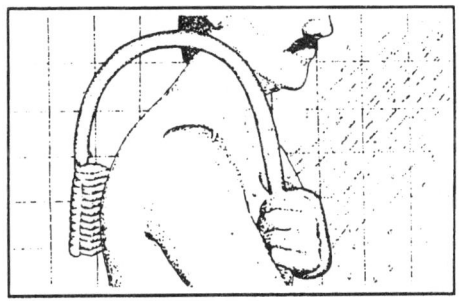

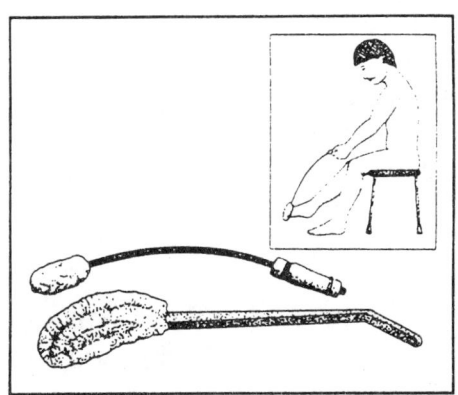

Source: "Cleanliness is Next to . . ." produced by the Iowa Program for Assistive Technology, University Hospital School, Iowa City, Iowa. Reprinted with permission from the Status of Disabled Persons Secretariat, Department of Human Resources Development Canada. Copies of the brochure are available from IPAT. Additional information may be obtained from the Canadian Clearinghouse on Disability Issues, 25, Eddy Street, Suite 100, Hull, Quebec, Canada, K1A 0M5.

Reaching and Mobility Aids

REACHING AIDS

Pushing, pulling, grasping, and turning are movements that can be easier for you with a reaching aid. The model shown here is designed to cover a wide range of activities and will help people with a weak or painful grip or a limited range of motion.

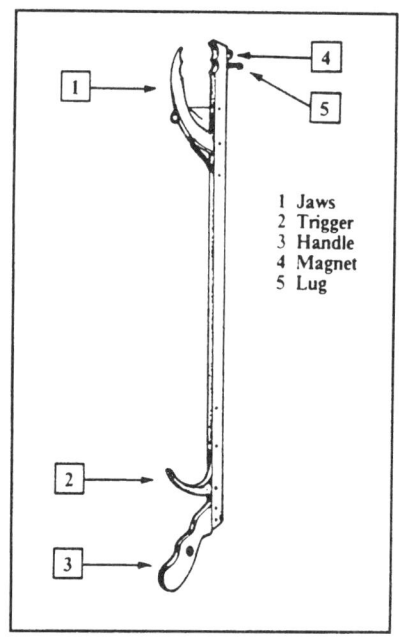

1 Jaws
2 Trigger
3 Handle
4 Magnet
5 Lug

The most common reachers consist of a pair of jaws controlled by a trigger mechanism. Made of lightweight aluminum and plastic, they are available in a variety of sizes and lengths. The desk-sized model, about 24" long, is useful for retrieving objects on your desk, kitchen counter, or bedside table. A mid-range length, about 28" long, is useful for everyday activities such as picking up objects from the floor or reaching high storage areas. An extra-long model (32") is also available if you need extended reach. Features you'll find useful include a magnet for catching and holding metal objects, and a projecting lug for pulling things toward you. Folding styles and reachers with toggle (rather than trigger) closing action, swivel heads, or forearm extension are also available.

Prices vary widely, depending on the size and features. Reachers are generally available at most medical supply stores.

MOBILITY

Mobility can be complicated by many factors, such as pain and weakness in the legs or back, uncertain balance or dizziness, muscular tremors or spasms, or paralysis. There are a variety of changes in your environment, as well as canes and walkers, that can enhance your mobility in and out of your home.

Modify Your Home

- Install grab bars in critical locations.
- Remove small rugs; avoid shag carpeting.
- Arrange furniture so that you can walk from solid piece to solid piece, using the furniture for support.

continues

continued

Clothing and Footwear

- Choose pants and tops that do not restrict motion and do not trail behind.
- Choose shoes with textured soles for better grip.
- Removable cleats can give you better footing on ice or snow.

Canes

Although canes can be purchased at many drugstores, you should consult with your doctor if you are having frequent or pronounced periods of weakness, dizziness, or poor coordination.

Consider the following factors in selecting a cane:

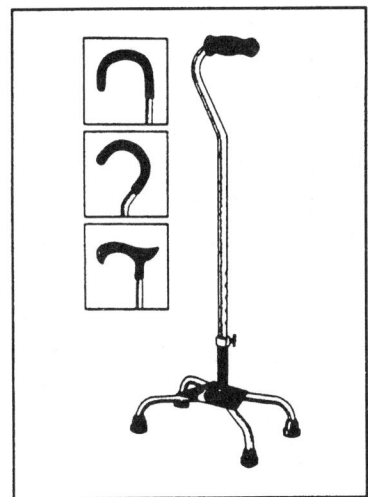

- **Height:** The handle should be at the height of your hip joint.
- **Weight:** You should have no trouble lifting it.
- **Handle:** The grip should be comfortable and secure.
- **Base:** Canes are available with single tips or four-legged, wide bases.

Other options available include a loop on the handle of the cane, which frees your hands for other activities, and a fold-down ice gripping tip, which can be attached to the side of the cane.

Walkers

The walker is particularly useful for individuals with balance problems, since it affords support through both arms at a fixed distance. Walkers come in a wide range of heights and weights, with a variety of handle styles. Ask your doctor or physical therapist for help in making a selection.

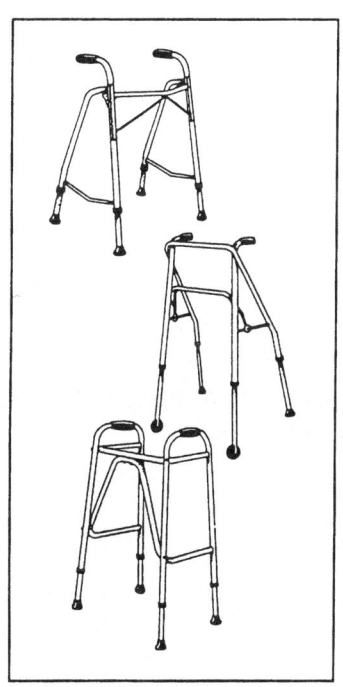

continues

continued

Grab Bars

Grab bars make the most of your strength by giving you extra support when and where you need it, such as climbing in and out of the bathtub or your bed.

A grab bar looks like a towel rack, but that's where the similarity ends. A grab bar is designed to be strong enough to support your weight and more. Flanges on the ends of the bar have sturdy screws for installation, preferably into wall studs. There is room between the bar and the wall for you to get a good grip, and the diameter of the bar will feel solid in your hand. Made of plastic or rust-resistant metal, the bar may have a rough surface to prevent slipping. Many shapes and sizes are available for different uses. Most are wall mounted, but some attach to the edge of your bathtub.

Some considerations in selecting a grab bar:

- Evaluate your physical abilities, and choose a bar and a location that lets you use your strongest muscles most effectively.
- Make sure the bar you select is long enough to carry a movement through to its conclusion. If you run out of support

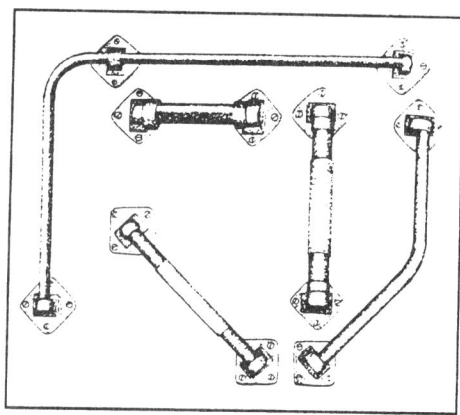

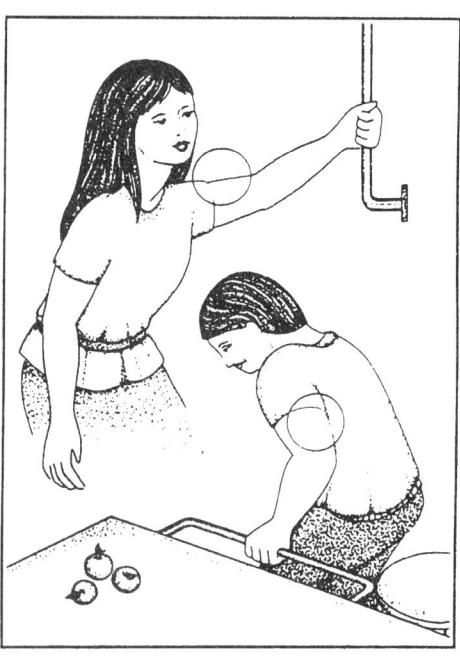

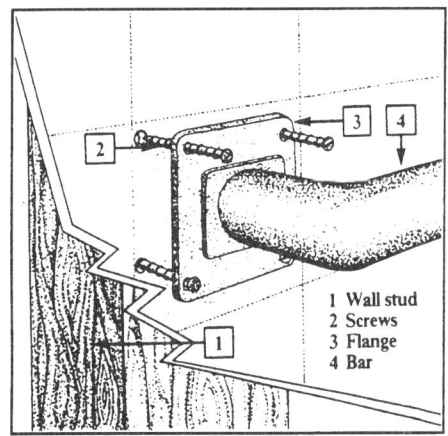

1 Wall stud
2 Screws
3 Flange
4 Bar

continues

continued

before you're fully standing, you could lose momentum and fall back, or fall forward from too much force.
- An occupational therapist can help you with decisions about where to place what kind of bar.

Some shapes and sizes of grab bars are illustrated here. They can be purchased at plumbing supply outlets, some department and hardware stores, and at medical/surgical supply stores. If you can't find one to suit your needs, some companies will custom design a bar for a somewhat higher price. Alternatively, you may be able to combine standard bars in sequence to give you the support you need.

Notes:

Source: "You Can Get There from Here," produced by the Iowa Program for Assistive Technology, University Hospital School, Iowa City, Iowa. Reprinted with permission from the Status of Disabled Persons Secretariat, Department of Human Resources Development Canada. Copies of the brochure are available from IPAT. Additional information may be obtained from the Canadian Clearinghouse on Disability Issues, 25 Eddy Street, Suite 100, Hull, Quebec, Canada, K1A 0M5.

WHEELCHAIRS

Wheelchairs for People with Spinal Cord Injuries

Your wheelchair is more than just an alternate means of mobility. It should be an extension of your personality. The right wheelchair with the correct fit can play an important part in whether you view yourself as being "confined to a wheelchair" or as someone who has adopted a "different way of mobility."

TYPES OF WHEELCHAIRS

Medical Model

The medical model wheelchair is the standard hospital or chromed version. It has few, if any, adjustments. Its total weight is usually 50 pounds, and it has poor maneuverability and a high seat back. Often, this is the first chair a person is exposed to because it may have the capability of reclining the back or elevating the footrests. These features are sometimes helpful when a newly injured person is first brought to a sitting position, but this chair should be treated as a piece of medical equipment, *not* as a means of mobility. It is essential at this phase of rehabilitation to realize that this kind of wheelchair is merely a "stepping stone" and that your personal equipment will be quite different.

Lightweight Wheelchairs/Sportschairs

The ultralight wheelchair was initially developed to be used in wheelchair sports. Its durability and maneuverability, however, provided extended freedom to its users, and the demand for these qualities moved from sports participants to the general population. Such a chair is highly adjustable and provides a custom fit. It weighs less than 30 pounds and comes in folding and rigid frame models. This chair is narrow and light (when fitted and equipped properly) and allows more freedom in tight quarters and when overcoming barriers. Optional equipment and adjustments allow the chair to grow along with your skills.

Some of the advantages of the lightweight chair, however, may cause you to feel less secure when first introduced to this type of chair. You must learn to use a wheelchair, just as a child learns to ride a bicycle, because it is not a "natural" means of mobility. As with shoes, the essential component of a good functional wheelchair is proper fit.

Motorized Wheelchairs

The motorized wheelchair was developed for the use of individuals with limited arm use. It is a battery-powered unit capable of speeds of 5 mph or more and may be controlled by the hand, mouth, head, or chin. It is extremely heavy (80 pounds or more), bulky, and very expensive. But it is often prescribed as a preventive measure against upper extremity muscle over-use syndrome.

Fortunately, in recent years there has been a tendency to prescribe both an electric and a manual wheelchair for people with very high level tetraplegia. As a rule, people with C5 and lower

continues

continued

injury can learn to push a lightweight wheelchair independently, which allows a high degree of independence and mobility. Longer distances, however, may require the electric wheelchair.

Depending on a motorized wheelchair alone often leads to a decrease in strength and self-care skills. However, it can also free up your time, allowing you to engage in other activities.

CHAIR FIT

There are five keys to proper wheelchair fitting:

1. **Seat width** is determined by measuring hip width. The frame width of the chair should be the same as the hip measurement (taken with no cushion). This hip width can be taken by placing a hardcover book on each side of the hips and measuring the straightline distance between the books. The misconception of allowing an inch on each side for "growing into the chair" is as ridiculous as it would be if attempting to properly fit shoes.
2. **Seat length** is the distance from the seat back to slightly behind the knee (when bent).
3. **Frame length** (different from seat length) is determined by the height of the person. Generally, persons 5 ft 8 in or shorter will use a short frame; those 5 ft 9 in to 6 ft 2 in will use a standard frame; and those 6 ft 3 in and taller will use a long frame. The frame length, to some degree, determines how easily the chair will maneuver in tight places. Therefore, it should not be overestimated. The shortest frame that is practical should be selected.
4. **Back height** should be taken from the seat of the chair to the bottom of the shoulder blade. This is a maximum height and should be taken with the cushion in place. Generally, most wheelchairs are ordered with backs that are too tall, with the mistaken justification that it will help balance. Backs that are too high cause poor posture by pushing the shoulder blades forward and rounding the back. To counter this effect, the individual either slides the hips forward, which causes rounding of the lower back and compression of the organs, or uses armrests to push on to prevent falling forward. If the chair back is below the level of the shoulder blade, it allows the upper back to extend slightly behind the seat back, which prevents the sensation of being "pushed" from the chair. Often instability is caused by cushion type rather than by a back that is too low.
5. **Footrest or foot support length** should be measured from the heel of the foot with the ankle at 90 degrees to the back of the knee, which is positioned slightly higher than the hip. When the knees are higher, maintaining balance is easier, and spasms may not be as severe. Allow the heel of the foot to extend beyond the rear of the support. This will prevent "foot drop" and maintain better contact to keep the feet from vibrating off the support.

EQUIPMENT OPTIONS

Cushions

There are three types of cushions:

continues

continued

1. **Roho:** Multichambered, air-inflated, rubber cushion. It is available in regular, low-profile, and mini-profile versions. This cushion is expansive and offers poor sitting balance. However, it does offer maximum protection from skin breakdowns while being lightweight.
2. **Gel:** Dense, gelatinlike semisolids that offer greater stability for balance. Such cushions are very heavy.
3. **Foam:** Dense, spongelike cushion that is relatively inexpensive and lightweight. It may be sculpted to provide both skin protection and sitting stability.

Footrests

Footrests can be classified into one of three categories:

1. **Swing-away:** As their name implies, these swing away from the front of the wheelchair and detach. They allow ambulatory wheelchair users to adopt a wider stance when assuming a standing position. Such footrests may become lost or may be damaged easily during sports or active use and may add weight to the wheelchair.
2. **Folding:** These platforms fold tightly against the frame of the wheelchair and offer many of the advantages of the swing-away footrests without adding weight or structural weakness.
3. **Rigid:** These supports are permanent extensions of the nonfolding wheelchair. These are the most durable type and also the most desirable type for sports use. They offer protection for the feet and add strength to the wheelchair.

Brakes

There are three types of brakes:

1. **High mount:** These are the most widely used and are mounted in front of the rear wheel, usually at seat level. They are the easiest to lock and unlock. Because of their position, however, they may cause injury to the hands when vigorous activities are pursued.
2. **Low mount:** These are located on the bottom frame member well below the level of the seat. This position requires the user to lean forward slightly to operate, but the location provides no hindrance in any activity.
3. **Hill climbers (grade aids):** These brake attachments prevent the wheelchair from rolling backward on a steep incline. They are only available with high mount brakes and therefore retain the same disadvantages for the active individual.

Armrests

Armrests can be divided into three categories:

continues

continued

1. **Nonremovable:** These come on the medical model wheelchair and are permanently attached to some part of the frame. They greatly hinder mobility and efficient pushing techniques and "hide" the individual.
2. **Removable:** These provide the same stability as the fixed type but offer greater versatility for transfers, pushing, and so forth.
3. **Swing-away:** These provide versatility but hinder efficient pushing techniques as does the nonremovable type.

Tires

Tires can be classified into one of two types:

1. **Hard/solid rubber:** These tires have the advantage of long wear with no flats. The disadvantages are poor ride quality, poor traction, and heavy weight.
2. **Pneumatic:** These air-filled tires have the advantages of good traction and good shock-absorbing ride quality and are lightweight. The disadvantage is that flats may occur (as on a car).

Notes:

Source: Sis Theuerkauf and Phil Carpenter, "Return to the Real World," *Journal of Home Health Care Practice*, Vol. 4:4, Aspen Publishers, Inc., © 1992.

Features to Consider When Purchasing a Wheelchair

Type	Advantages	Disadvantages
Backrests		
Fixed	Strong, durable.	More difficult to transport.
Folding	Easier to transport.	May release accidentally.
Armrests		
Padded tubular	Easily moved/removed. Allows easy access to tables/desks. Lightweight.	Minimal height adjustability. Does not protect clothing or skin or keep cushion in place. Less stable than others. May not provide appropriate positioning for persons with high tetraplegia.
Height adjustable		
Single post	Provides support and positioning options for upper extremities. Protects clothing and skin, and keeps cushion in place.	Less stable than a double post. Not durable. May be difficult for persons with tetraplegia to manage.
Full length	Allows for support and positioning options. Helpful during sit-to-stand transfers.	Difficult to access work/table surfaces closely.
Desk length	Easy to access work surfaces.	May not provide enough support or positioning options.
Double post (height adjustable or standard model)	Greater stability than others. Some models help protect clothing and skin and keep cushion in place.	May be difficult to remove and insert.
Pivot arm	Easy to swing away. Stable.	Some styles are not height adjustable. May be difficult to manage with decreased hand function.
No armrest	Ease of transfers. Cosmesis.	No upper extremity support. Not recommended for higher-level injuries because of safety and posture concerns.

continues

continued

Type	Advantages	Disadvantages
Lightweight Frames		
Rigid	Greater push efficiency. Greater strength and durability.	Overall folded size is bulkier.
Folding	Folded size is compact to increase ease of transport. Increased play in frame allows it to fit in tighter spaces.	Decreased durability. Less push efficiency.
Front Rigging		
Rigid	Strong, durable. Advantageous for wheelchair sports.	May interfere with transfers and ambulation. May limit access to tight spaces. May not provide adequate foot support.
Swing away	Can be moved out of the way for transfers and ambulation. Can be removed for easier access in tight spaces.	May add weight. Less durable than rigid type. Release mechanism may not be accessible to user.
Elevating	May decrease edema in elevated position. Minimizes orthostatic hypotension in elevated position.	Increases overall length of chair. Adds weight. Length of legrest needs adjustment each time hanger angle is changed.
Fixed front rigging with flip-up foot plates	Strong, durable. Foot plates can be flipped up for transfers and ambulation.	May limit access to tight spaces.
Fixed hanger angles*		
Closer to 60°	Allows for more foot plate clearance.	Increases overall length of chair.
Closer to 90°	More anatomically correct sitting posture. Decreases overall length of chair.	May not allow adequate foot plate clearance. Need adequate knee range of motion.
Tapered	Cosmesis. Can get closer to furniture.	May touch the legs.
Back Posts		
Angled	More comfortable.	—
Straight	—	Person may feel as if he or she is falling forward.

*Wheelchair manufacturers produce different hanger angles. Check with the manufacturers for the specific angles they provide.

continues

continued

Type	Advantages	Disadvantages
Brakes		
High mount	Easy to reach.	May interfere with pushing.
Low mount	Do not interfere with pushing.	Hard to reach. Need good hand function to use.
Front Casters (2 to 8 inches)[**]		
Small	Small turning radius.	Less stable. Less shock absorption.
Large	More stable. More shock absorption.	Less maneuverable.
Pneumatic	Good ride.	Gets flat tires. Needs maintenance.
Semipneumatic	No flat tires.	Better ride than poly, not as good as pneumatic.
Poly	No flat tires.	Less shock absorption.
Rear Wheels (24 inches)		
Spoke	Lighter.	Needs maintenance.
MAG	No maintenance.	A few ounces heavier than spokes.
Tires (Rear)		
Pneumatic	Good ride. Absorbs shocks.	Gets flat tires. Needs maintenance.
Pneumatic with solid inserts	No maintenance. Ride is better than with poly.	Ride not as good as with pneumatic.
Poly	No flat tires.	Hard ride. Less shock absorption.

[**]Sizes available vary among manufacturers.

Source: Robert Harold Jackson, *Spinal Cord Injury: Medical Management and Rehabilitation*, Gary M. Yarkony, ed., Aspen Publishers, Inc., © 1994.

Wheelchair Accessories Glossary

- **Anti-tippers.** Also called wheelie bars. These devices prevent the wheelchair from tipping over backward. They usually are found on the back of the wheelchair near the floor. Most have tiny wheels on the ends.
- **Brake extension.** An attachment to extend the brake applicator arm. Allows the patient to reach and apply brakes with increased ease. They are available from approximately 6 to 9 inches, and are usually removable for transfers.
- **Camber.** An angling of the wheel from top to bottom, usually done by inserting washers between the axle plate and the wheelchair frame. The angling increases the base of support (BOS) of the wheelchair and its stability and push efficiency; it also increases the width of the wheelchair.
- **Caster pin lock.** Located just over the caster housing, its purpose is to keep the caster in a forward position. It must be removed to turn a corner. This device is useful when propelling over a slanted surface.
- **Clothing guards.** Guards sit on each side of the seat to protect the user from debris on the wheels. Guards can be made of any number of fabrics or plastic. Guards can be fixed (nonremovable) or removable.
- **Grade aid.** Usually located near the brake, this device, when applied to the wheel, will allow the wheel to roll forward but not backward. It helps the individual on inclines. It is also referred to as a hill holder.
- **Heel loop.** Usually present as a cloth strap placed across the back of a single foot plate. It prevents the feet from sliding off the back of the foot plate.
- **Leg strap.** Any type of strap used across the front rigging to prevent legs from getting caught underneath the wheelchair.
- **Push handles.** Found on the back of the wheelchair, either attached to the back posts or mounted separately. They are used by a non–wheelchair user to push or manipulate the wheelchair. The push handles also are useful to hook with a user's arm as a point of stability while doing functional activities.
- **Rear wheel sizes.** Sizes range from 20- to 26-inch diameters. The standard is 24 inches. Smaller sizes usually are used for hemiheight wheelchairs. With increased wheel diameter, the turning radius of the wheelchair is larger, so the wheelchair may be harder to maneuver for some users.
- **Retractable armrests.** Useful on wheelchairs that will recline because they recline with the backrest. This provides constant support for the user's upper extremities.
- **Seat belts.** Depending on the attachment (45° or 90°), seat belts can be for safety and/or positioning of the individual in the wheelchair. Clasp styles include wraparound, auto style, and airline style.
- **Spoke guard.** This device rests over the spoked part of the wheel to prevent an individual's fingers from getting caught in the spokes.

Source: Robert Harold Jackson, *Spinal Cord Injury: Medical Management and Rehabilitation*, Gary M. Yarkony, ed., Aspen Publishers, Inc., © 1994.

Important Information about Your Wheelchair Cushion

HIGH-DENSITY FOAM CUSHION

- **Average lifespan:** 6 to 12 months.
- **Warranty:** There is no warranty on this cushion.
- **Weight:** Approximately two pounds.
- **Maintenance:**
  - Keep covered to prevent sunlight from breaking down the foam.
  - Rotate the cushion weekly to prevent wear in one area.
  - Do not wash cushion (and do not sit on wet cushion).
  - Wash cover in washing machine as needed; line dry.
- **Important tips:**
  - Always use the cover that comes with the cushion for maximum effectiveness. **Do not** use Chuxs, sheepskins, towels, or cushion covers provided with ultralight wheelchairs over your cushion.
  - If you or lose a significant amount of weight, return for reevaluation by a rehabilitation professional to determine the appropriateness of your cushion.
  - **Remember**, even the best cushion does **not** replace weight shifts.
  - If skin breakdown or red marks occur while using your cushion properly and performing weight shifts as recommended, contact your doctor immediately.

JAY CUSHION

- **Average lifespan:** Three to five years.
- **Warranty:** 18 months from date of purchase. Warranty covers defects in materials or workmanship not due to misuse or accidents.
- **Weight:** Six to nine pounds.
- **Maintenance:**
  - To clean cushion, sponge wipe with warm soapy water. Flolite Pad (jelled portion) may be removed from base for ease of cleaning.
  - Cover may be machine washed and dried.
  - If Flolite Pad is punctured, repair immediately with patch kit provided with the cushion.
- **Important tips:**
  - Jelled portion can be removed from base and used when sitting in a chair other than your wheelchair for long periods of time (e.g., driving, at the movies, etc.)
  - Make sure the Flolite Pad is placed in the cushion according to instructions clearly marked on the pad itself.
  - Always use the cover that comes with the cushion for maximum effectiveness. **Do not** use Chuxs, sheepskins, towels, or cushion covers provided with ultralight wheelchair over your cushion.

continues

continued

- —If you gain or lose a significant amount of weight, return for reevaluation to determine the appropriateness of your cushion.
- —**Remember**, even the best cushion does **not** replace weight shifts.
- —If skin breakdown or red marks occur while using your cushion properly and performing weight shifts as recommended, contact your doctor immediately.

ROHO CUSHION

- **Average lifespan:** Approximately three years.
- **Warranty:** One year from date of purchase. Warranty covers defects in materials or workmanship not due to misuse or accidents.
- **Weight:** Three pounds, six ounces (3 lb. 6 oz.).
- **Maintenance:**
  - —Air pressure should be checked daily to ensure proper skin protection. Instructions for checking air pressure are located on the back of the cushion.
  - —To clean cushion, sponge wipe with warm soapy water.
  - —Cover may be machine washed in cool water and, for best results, line dried.
- **Important tips:**
  - —Overinflation may cause bladders to burst.
  - —For small leaks, repair immediately with patch kit provided with your cushion.
  - —Rubber can pop, tear, or melt; therefore, use caution with sharp objects or cigarettes.
  - —Refer to the back of the cushion for more specific information.
  - —Always use the cover that comes with the cushion for maximum effectiveness. **Do not** use Chuxs, sheepskins, towels, or cushion covers provided with ultralight wheelchairs over your cushion. Covers can be ordered separately if original is damaged.
  - —If you gain or lose a significant amount of weight, return for reevaluation to determine the appropriateness of your cushion.
  - —**Remember**, even the best cushion **does not** replace weight shifts.
  - —If skin breakdown or red marks occur while using your cushion properly and performing weight shifts as recommended, contact your doctor immediately.

Source: Shirley S. Paulson, *Spinal Cord Injury Home Care Manual*, Norman B. Nelson Rehabilitation Center, Santa Clara Valley Medical Center, San Jose, California, © 1994.

Wheelchair Information Sheet

Date Received: _____

Serial Number: _____

VENDOR:

Name: _____

Address: _____

Phone: _____

Type: _____
Seat Width: _____
Seat Depth: _____
Armrests: _____
Footrests: _____
Tires: _____
Casters: _____
Brakes: _____

OTHER ATTACHMENTS:

_____
_____
_____
_____

Therapist: _____
Date: _____

Source: Kelly B. Wascher, ed., *Patient Education and Discharge Planning Manual for Rehabilitation*, St. Joseph Rehabilitation Hospital and Outpatient Center, Aspen Publishers, Inc., © 1995.

Wheelchair Maintenance

Proper maintenance is essential for a wheelchair to be useful. Basic maintenance involves keeping the chair clean, dry, protected from weather, and repaired when needed.

Following simple measures, plus getting a yearly checkup by a reputable wheelchair dealer, can help prevent costly repairs.

CLEANING

- To clean a wheelchair, use a mild soap and water solution and be sure to wipe dry.
- Never use an abrasive on the chrome, and pay special attention to the wheels and casters to keep them free of lint, string, hair, and dirt.
- Rub the telescoping parts with paraffin to prevent sticking. Do not use oil on these parts, because it collects dirt.

HANDLING

- Never force a wheelchair to open or close.
- To close most wheelchairs, pull up on the seat by placing your hands on the front and the back of the upholstery.
- Some wheelchairs have upholstery handles provided on the sides of the seats; to close these wheelchairs, pull up on the handles.
- To open, push down on the sides of the seat. Never push *out* on the arms of the chair. This can "spring" the frame of the chair.

Notes:

Source: Georgianna Burbidge Wilson and Virginia L. Kerr, "Wheelchairs: Selection, Uses, Adaptation, and Maintenance," in *Basic Rehabilitation Techniques*, ed 3, Robert D. Sine et al., eds., Aspen Publishers, Inc., © 1988.

Charging Guidelines for Power Wheelchairs: Lead Acid Batteries

BASIC INFORMATION

- **Wear protective eye shields when working with batteries.**
- The batteries consist of two 12-volt deep-cycle batteries (boat batteries).
- Use grounded outlets.
- Charge batteries in well-ventilated areas due to release of gases.
- Charge batteries in dry areas away from water.
- The usual recharging time is 8 to 12 hours. It should never take longer than 18 hours.
- The charger will automatically stop when batteries are fully charged. Do not keep them plugged in for more than two days (shortens life of batteries).
- Monthly, check water level in batteries **after** the batteries have been fully charged. Add **distilled** water to levels as marked. **Do not** overfill.

To Charge Batteries

1. Make sure wheelchair is turned off.
2. Plug charger into wall.
3. Plug charger into wheelchair. Charger should turn on automatically.

To Unplug Charger When Charging Is Complete

1. Unplug from wheelchair first.
2. Unplug charger from wall next.

To Unplug Charger BEFORE Charging Is Complete

1. Unplug charger from wall first.
2. Unplug charger from wheelchair next.

BATTERY LIFE

- A battery can last 6 months to 2 years. The average life of a battery is 1 to $1\frac{1}{2}$ years.
- Batteries will last longer if:
  - They are not overcharged.
  - They are not run all the way down.
  - *Distilled* water is added monthly as needed.
- Usually, lead acid batteries will last through one day of heavy use. Batteries should be charged every night.
- Lead acid batteries are not allowed on commercial airlines (use gel batteries for traveling).

Source: Kelly B. Wascher, ed., *Patient Education and Discharge Planning Manual for Rehabilitation*, St. Joseph Rehabilitation Hospital and Outpatient Center, Aspen Publishers, Inc., © 1995.

Wheelchair Positioning

WHAT IS WHEELCHAIR POSITIONING?

Wheelchair positioning is sitting correctly in a wheelchair. It involves using the right equipment and wheelchair. A physical or occupational therapist looks at wheelchair positioning needs.

WHY IS PROPER WHEELCHAIR POSITIONING IMPORTANT?

Proper wheelchair positioning prevents:

- skin breakdown (pressure sores)
- shortening of muscles (contractures)
- bony changes (deformities)

Proper wheelchair positioning also:

- allows the wheelchair user to get around easily
- keeps lungs clear
- allows for safe swallowing
- manages abnormal muscle tone (too much or too little tension in the muscles)
- provides comfort

HOW TO MAINTAIN GOOD WHEELCHAIR POSITIONING

- Keep thighs parallel to the wheelchair seat.
- Keep two- to three-finger spacing between the back of the knees and the end of the wheelchair seat.
- Place feet flat on the footrests.
- Place elbows on the armrests.
- Keep $\frac{1}{2}$-inch spacing on each side between the hips and the sides of the wheelchair.
- Place buttocks against the back of the chair. Sit straight—**do not** slouch.
- Point legs forward, not upward or outward.
- Keep bony areas free from pressure.
- Keep brakes and driving mechanism (wheels for a manual chair, hand or chin controls for an electric chair) within reach.

Source: Kelly B. Wascher, ed., *Patient Education and Discharge Planning Manual for Rehabilitation*, St. Joseph Rehabilitation Hospital and Outpatient Center, Aspen Publishers, Inc., © 1995.

Basic Wheelchair Transfer Considerations

When helping a person who uses a wheelchair to perform a transfer, you should keep the following considerations in mind:

- Lock the brakes of the wheelchair and swing the foot pedals out of the way.
- Put shoes or nonslip slippers on the person. If a brace has been prescribed, this also must be worn.
- Place a transfer belt around the person for the protection of the person and the caregiver. This also discourages the tendency to grasp the person at painful joints, especially the shoulders.
- Explain and demonstrate the initial transfer to the person who is aware, and repeat if the person is confused.
- Position the wheelchair so that the edges of the two transfer surfaces form an angle of 60 degrees.
- Position the wheelchair so that the person moves toward the strongest side—if the individual has a strong side.
- Stand close to the person for maximum support and safety during a transfer.
- Bend your hips and knees and keep your back straight. Lifting should be done with the leg muscles, not the back. Assist the person to the standing position by straightening his or her hips and knees.
- Stand with a broad base of support. Keep your feet apart, with one foot ahead of the other. This improves balance and permits easy weight shifts.
- Allow the person to see the surface to which he or she is being transferred.
- Allow the person to practice the entire transfer preparation independently. The person and the caregiver must learn the importance of the safety factors of locking the brakes and positioning the chair.

Source: Ruth L. Di Domenico and Wilma Z. Ziegler, *Practical Rehabilitation Techniques for Geriatric Aides*, ed 2, Aspen Publishers, Inc., © 1994.

Wheelchair Safety: How to Handle and Push a Wheelchair

IS IT DIFFICULT?

Some people are apprehensive about taking an individual who uses a wheelchair on an outing. Other people are overly confident. Both approaches are wrong. Once aware of the general rules, the actual act of pushing a wheelchair is no more difficult than pushing a baby carriage. On the other hand it is not quite as simple, for the person you are pushing may be cumbersome and may have ideas of his or her own.

BASIC PARTS OF STANDARD WHEELCHAIR

Armrests

Armrests are usually removable. Many a novice has attempted to lift or fold a wheelchair by grabbing the arms and pulling upward, only to find the chair still stationary, and the two armrests in midair. The surprise is often amusing, and sometimes dismaying. Any attempt to lift the arms of the wheelchair when its user is in it is most dangerous. Wheelchair arms free themselves, and people with disabilities may not have the muscle control and balance to prevent a bad fall. They may also be startled to have the source of support on both sides suddenly removed. Never lift a wheelchair by its armrests.

Footrests

Some footrests are removable. They are attached to each side of the chair and usually swing outward and fold upward on hinges. When you push a wheelchair, they are out of your vision, so take care to keep an ample distance between the wheelchair and any pedestrians in front of it. Being bumped by footrests can be both annoying and painful to an innocent pedestrian.

Some people don't have, or don't use, footrests. Always allow enough foot room for the person in the chair. Be careful not to run the person's feet into objects or cause objects to get caught in the front wheels.

Brakes

There is a separate brake for each side of the chair. Be sure to find out how the brakes are used. Some lock when pushed back in toward the chair and others when pushed forward.

continues

continued

SAFETY SUGGESTIONS

Curbs

When getting a wheelchair from the curb to the street, turn yourself and the chair backward. After you have stepped into the street, ease the chair down until the large wheels hit the pavement. To get the wheelchair onto the sidewalk from the street, put the chair in front of you and tilt the chair back far enough so that you are sure the small wheels are on the sidewalk first. It will then be easy to lift the rest of the chair up onto the sidewalk.

Ramps

Descending a long ramp can be more difficult than you think. No matter how short or long a ramp is, always turn yourself and the chair around and *go down backward*. Your body will then keep the chair from picking up momentum. A second person is sometimes needed to grasp the lower part of the chair to help keep the chair under control.

It is not difficult to push a wheelchair up a gradually sloped ramp, but a long, steep ramp may be very difficult and require two people—one to push the chair and the other to back up and pull while grasping some secure part on the front of the chair.

Stairs

At least two people are needed to lift a person in a wheelchair up and down stairs.

- **Going upstairs.** Always take a wheelchair up a flight of stairs backward. One person should firmly grasp the handgrips, tilt the chair quite far back, and pull the chair up one step at a time, resting the large back wheels on each step. The second person should face the chair and grasp the rods to which the footrests are attached. This person lifts the front of the chair and provides balance. Be careful: Some footrests are detachable. Be sure all parts used in lifting are securely attached. The wheels should never be used for lifting purposes.
- **Going downstairs.** Always take a wheelchair downstairs forward (the chair faces the stairs). One person should firmly grasp the handgrips and tilt the chair quite far back. The second person goes down backward while grasping the rods to which the footrests are attached. Gently ease the chair down one step at a time, resting the large back wheels on each step. Keep the chair tilted in the same position throughout the descent. The person in front should provide balance and help control speed.

If a very heavy person is being taken up or down stairs, it is advisable to use three people—one to hold the handgrips and two to hold the front rods, with one person on each side of the chair. If three people are used, lifting up or down stairs is done with ease.

continues

continued

Automobile Trips

To move a person who can sit in a regular automobile seat from the wheelchair to a car, first be sure the car is parked away from the curb. Place the wheelchair close to the car so that the lifter will be able to move the person from the chair into the car and not have to bend way over in doing so. A person who can move from a wheelchair into a car without help usually finds it easier if the car is parked closer to the curb. In either case, it is best to place the person in the seat next to the driver. Some support may be needed if the person does not have adequate balance; this can be supplied by having someone sit next to the person. The driver should always be cautious in starting and stopping so there are no unnecessary jerks. Always use seat belts.

Always be sure to put the brakes on when stopping the chair, even for a brief pause, or when the person is being moved in or out of the wheelchair. The brakes must be locked into place when a person remains seated in the wheelchair while being transported in a motor vehicle.

Wheels

Take care that nothing gets caught in the spokes of the wheels. Dangling ends of clothing worn by the person in the chair and objects hung onto the back of the chair should all be kept away from the moving wheels.

When putting a wheelchair into the trunk of a car, grasp the rim or the center of one of the large wheels and any stationary part of the front of the chair. Lift as you would any other bulky object. Be sure to lift the chair high enough to clear the license plate and bumper, which often extend above the openings of a car trunk.

Seat Belts

It is a desirable safeguard for everyone in a wheelchair to use a seat belt, although some say they feel more comfortable without one. Those whose disability does not allow them to make immediate, automatic adjustments of balance while moving should *always* use a seat belt.

Seat belts can be purchased at any surgical supply store. Good substitutes for the manufactured item are trunk or suitcase straps or regular leather belts. Any substitute must, of course, be large enough to go around the person's waist or lower chest and the back of the wheelchair. It should be comfortable and of strong material and should have a sturdy buckle.

In circumstances when improvisation becomes necessary, a large square scarf may be used. Fold the scarf diagonally and tie it securely to prevent sliding and sudden constriction, which can cause discomfort or pain.

Tilting Rods

Modern wheelchairs have two rods close to the ground in the rear. These rods serve as foot pedals for the pusher, and it is extremely important to know how to use them. After getting a good

continues

continued

grasp on the handle, the pusher puts one foot on one of the pedals, applies a downward pressure that raises the front wheel of the chair from the ground; the chair is then tilted back slightly and can be maneuvered safely over bumps and holes in the street, door sills, and any other gradation in levels, such as from the street to a curb. Using the tilting rods may require more caution, but no more energy, on the part of the pusher. Occasionally, a chair-bound person may wish you to negotiate differences in levels in another way, but in most cases the above method is safe and satisfactory.

CLOSING AND OPENING A WHEELCHAIR

- **Closing.** Do not try to close the wheelchair by lifting up on the armrests. Lift the seat up by the leather handles attached to the seat of the chair, by the seat frame, or by the front and back of the seat. Be sure that the footrests are up, or the chair will not close. If the wheelchair has a high backrest, always remember to unlock the bars behind it.
- **Opening.** Grasp the seat frame on both sides. The seat will flatten as you push down on the frame. Do not try to open it by pulling or pushing it apart by the armrests. If there are footrests, they should be upright when you start. Don't lower them until the chair is open and/or the person is seated in the wheelchair. Wheelchairs with high backs have two locking bars behind the backrest that must be locked in place when the chair is open to keep the backrest firm.

MAJOR RULES: CONSIDERATION OF THE RIDER

- Always consult with the person you are to push as to the "dos" and "don'ts" that pertain to that particular person and wheelchair.
- Ask the person you are to push exactly how his or her wheelchair works, because each wheelchair is as different as the person who uses it. The user knows best, since that wheelchair is his or her "better half" and is as important to the person as a seeing-eye dog is to its master. This applies to children as well as adults.
- Ask how the person wishes to be pushed—not only on level ground, but up and down curbs, on stairs, and so forth. Do not try to impose unfamiliar ways of doing things.
- The person has probably developed safe and efficient routines in which he or she has the greatest confidence. Follow those routines not only in pushing the chair, but also in moving an arm or a leg to a more comfortable position, or getting the person into and out of clothing, automobiles, etc.
- Ask the above questions repeatedly, if necessary.
- In cold weather don't push the wheelchair too slowly, for people in wheelchairs are apt to have poor circulation and, even when well wrapped up, may get chilled easily.

continues

continued

TIPS FOR THE WHEELCHAIR PUSHER

When pushing a wheelchair, women will feel more secure and have better footing if rubber-soled, low-heeled shoes are worn. This is especially true when pushing a chair for some distance or going up and down ramps or stairs.

If one is not used to it, pushing a wheelchair for long distances can leave wrist muscles (ordinarily not used in this way) stiff and the palms of the hands sore. Not much can be done to ease the wrists, but pressure on the palms can be eased by wrapping a piece of foam rubber around the handles of the wheelchair, even though they may already have hard rubber covers.

Just one word of caution: Do not let your concern make you overly zealous and lead you into doing more than is necessary. A person with a disability likes to be as independent as his or her physical limitations allow.

Notes:

Source: *Developmental Disabilities Review Course*, Children's Association for Maximum Potential, San Antonio, Texas, 1992. Reprinted with the permission of the Easter Seal Society of Nebraska.

Switching to a Power Chair

For many spinal cord injury survivors, recapturing independence is their single most significant achievement. They view any concessions to that independence—accepting more help, using more or different equipment—as giving up, as failure, as the ultimate defeat. But it's hard to deny the fatigue and pain that may come from years of pushing a manual chair. Switching to a power chair could be the way to actually maintain that independence.

SYMPTOMS AND SIGNS

Accepting change is rarely easy. Many survivors choose to ignore the signals that indicate that a power chair would be appropriate for them. Picturing themselves in a power chair or admitting they might need one can be one of the most difficult adjustments for those with spinal cord injury. Physical therapists say three major issues result in symptoms that cause people to make equipment changes: level of injury, number of years postinjury, and age. These three factors often interact and result in:

- lower strength or function
- increased pain
- decreased mobility
- weight gain or loss
- less activity
- skin sores
- posture problems
- fatigue
- aging of the primary caregivers

STIGMA

The stigma of disability keeps many people from increasing or changing equipment. Some find they must let go of the "live for the moment" kind of attitude. Others, some of whom were injured during "the super quad" era when more equipment meant more disabled, sometimes struggle to accept the idea that changing equipment doesn't mean going backward.

Even caregivers, family, or friends struggle with stigma issues. Some family members or friends need to be needed. Others may not understand the necessity or wisdom of conserving energy and function in order to preserve quality of life. They may need to hear that equipment changes such as power chairs can save shoulder muscles and joints, thus making more things possible in life.

continues

continued

IT'S NOT ALWAYS OBVIOUS

Sometimes fatigue and pain can get in the way too slowly and gradually to notice. People may eliminate errands in order to avoid the car transfers, or they may skip certain chores at home. They don't have the energy to do the things they want or need to do, like playing with their kids or stretching each night. Quality of life becomes the issue. Power chairs allow people to do more things with less pain, less fatigue, and more mobility, resulting in more independence.

IT'S FOR REAL!

New research is indicating that over half of long-term spinal cord injury survivors are making equipment changes to preserve their mobility, their function, their independence, or the well-being of their caregivers and attendants.

In a study of 279 British spinal cord injury survivors, all of whom had been injured at least 20 years, 59 percent reported having made changes in durable medical equipment, such as new wheelchairs, cushions hoists, and lifts to ease transfers. Almost 25 percent listed fatigue and/or weakness as the cause for change. The same number listed medical problems. Others cited stiffness, pain, other injuries, or their age.

In this British research group, over 31 percent of all those interviewed reported shoulder pain. Forty-seven percent had experienced postural changes, while 54 percent were dealing with fatigue. The changes come because spinal cord injury is not the static condition it was once thought to be.

Forty percent of the 180,000 spinal cord injury survivors in the United States already are over 45; one in four has lived with injury for over 20 years. Some feel that the changes of aging come sooner to people who have spinal cord injuries. And, findings from the British study, where functional declines appeared, on average, in subjects in their late 40s and early 50s, certainly support the belief of accelerated aging.

WHEN IS IT TIME TO CHANGE?

A personal inventory can be helpful in determining if a switch to a power chair is worth thinking about.

- Do you find yourself avoiding going certain places—places you used to go or want to go but don't—because it's just too hard or simply not worth it?
- Do you have persistent shoulder pain when wheeling?
- Do you find yourself using more energy wheeling and not doing those things you want to do, like working, going out, entertaining, or playing?
- Do you have noticeably less fatigue and pain on days when you don't wheel much?

continues

continued

ROADBLOCKS TO CHANGE

But power chairs *are* big and bulky. Most don't jump curbs. They do cost a lot of money. They are a hassle to travel with. But the hassles of lifts and power chairs may be small potatoes compared to the hassles of needing an attendant or simply not being able to work or play at all.

People use lots of reasons to avoid changing to a power chair—money, exercise, strength, travel. Often their reluctance is really about not wanting to give in to aging and decline of function. Used equipment, family help, charitable organizations, Medicare, or Medicaid can help pay for equipment. Different types of exercise can be less destructive to shoulders and arms, while preserving strength and stamina. Travel can be more fun without fatigue.

The costs of "hanging in there" and putting off getting new equipment may be greater than imagined, not just in money but in muscle pain, strength loss, and general quality of life.

PREVENTION, TRADE-OFFS, AND THE FUTURE

Sometimes more equipment can prevent future problems and can mean more independence. Equipment changes in response to warning signals can help control or prevent chronic conditions such as scoliosis, carpal tunnel syndrome, degenerative shoulder disease, or major muscle imbalances. Power wheelchairs and other equipment changes can also serve to project a more positive, independent, and functional image, as they are faster, more maneuverable, and energy conserving.

Taking action prior to major problems can also help prevent skin problems or the onset of some chronic pain. Some survivors are little more than a shoulder injury away from major dependence on others. They may need permission not to work so hard, not to be in so much pain, not to be so independent. While changes in durable medical equipment cannot totally prevent functional decline in all spinal cord injury survivors, they can delay or minimize decline or the need for additional help.

Change rarely comes overnight and is often the result of trade-offs that are not readily apparent, like paying for fatigue with less time for kids, friends, or other obligations; fewer hours on the job; or a major decline in social life. Sometimes a person simply needs overwhelming evidence in order to know just how necessary change is.

When the price for not changing is a clear decline in quality of life, then change may be easier to accept. No one has a formula for how to figure this out, since everyone is different. What is clear, though, is that survivors who have made the change to a power chair clearly report less pain and fatigue. If pain and fatigue from pushing a manual chair are ongoing problems and threats to independence in your life, a power wheelchair may be a logical and appropriate response.

Source: The Rehabilitation Research and Training Center on Aging with SCI, a joint project of Craig Hospital and the Department of Rehabilitation Medicine at the University of Colorado Health Sciences Center. Funded by the National Institute on Disability and Rehabilitation Research. For more information about the "SCI & Aging" publications, contact the RRTC at 800-5-REHAB-8.

ADAPTIVE DRIVING

Adaptive Driving: The Basics

Driving is an important aspect of our lives. It allows us greater independence. Many people with spinal cord injuries can relearn this skill with the assistance of a qualified driver training instructor. These individuals can assist with evaluating the need for adaptive equipment and provide the training needed to become a safe driver.

HOW TO OBTAIN A LICENSE

The first step in obtaining a license is to contact your local Department of Motor Vehicles. Each state differs slightly in its policies, but most require that you have your doctor complete a form stating that you are medically stable to drive. They may also comment on your current medication, history of seizures, or need for adapted equipment. Even if your current license will not expire for years, you are responsible for having your driving record updated to reflect your change in medical condition.

The next step in obtaining or updating your license is to complete an evaluation with a qualified driver trainer. He or she will assist you in determining your specific equipment needs and ensure that you can resume safe driving.

Finally, if you are driving with adapted equipment, you can expect to be required to retake the driving test. This will ensure that your license is updated. In most states, it is illegal to drive with adapted equipment that is not reflected on your license.

FINDING A QUALIFIED DRIVER TRAINER

Many of the well-known driving schools are unable to offer the specialized equipment and evaluation that you require to resume safe driving. There are, however, major rehabilitation medical centers and Veterans Affairs hospitals that have driving programs for people with disabilities. The instructors are often therapists who have received additional training and experience to become driver trainers.

If you are unable to find a qualified driver trainer in your area, contact The Association of Driver Educators for the Disabled, P.O. Box 49, Edgerton, WI 53534; (608) 884-8833.

WHEN YOU SHOULD BEGIN DRIVER TRAINING

In the initial months after your injury, you are very busy focusing on the medical and therapeutic aspects of your rehabilitation. Often, driver training isn't addressed until you are closer to discharge. If you have tetraplegia, you may want to wait at least a year or more before driving. People with tetraplegia may make additional improvements in strength and abilities within the first two years of their injury. The expensive equipment and training you purchase could become

continues

continued

obsolete in a matter of months. The decision of when to start training should be made with the help and ideas of your doctor and therapist.

If your injury included a loss of consciousness, seizure, head injury, or stroke, there may be a mandatory waiting period before you resume driving. Contact your state's Department of Motor Vehicles for complete details.

DRIVER TRAINING

Before you actually get behind the wheel, your instructor will need to complete an in-clinic assessment. This usually consists of a visual and perceptual screening, strength and sensory evaluations, and time reaction tests. In addition, he or she will ask you about your previous driving experience and what type of driving you wish to resume. This will allow the instructor to tailor the lessons to your specific needs.

After the in-clinic assessment, the instructor will determine the type of adaptive equipment needed. He or she may set up this equipment on a driving simulator to determine your ability to drive safely.

Once the appropriate equipment is determined, you will be given personalized training in its use. The instructor will begin teaching you to drive in a parking lot or another safe practice area. As you progress in developing your skills, the instructor gives you more complex driving instructions. In addition, you may be instructed in defensive driving techniques.

At the completion of training, you will be ready to take the road test at your local Department of Motor Vehicles. Often you can use the driver training vehicle, since you will rarely have the time or finances to already have your own vehicle modified.

CAR INSURANCE

You will want to inform the insurance company of your change in driving methods. The company may require proof that your license has been updated with adapted equipment and that your doctor feels you are medically safe to drive.

Although your insurance company cannot cancel your policy because of a spinal cord injury, it may increase your rates for the first year of driving. After one to three years of driving with adapted equipment accident free, you should no longer be considered a high-risk driver. It is also important to tell the company about any adapted equipment you have installed on your vehicle. This will ensure that it is covered under your policy.

HOW TO GET A DISABLED PARKING PERMIT

Most states require that your doctor sign a form indicating your need for this type of parking. Contact your local Department of Motor Vehicles for an application. Many states are beginning to issue removable placards that you can place on the dashboard or rearview mirror. Placards are more versatile than the license plates because they allow you to use disabled parking when

continues

continued

you are in a car other than your own. If you travel, make sure that other states will honor your parking permit.

You may also want to ask if your state has legislated a policy pertaining to gasoline stations. In many states, your disabled parking permit entitles you to purchase gas at self-service prices while having the full-service attendant dispense the gasoline. This is meant to prevent price discrimination against those who are physically unable to complete this task.

THE IMPORTANCE OF TIEDOWN SYSTEMS

If you are ever transported by a Cabulance service, take public transportation, or even ride in your van, then you need to know about tiedown systems. These are the straps that are secured to your wheelchair to keep it (and you) safe. When secured properly, tiedowns will prevent the wheelchair from moving around. Your wheelchair brakes are not sufficient, especially in an accident.

It is your responsibility to instruct people in how to best attach the tiedowns to your specific wheelchair. Review it with your driver trainer or therapist.

Some general guidelines include the following:

- Tiedown systems should be attached to the frame of the wheelchair. Never secure them to removable parts such as footrests or armrests.
- A four-point tiedown system is the safest. This system is secured at all points of the wheelchair—two in the front and two in the back.
- In addition to securing your wheelchair, you will want to have a separate wall-mounted shoulder/lap harness. This will keep you in the wheelchair in case of a sudden stop.
- Whenever possible, tiedowns should be positioned so that you are facing forward. You do not want your back lined up against a wall or window.
- All systems should be safety tested at speeds up to 30 mph/20 G force.

Source: Margaret Hammond, et al., eds., *Yes, You Can! A Guide to Self-Care for Persons with Spinal Cord Injury*, Paralyzed Veterans of America, Washington, DC, © 1989. Original body of text produced by the Seattle Veterans Affairs Medical Center.

How to Select a Vehicle

Your first decision in selecting a vehicle is whether you will need a car or a van. If you use an electric wheelchair, a van equipped with a lift is usually indicated. Although there are "portable" electric wheelchairs available, they usually require assistance for disassembly and trunk storage.

If you use a manual wheelchair, you need to choose a vehicle that suits your transfer and wheelchair storage ability. For example, the seating height of some cars may make for a level wheelchair to driver seat transfer. Conversely, however, the seating height of a truck may mean transferring up 10 or more inches.

WHAT TO LOOK FOR IN A CAR

Certain vehicles are better suited for transfers, wheelchair storage, or installation of hand controls. Your driver trainer can provide you with specific equipment and selection criteria. The following list offers general guidelines on purchasing an accessible car.

- A two-door vehicle is recommended for ease of access because the doors open wider. This means that you can position the wheelchair closer for transfers.
- An intermediate or large car is generally recommended because hand controls take up space in the driver area. When in doubt about a specific car, call a hand-control vendor and ask.
- Bucket seats can provide improved balance and stability by "cupping" the driver. A bench-type front seat will enable the driver to enter from either side of the vehicle and slide to the driver's position.
- A center armrest/console is desirable for long-distance driving, as well as driver stability, balance during turning maneuvers, and assistance with pressure relief.
- If using a folding wheelchair, there should be enough room between the front and back seats to allow for storage. Also, check that seat belt anchors do not interfere with access.
- Seat belts are required to be worn in all vehicles. In addition, seat belts and shoulder harnesses help maintain stability and balance on stops, during turns, etc.
- Four-wheel drive is recommended for those driving on snow and ice and is now available on many different makes and models.
- Automatic transmission is required to operate hand controls.
- Power steering is recommended for improved turning and to avoid over-fatiguing your arm(s).
- The steering column must be designed so that standard hand controls may be attached.
- A tilt steering wheel allows more space when entering and exiting and when operating the hand controls.
- Power brakes allow a faster response with less strength required to operate the controls.
- Cruise control allows the driver to maintain a steady speed without having to constantly operate the accelerator. It will also prevent unnecessary arm fatigue during long-distance driving with hand controls.

continues

continued

- Power windows are recommended for drivers with limited hand function. It is also a good idea for hand-control users because it is a faster method of operation.
- Power door locks are recommended for drivers with limited hand function and/or limited mobility so that doors can be locked and unlocked from the driver's seat.
- Air conditioning is recommended for drivers with low-level respiratory problems, or as a medical necessity for temperature regulation.
- Remote adjustable outside mirrors enable the driver to obtain optimum rear vision without being outside the vehicle.
- Rear window defroster and rear window wipers will improve overall vision and safety while driving.

WHAT TO LOOK FOR IN A VAN

Buying a modifying van can be very expensive. General guidelines are difficult to provide, since the equipment and type of van that you require is very personalized. You must work closely with your driver trainer before making this purchase. In addition, the vendor who will install your equipment is invaluable. Ask the vendor if he or she is certified to install specific equipment and if he or she carries liability insurance to cover the equipment and work performed.

To find a qualified vendor, ask your instructor or contact the National Mobility Equipment Dealers Association, 909 East Skagway Avenue, Tampa, FL 33604; (813) 932-8566.

Notes:

Source: Margaret Hammond, et al., eds., *Yes, You Can! A Guide to Self-Care for Persons with Spinal Cord Injury*, Paralyzed Veterans of America, Washington, DC, © 1989. Original body of text produced by the Seattle Veterans Affairs Medical Center.

Am I Ready for a Van?

Most spinal cord injury survivors who are used to driving a car aren't too excited about switching to a modified van. "They're too big. They're too expensive. They're not very sporty or fun. They're too hard to drive." Sound like you? If so, you may have even more reasons not to switch. Yet, increasing hassles, pain, and fatigue may be telling you otherwise.

People offer many reasons for staying away from modified vans:

- What I drive is a reflection of my personality. A seven foot high van isn't who I am.
- Meeting the challenge of transferring to my car and hauling my chair in behind me makes me feel good about myself.
- I simply don't have money for a lift and all the modifications I'd have to do to a van.

THE I'M NOT READY SYNDROME

Mostly what keeps people in their cars is the "I'm Not Ready Syndrome":

- I'm not ready to give up the fun car.
- I'm not ready to give up the challenge.
- I'm not ready to spend the money.

Eventually, two or three primary factors—preserving function, maximizing options and flexibility, looking into the future in order to plan for and anticipate change—drive the decision and help clarify the choices.

Despite all the good, logical reasons for continuing to drive those cars, many find it difficult to deny nagging shoulder pain, decreased tolerance for the hassles of car transfers and chair loading, or the simple fact that they don't have the energy they once did. Making a change is a dilemma many survivors confront each day.

MAKING A CHANGE

Reason 1: The Shoulders

The first consideration mentioned by many in the rehabilitation field for making the change from car to van is maintaining and preserving physical function. Research with those injured more than 20 years indicates that the biggest predictor of pain and fatigue—two things that can get in the way of function—was having experienced pain and fatigue three years earlier. Not making changes when problems first arise is an almost sure way of having them get worse.

The pain and fatigue can come from the *distance* of the transfer, because getting as close to the car seat as to a bed is difficult. Another consideration is the *height* of the transfer. Having to lift up or down in the process of doing a transfer adds considerable extra stress to shoulders. Also, muscling the chair itself in and out of the car can cause more pain and do damage. And just the

continues

continued

sheer number of transfers *continues to accumulate* over time. What results from all this is usually joint pain—from the neck all the way down to the wrist—often arthritic in nature, and often accompanied by tendinitis. The joint pain, the arthritis, and the tendinitis are the body's way of saying that what you're doing isn't working very well and is causing some harm.

Researchers have also linked fatigue to *future* problems, including depression, lower quality of life, and, in some survivors, the need for both more durable medical equipment and more help from others. As car transfers and chair loading become more difficult, many people report curtailing activities in order to avoid the transfers. Too often therapists encounter aging clients who are giving up things they enjoy—fishing, traveling, even working—because of pain and fatigue.

Still, even though people find themselves giving up activities, they resist making the changes necessary to avoid the hassles, the pain, and the fatigue. For many it comes down to wanting to fight off the realities of aging with a disability for as long as possible. The arguments are predictable, in part because they're so valid: big vans are inconvenient and hard to drive, they cost too much, people like the physical challenge of doing transfers. Often it's an image thing.

Reason 2: Image

A vehicle is often an extension of one's personality. Giving up part of one's personality—rugged or adventurous individual; sporty, fun kind of guy; or sedate, respectable, suburban family person—isn't easy. Most everyone who buys a vehicle gives some thought to image. Not everyone feels comfortable driving a big van. Vans can be too big or not sporty enough, or they simply don't fit people's self-image. While minivans are an option for some individuals, many—especially big people who use big chairs—find minivans too small for the lift they need and too tight inside for the necessary maneuverability.

Regaining independence following injury and rehab is, for many people, the single most significant achievement of postparalysis life. Giving up the car may be viewed as giving up—not only by the survivor but also by those around him or her. Yet, making the changes and using the lift may be necessary to maintain that highly prized independence: Isn't *getting* there far more important than just exactly *how* it's done?

Reason 3: Somebody Else

Decisions about what to drive affect more than just the survivor, especially if someone else is doing the chair loading. A change to a van with a lift could be necessary even if your back or shoulders are just fine. Wives, husbands, and caregivers age too, and they are often called on to help with many transfers, chores, and tasks requiring heavy or awkward lifting. Survivors need to be not only aware but also sensitive to their needs.

continues

continued

Reason 4: Expense

A switch to a modified van can add $10,000 to $20,000 or more to the cost of a vehicle. Insurance and fuel costs usually go up, and some modified vans—even ones without raised roofs—won't fit in standard garages and may require modified garage arrangements as well. Yet there are costs involved in becoming less active, not going out as much, and staying home more. Active people tend to be healthier, happier, and less depressed. Going too long on deteriorating shoulders can leave people even more dependent, eventually making hired help more necessary.

People—even some who are unemployed and on Medicaid—buy vans and somehow find ways to pay for them. Workers' compensation, Medicaid waivers, vocational rehabilitation, and Veterans Affairs are all government programs that may help with funding. Charitable organizations such as Easter Seals are a possibility. Fraternal organizations may provide help. Some banks issue extended loans and independent living centers may offer low interest loans. Lower cost home equity loans may also be an option. There are always fund raisers through church, civic, or community organizations. And used equipment or used modified vans are also possibilities. People tend to figure out ways to secure necessities.

THINKING AHEAD

Sound decisions that will provide flexibility for five to eight years need to be based on a realistic assessment of present function and trends in your strength, stamina, lifestyle, pain, and function. Is it practical to stick with a car if strength has been decreasing and pain has been increasing for the past three years? Transfers may not be much of a problem now, but is it realistic to expect they'll still be as easy in five years, when you're 56? Can you afford *not* to change?

More often than not, the decision to switch from a car to a van is one of many decisions that contribute to the lifelong process of adaptation to disability. Adaptive equipment helps narrow the gap between aspiration and ability, between wants and needs, and allows spinal cord injury survivors to do so comfortably and safely. Adaptive equipment can help avoid pain, preserve energy, and prevent future problems. New equipment can preserve time and energy and help enhance as well as maintain both independence and quality of life.

Quality of life may be the prime consideration for switching from car to van. The switch is a matter of preventive maintenance—a change that may allow you to keep the function you have and to maintain the quality of life you desire. *How* you regard these changes can be as important as the changes themselves.

Source: The Rehabilitation Research and Training Center on Aging with SCI, a joint project of Craig Hospital and the Department of Rehabilitation Medicine at the University of Colorado Health Sciences Center. Funded by the National Institute on Disability and Rehabilitation Research. For more information about the "SCI & Aging" publications, contact the RRTC at 800-5-REHAB-8.

13
Maintaining Optimal Health

> Most materials in the *Spinal Cord Injury Patient Education Manual* are intended for the health care professional to share with the patient. Materials that are intended solely for the professional are labeled "Exhibit" in the table of contents.

Nutrition

After Spinal Cord Injury: Changes and Concerns	453
The Food Guide Pyramid	456
What Nutrients Do for You	458
The Battle of the Bulge	461

Physical Fitness

What Is Physical Fitness?	464
What Should I Do Before I Start My Fitness Program?	466
General Exercise Guidelines	467
Fitness Recommendations According to Level of Spinal Cord Injury (Exhibit)	468

NUTRITION

After Spinal Cord Injury: Changes and Concerns

Basic good nutrition is important for everyone. The foods you eat affect how you look, how you feel, and how your body systems work. Eating the right foods each day provides your body with all the nutrients it needs. A proper diet helps to

- give you energy
- fight infections
- maintain proper body weight
- keep all your body systems working properly

This does not change after having a spinal cord injury (SCI). However, because of changes that occur to the body after an SCI, you need to understand the role that nutrition plays in keeping you healthy. The foods you include in your daily meal plan are important to your overall health following an SCI.

After an SCI most individuals normally lose some weight. Men usually lose more than women. Immediately after the injury the body requires energy and nutrients to repair itself and fight infection. The SCI puts stress on the body. When the body is stressed, the heart beats faster. This means that the body burns calories faster. Often during this time newly injured patients are not able to eat a regular diet. Paralyzed muscles also atrophy, which causes additional weight loss. The loss of weight slows after three to four weeks.

Individuals with SCI experience changes in how their different body systems work. Many of the changes that the body experiences can be managed by eating healthy meals and snacks. Eating the proper foods, in the correct amount, every day provides the body with the essential nutrients.

SPECIAL HEALTH CONCERNS FOR INDIVIDUALS WITH SCI

Bowel Management

Individuals with SCI may have neurogenic bowel. This means the messages from the brain that control the downward muscular movements of the bowel are either absent or not working properly. This makes it difficult for stool to move through the intestines.

A healthy diet that includes high fiber and plenty of fluids is the way to regulate your bowel program. The fiber helps move the stool through the bowel. The fluid keeps the stool soft. Foods high in fat may make it difficult to regulate your bowel program.

- Eat 25–35 grams of fiber every day. Foods high in fiber include whole-grain breads and cereals, peas and beans, and fruits and vegetables (with edible skins left on for extra fiber).
- Drink 8–10 (8 oz.) glasses of liquid each day.

continues

continued

Heart Problems

Individuals with SCI are now at greater risk for cardiovascular and heart problems since they are now living longer. Too much cholesterol can increase your risk of heart disease.

- Watch the amount of cholesterol that you eat each day. Have your cholesterol checked when you go for your annual medical checkup.
- Avoid foods high in cholesterol. Cholesterol is found only in animal products (meats, eggs, cheese, and whole milk dairy products).

You also may need to limit the amount of salt in your daily food plan. Too much salt is a hazard if you have high blood pressure or heart problems.

Pressure Ulcers

Pressure ulcers are always a concern to individuals with SCI. Your skin is more likely to break down when you do not eat healthy meals and snacks. A healthy diet helps keep your skin healthy and prevents the risk of pressure ulcers. If you should develop a pressure ulcer, a diet high in protein, vitamins, and minerals is recommended.

- Eating foods rich in vitamins and protein helps pressure ulcers heal quickly.
- Remember, do your pressure releases frequently!

Kidney or Bladder Stones

Individuals with SCI may be prone to developing calcium stones. Certain beverages can cause crystals to form in the urine. Ask your doctor if you should watch your consumption of dairy products (milk, cheese, yogurt, ice cream).

- The best way to avoid kidney or bladder stones is to make water your beverage of choice.

Urinary Tract Infection

The loss of normal bladder function after SCI places an individual at risk for urinary tract infection (UTI). A high fluid intake every day reduces the problem of infections and stones forming. The fluids that pass through the kidneys help keep the bladder and catheter relatively clear. You need to understand how much fluid to drink each day to manage your bladder program.

Drinking carbonated beverages (soda pop), orange juice, and grapefruit juice can cause the urine to become alkaline. When urine becomes alkaline it can have a strong, unpleasant odor.

continues

continued

Alkaline urine is a breeding ground for bacteria that can cause UTI. Limit the amount of these beverages you drink each day.

- Make WATER your beverage of choice.

Notes:

Source: Developed by Michelle C. Jeffcoat, MS, RD, and Linda Lindsey, MEd, Medical RRTC in Secondary Complications in SCI, Department of Physical Medicine and Rehabilitation, University of Alabama at Birmingham-Spain Rehabilitation Center, Birmingham, Alabama, © 1996. Supported in part by a grant (#HI33B30025) from the National Institute on Disability and Rehabilitation Research, U.S. Department of Education. Opinions expressed in this document are not necessarily those of the granting agency.

The Food Guide Pyramid

There are approximately 50 different nutrients needed by a cell for it to live. A basic diet plan following the food guide pyramid provides these needed nutrients. Use the food pyramid as your daily eating guide.

The foods at the bottom or the largest part of the pyramid should be eaten in the largest amounts.

The foods at the top or the smallest part of the pyramid should be eaten in the smallest amounts.

The base of the pyramid is made up of breads and starches. These foods should form the base of your diet. Foods in this group include breads, cereals, pasta, and grains. They are usually low in fat and high in carbohydrates and are the body's favorite energy source. They are also high in vitamins, minerals, and fiber. Plan 6–11 servings in your daily food plan.

The next pyramid level contains fruits and vegetables. As with the breads and starches, foods from this group should be eaten in large amounts. Fruits and vegetables are packed with vitamins, minerals, and fiber. They are fat free and make great snacks during munchy attacks. Plan for 3–5 servings of vegetables and 2–4 servings of fruits each day.

The third level of the pyramid includes dairy products and meats and meat substitutes. These foods are great sources of high-quality protein. Unfortunately, they also tend to be high in fat, so choose carefully. The best choices include skim or 1% milk, low-fat or nonfat cheeses, and yogurt. Low-fat meats include skinless chicken, fish, lean beef, fresh pork, and lean ham.

The top of the pyramid is occupied by fats, oils, and sweets. Since this is the smallest part of the pyramid, these foods should make up the smallest part of your diet.

continues

continued

Does your diet look like the food pyramid? Think of ways you can increase breads, starches, fruits, and vegetables in your diet.

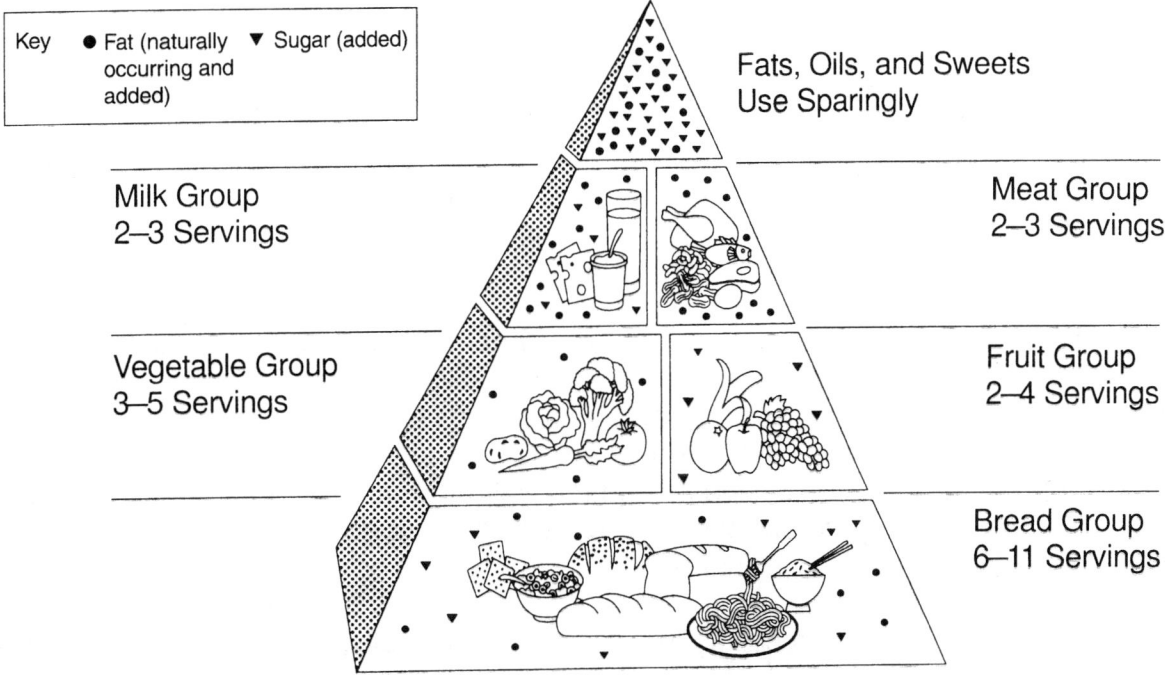

The Food Guide Pyramid: A Guide to Daily Food Choices. Reprinted from *Home and Garden Bulletin*, No. 249, U.S. Department of Agriculture, 1992.

Source: Developed by Michelle C. Jeffcoat, MS, RD, and Linda Lindsey, MEd, Medical RRTC in Secondary Complications in SCI, Department of Physical Medicine and Rehabilitation, University of Alabama at Birmingham-Spain Rehabilitation Center, Birmingham, Alabama, © 1996. Supported in part by a grant (#H133B30025) from the National Institute on Disability and Rehabilitation Research, U.S. Department of Education. Opinions expressed in this document are not necessarily those of the granting agency.

What Nutrients Do for You

Eating a healthy variety of foods is the key to good nutrition. There are eight main nutrients that the body needs each day to stay healthy and keep your body working properly.

Carbohydrates

Carbohydrates are the body's main source of energy. They also help to give the stomach a full feeling.

Foods rich in carbohydrates include breads, pasta, potatoes, rice, fruits, and vegetables. Carbohydrates do not contain a significant amount of fat, unless it is added.

Fats

Fats provide the body with energy, help insulate the body, and help in cell and membrane growth.

There are two types of fats, *unsaturated* and *saturated*. Unsaturated fats (monounsaturated and polyunsaturated) are liquid at room temperature. They can actually help reduce the cholesterol level in the blood and are considered "heart healthy." Saturated fats are solid at room temperature. These fats are generally bad for your heart and arteries and should be avoided.

Examples of the two types of fat include

- *Saturated* (solid): whole milk products, butter, lard, coconut oil, palm oil, poultry skin, bacon grease
- *Unsaturated* (liquid):
  —Polyunsaturated—safflower oil, sunflower oil, soybean oil, corn oil
  —Monounsaturated—canola oil, olive oil, peanut oil, nuts

WARNING! Avoid hydrogenated fats. These are liquid fats that are processed into hard fats (read the food labels).

Fats are also present in many different foods—margarine, salad dressings, mayonnaise, bakery goods, meat, and dairy products.

Protein

Protein builds and repairs body cells, helps prevent skin breakdown (pressure ulcers), helps fight infection, and helps heal wounds.

Food containing protein includes meat, fish, poultry, cheese, eggs, dried peas and beans, nuts, and peanut butter.

Remember, foods high in protein may be high in fat!

continues

continued

Vitamins

Vitamins help with certain chemical reactions in the body.

- Vitamin A keeps skin and nerves healthy and helps the body resist infection. Foods high in vitamin A include dark green and yellow fruits and vegetables (carrots, squash, sweet potatoes, apricots, and spinach) and egg yolks.
- B vitamins help with digestion, provide energy, and keep eyes, skin, and nerves healthy. Foods rich in B vitamins include whole-grain cereals and breads, pork, peanuts, meats, and green leafy vegetables.
- Vitamin D helps the body use calcium and phosphorus. It also works with calcium to form bones. Sources of vitamin D include fortified milk, fish liver oils, and exposure to sunlight.

Minerals

Minerals aid in wound healing and tissue repair.

- Calcium helps build bones and teeth, aids in blood clotting, and helps develop muscle tone. Foods rich in calcium include milk, cheese, yogurt, dried peas and beans, salmon with bones, sardines, dark green leafy vegetables, and broccoli.
- Iron helps build blood cells and carries oxygen to all cells. Foods rich in iron include liver, lean red meats, fortified breads and cereals, dried peas and beans, green leafy vegetables, dried fruits, and nuts.
- Potassium regulates muscles and nerves. A good source for potassium is bananas.

Fiber

Fiber, or "roughage," is found in foods that come from plants. It is the part of fruits, vegetables, and grains that cannot be digested. There are two kinds of fiber, *soluble* and *insoluble*.

- Insoluble fiber (like wheat bran) speeds up elimination.
- Soluble fiber (oats and fruits) binds with fats like cholesterol and carries them out of the body. It also keeps bowel movements regular, holds food in the stomach longer, slows down calorie absorption, and helps keep you from feeling hungry.

Foods high in fiber include fresh or dried fruits, vegetables (fresh is best), brown or wild rice, dried beans and peas, wheat germ, popcorn, and whole-grain breads and cereals.

Fiber cannot do its job without fluid!

continues

continued

Water and Fluids

Water is an important nutrient that most people do not think about when planning their diet. Water regulates body temperature, carries food nutrients through the body, and carries food waste out of the body.

After spinal cord injury it is recommended that you drink 8–10 (8 oz.) glasses of water or other liquids every day. This amount helps prevent urinary tract infections, helps prevent kidney and bladder stones, keeps stools soft for regulating your bowel program, and aids with digestion and elimination.

There are many fluids that you can drink, but water should be your number one beverage choice. When selecting your beverage remember to:

- Limit carbonated beverages (soft drinks) to one a day. They cause the urine to become alkaline and have an unpleasant odor.
- Avoid fluids with calories (juices, milkshakes, soft drinks) if you are watching your weight.

Fluids include water, lemonade, Kool-Aid, decaf tea, and nonfrozen cranberry or apple juice.

Notes:

Source: Developed by Michelle C. Jeffcoat, MS, RD, and Linda Lindsey, MEd, Medical RRTC in Secondary Complications in SCI, Department of Physical Medicine and Rehabilitation, University of Alabama at Birmingham-Spain Rehabilitation Center, Birmingham, Alabama, © 1996. Supported in part by a grant (#H133B30025) from the National Institute on Disability and Rehabilitation Research, U.S. Department of Education. Opinions expressed in this document are not necessarily those of the granting agency.

The Battle of the Bulge

So you gained five pounds in the last year. No big deal. It's probably not enough for anyone to notice. But think about it: What's five pounds a year? It's 20 pounds in four years, 50 pounds in 10 years, and 100 pounds in 20 years! Were you planning to be around in 20 years? Imagine carrying 400 Quarter-Pounders around on your back every minute of your life. Yikes!

HOW BIG A PROBLEM?

Don't get the wrong idea. Every spinal cord injury (SCI) survivor is not becoming obese. In fact, according to one study of almost 300 survivors—all injured between 20 and 50 years ago—the average weight gain was only about one pound a year. But some individuals had gained as much as 40 pounds in just three years. For them, and for others who do gain a lot of weight, the results can be very serious.

What happens when people with disabilities gain weight? They have all the same problems that nondisabled people have. They face a much greater risk for heart attacks, strokes, and other complications from clogged arteries; respiratory or breathing problems; diabetes; kidney and gallbladder diseases; arthritis; and some kinds of cancer. Obese people become less active, and they may lose self-esteem.

And there's more. Probably most important are all the side-effects of obesity, which plague the SCI survivor more than the nondisabled person, such as loss of function, skin problems, decreased mobility, less independence, higher costs, and a decreased quality of life. Probably all of these problems occur sooner in the SCI survivor, and with less actual pounds gained.

WEIGHT GAIN IS A REAL PROBLEM

Besides putting you at risk for some very real health problems, excessive weight gain can create other kinds of dilemmas, ones that only are magnified when the bigger body is paralyzed or weak.

First, there's the increased risk of injury you face if you're overweight. SCI survivors use their arms to do the work that legs once did, and arms start aching, paining, and giving out long before legs do. Research is showing that SCI survivors are at risk for shoulder pain, joint deterioration, even things like rotator cuff tears, simply because of the amount of stress they place on their arms. This problem is not limited to people with paraplegia. A 1993 study found that over half of its participants with long-term quadriplegia also had pain in the shoulders. A few had it in the elbows, wrists, and hands too.

In addition to the risk of injury, there's also the risk your skin faces. If your bulkier body can't avoid hitting that wheelchair tire when you transfer, or if you just can't turn yourself in bed, your skin may pay the price. Excess weight also puts more pressure on the skin. As people gain weight, skin folds develop that trap moisture, greatly increasing the risk of skin ulcers.

continues

continued

Then there are the cost, comfort, and convenience issues. A bulkier body may not fit in those awful, tiny airplane seats. Wide, first-class seats cost more. If you need to get a wider wheelchair, more doors, hallways, and aisles will become inaccessible. Special equipment costs more. And, if you're not able to do all of your own care, it's harder on your attendant too. In fact, it may be even harder to *find* attendants. If attendants think that lifting you will cause them back problems, they won't be eager to sign on. Then you have another problem that may mean more expense.

DOES ANYONE EVER WIN THE BATTLE OF THE BULGE?

Millions of nondisabled people struggle with unwanted weight. For SCI survivors, the struggle may be even harder. First, following SCI, the body's metabolism changes; how SCI survivors use food they eat and the fat they store is altered. In short, they use up less energy than they did before their injuries, and the higher the level of SCI, the less energy they seem to need.

Lean body mass—meaning muscle tissue—*decreases* after SCI. At the same time, the amount of body fat *increases*. In fact, much of the muscle tissue below the level of the injury may be replaced by fat. This happens even if you don't look or feel like you've gained weight or gotten "wider." This is partly because you're less active than before your injury, and partly because how your body itself works is changed by the injury. The result: It's much easier to become obese, even by overeating just a little.

This combination of changed metabolism and decreased muscle mass, along with an often lower activity level, means that even the "ideal body weight" charts used by doctors and insurance companies may not be the best guides. Several authors have reduced the guidelines in those charts by 10 percent to 15 percent. Using their suggested guidelines, the average 5'4" woman with a SCI should weigh between 110 and 125 lbs.; the average 5'11" man with a SCI should weigh between 145 and 160 lbs. To figure your own ideal body weight, find your height and frame size on an insurance chart, and subtract at least 10 percent from the weight that's given.

WHAT TO DO

Move past the denial. In one study of long-term SCI survivors, only half of those who had gained 20 or more pounds felt that their weight was a concern. The truth is that very few people can afford to gain 20 pounds!

Weight control—not gaining in the first place—and, if necessary, weight loss, are what is needed. The two standard components of responsible weight management are exercise and diet. They work the same for nondisabled people and for most people with SCI.

Yet for some people, especially those aging with overuse injuries, exercise can be a problem. It just may not be possible to maintain an exercise program capable of shedding excess pounds without risking new overuse injuries or aggravating old ones.

continues

continued

Diet, then, is your basic tool, and a sensible diet, though difficult, is possible.

- Low-fat, high-fiber diets are best; some may need a little modifying if other medical conditions like diabetes, skin breakdown, and high cholesterol are problems. You should cut back on fat and empty calories like those found in alcohol, soft drinks, and sweets.
- Fruit juices are also a threat. If you drink quarts of cranberry or other juices every day, you're getting too many calories from fructose. Don't cut down on all fluids, just those full of calories.
- Eat two or three small meals each day. When you fast or routinely skip meals, your metabolism, which is already lowered by your SCI and lack of exercise, tends to be lowered even more. The result is that you burn fewer calories and store more fat.
- Learn to read labels. Even foods labeled "fat free" may not be low calorie. Fat-free bakery goods, for example, can be loaded with sugar.
- Keep track of your eating habits: Do you go back for seconds, even when you're not hungry? Do you snack while watching TV? These are behaviors you can change once they're identified.
- Many people eat because of stress, boredom, or anxiety. Finding other ways of dealing with these emotions is a way to deal with overeating.
- If you need more advice or if you have other medical issues that might be complicating the picture, see a registered dietitian.

MOTIVATION

People who are highly motivated can go straight to a strict low-cholesterol, low-fat, low-calorie diet. But most people are better at negotiating: Keep the pie for dessert, but give up fast food burgers for lunch. Have one beer with dinner, but then drink water instead of soft drinks during the day. Pick one or two things you're willing to do, and stick with them. Add others later. Most motivated people, even those who don't—or can't—exercise, still can lose weight with diet alone. Finding that motivation is up to you.

You can call:

- The Consumer Hotline at the American Dietetic Association (800-366-1655)
- The National Dairy Council (800-426-8271)

Or write to

- The Food and Drug Administration, Consumer Affairs, H7E-88, 5600 Fishers Ln., Rockville, MD 20857
- American Heart Association, National Center, 7320 Greenville Ave., Dallas, TX 75231

Source: The Rehabilitation Research and Training Center on Aging with SCI, a joint project of Craig Hospital and the Department of Rehabilitation Medicine at the University of Colorado Health Sciences Center. Funded by the National Institute on Disability and Rehabilitation Research. For more information about the "SCI & Aging" publications, contact the RRTC at 800-5-REHAB-8.

PHYSICAL FITNESS

What Is Physical Fitness?

Fitness must be defined for each person individually, whether the person is disabled or not. In general, fitness means that a person has the cardiorespiratory endurance, muscular strength, and flexibility to perform all desired activities without undue physical stress. Living with a spinal cord injury (SCI) presents many challenges. Maintaining a healthy body is one of the necessary strategies for functioning well. A safe and effective fitness program to promote a healthy body can usually be designed for an individual based on his or her level of injury, lifestyle, and motivation.

The three principal components of physical fitness—cardiorespiratory endurance, muscular strength and endurance, and flexibility—are reviewed below.

Cardiorespiratory endurance, the ability of your heart and lungs to withstand long workouts, is an important component of physical fitness. For cardiorespiratory endurance you need to use the largest muscles available in a continuous and rhythmical motion. This activity results in an increased heart rate, increased oxygen consumption, and an increased rate of breathing. Individuals with levels of injury T6 and above typically show less improvement in cardiac and respiratory responses to endurance exercise, partly because of impairments in the autonomic (sympathetic) nervous system caused by SCIs at these levels.

Endurance activities that are recommended include:

- wheelchair endurance runs
- arm-cycle ergometry
- handcycling
- wheelchair aerobics
- wheelchair racing
- swimming
- rowing

Regular participation in endurance activities brings you the following gains:

- It improves blood circulation throughout your entire body. Lungs, heart, and muscles work together more efficiently, thus enhancing daily functional skills.
- It helps you handle stress. Regular exercise can bolster enthusiasm, energy, and optimism.
- It helps with weight control and helps maintain healthy muscles.
- It can help with reintegration into community life and increase opportunities to socialize when you participate in community-based programs or use community-based facilities.

continues

continued

Muscular strength and endurance are probably the most familiar components of fitness to the person with spinal cord injury because they are so much needed for wheelchair pushing, transfers, and dressing. Muscular strength is the ability of the muscle to work against resistance. Muscular endurance is the ability of the muscle to work over a period of time without fatigue. Muscular endurance is essential for wheelchair pushing over a long distance or up a hill. Even daily living activities such as washing dishes or cleaning house can require significant muscular endurance. For many people, significant musculature strength and endurance is required for doing transfers, dressing, and completing other self-care activities.

Exercising for muscular strength and endurance can help prevent injuries, improve the ability to transfer independently, and ease the strain of daily activities. Recommended resistance training activities include:

- free weights (dumbbells, cuff weights)
- weight machines (Universal, Equalizer, Versa Trainer)
- pulley system exercises
- stretch bands
- medicine balls

More information about resistance training exercises may be obtained from your rehabilitation professional.

Flexibility is the ability to use a muscle throughout its maximum range of motion. It's your ability to move your joints—to bend, stretch, and twist them easily. Stretching exercises are useful in maintaining or improving flexibility. Incorporate stretches into warm-up and cool-down activities, or do them as part of a daily workout.

Source: Indira S. Lanig, et al., *A Practical Guide to Health Promotion after Spinal Cord Injury*, Aspen Publishers, Inc., © 1996.

What Should I Do Before I Start My Fitness Program?

- **Consult Your Doctor.** A medical checkup prior to the start of any exercise program is advisable. Your doctor can identify any exercises you should not do because of medical problems, skin issues, or orthopaedic/neuromuscular limitations. Particular consideration will need to be given to any evidence of shoulder problems or carpal tunnel syndrome–related problems that could be aggravated by certain exercise activities. Any low blood pressure–induced dizziness problems should also be discussed. Your doctor can discuss the specifics of these issues with you.

- **Set Reasonable Goals.** Write down specific short-term and long-term goals. Usually, setting short-term goals will lead you to your long-term goals.

- **Progress Slowly.** Physical fitness is not something that can be accomplished in a hurry. Don't rush your conditioning program. Start easy, and gradually increase time and intensity of your physical activity.

- **Make Exercise Convenient.** Make physical activity a part of your daily routine. Find a convenient time and place so that exercise becomes a part of your daily routine. Enlist the support of family or friends. Exercising with a buddy increases motivation and can be more fun than exercising alone.

- **Enjoy Yourself.** Human beings have a tendency to stick with activities that are enjoyable and offer some pleasure in their lives. The same principle applies to exercise. When devising your workout plan, make sure to select activities you will enjoy doing. Vary your activities as much as possible. Exercise with a friend or join a class.

Source: Indira S. Lanig, et al., *A Practical Guide to Health Promotion after Spinal Cord Injury*, Aspen Publishers, Inc., © 1996.

General Exercise Guidelines

- **Frequency**: Making exercise and activity a regular occurrence in your daily life is very important. Occasional exercise will not improve endurance, strength, or flexibility capacity. Exercising at least three to five times per week is advisable, allowing at least one day between workouts for rest.

- **Intensity**: For your fitness level to improve, you must perform an activity at or above the activity levels you encounter during everyday life. You can determine intensity levels during cardiorespiratory endurance exercise by monitoring heart rate or by monitoring your own perception of exertion during exercise activities.

- **Duration**: The appropriate length of an exercise session will depend on your initial fitness level and your goals for the workout. Working up to a minimum of 20 minutes of continuous vigorous exercise is a good goal if you have not been exercising regularly.

- **Drink Plenty of Water**: Drinking sips of water before, during, and after exercise is recommended. This lessens the chances of dehydration. Remember, if you are thirsty, you may already be dehydrated. Individuals who perform intermittent catheterization (IC) will need to balance fluid intake and frequency of catheterizations carefully to ensure that bladder volumes do not become too high while they are drinking water during exercise.

- **Dress for Success**: Wear loose-fitting, absorbent clothing when exercising indoors and in hot weather. During cooler weather for outdoor workouts, year-round recommendations include the following: Remember to dress in layers. Be sure to use a proper wheelchair cushion, and wear padded gloves on hands to avoid skin irritation and pressure ulcers. Perform weight shifts periodically, and check for signs of skin irritation. Finally, gloves with extra padding on the palms will help decrease shock to hands and wrists during strenuous wheelchair-pushing sessions.

- **Listen to Your Body**: The important thing to remember in any exercise program is to listen to the reaction of your body in response to the increase in activity. Even if you choose not to listen, your body will have the last word. It's up to you to heed warning signs to prevent injury. Here are some of the warning signs to remember:
  —Stop exercising if you experience chest pain, dizziness, or excessive shortness of breath.
  —Pain in the wrist, elbow, or shoulder joints that won't go away is usually a sign that you need a rest or should decrease the intensity of your workout.
  —Pay attention to how you feel before and after exercise. If you are exhausted, sluggish, or even uncoordinated, you have been exercising too hard. You should feel a little tired yet exhilarated after a properly balanced workout.

Source: Indira S. Lanig, et al., *A Practical Guide to Health Promotion after Spinal Cord Injury*, Aspen Publishers, Inc., © 1996.

Exhibit
FITNESS RECOMMENDATIONS ACCORDING TO LEVEL OF SPINAL CORD INJURY

The level and completeness of spinal cord injury (SCI) determines the functional goals attainable by the client. The following information provides a framework from which to develop a physical activity program based on the individual's level of SCI, functional capacities, and potential for improvement. Individuals who manifest incomplete SCIs may have capacities beyond those stated in this section.

C4 AND ABOVE

The individual with a level of injury C4 or above has severe motor and sensory loss. Functional expectations include independent mouthstick activity and independent electric wheelchair propulsion with pneumatic or chin controls. He or she is dependent in all other activities of daily living (ADLs), though he or she should be able to direct his or her own care. Individuals with levels of injury at C1 to C2 are ventilator dependent. Those with injury levels at C3 to C4 may be partially or completely ventilator-free.

A "physical fitness" plan for these individuals will be limited to range of motion and postural exercises. Physical health and fitness must be approached in the broadest context, considering the unique challenges of high tetraplegia, and should be aimed at fostering as much independence and sense of mastery as possible.

Fitness recommendations are as follows:

- Promote an active role in planning the daily schedule and making life decisions such as hiring and training of attendants.
- Encourage use of a computer with software modifications (if resources allow) for correspondence, budget planning, distant communication, and so on.
- Encourage a proactive stance in planning nutritious, healthy meals.
- Teach breathing exercises for lung expansion and accessory muscle development in those who are partially or completely ventilator-free.
- Review flexibility and range of motion activities that can be done by a family member or attendant.
- Promote the pursuit of mental fitness activities (i.e., intellectual, social, and spiritual health activities) such as reading, planning projects, attending movies, cultivating relationships, and so on—anything that will help stimulate the mind and contribute to self, family, and community.

C5

Persons with a C5 tetraplegia have more mobility and independence than those with C4 and above levels of injury due to muscle strength primarily in the biceps, deltoids, and shoulder external and internal rotators. Self-feeding, facial hygiene and grooming, and writing can be accomplished with utilization of a universal cuff, adapted equipment, and setup assistance. Independent electric wheelchair propulsion with a joystick or chin control can be expected. Dependence in other ADLs is expected, and attendant/caregiver assistance is required. Some individuals with incomplete motor sparing into C6 can propel a manual wheelchair with oblique projections for very short distances indoors. Dependent transfers out of the wheelchair can be conducted with a transfer board or a one-person pivot transfer technique.

Fitness recommendations are as follows:

- Promote endurance manual wheelchair pushing on hard, level surfaces for short distances.
- Promote deltoid and biceps endurance and strengthening exercises with setup assistance using strap-on low weights and high repetitions.
- Use arm-crank ergometry with adaptive hand grips for increasing endurance levels. An attenuated heart rate response during endurance exercise will be noted.
- It may be possible to use rickshaw or shoulder depressor exercises for increase in functional strength during assisted transfers.
- Emphasize strengthening of intact scapular muscles, chest flexibility, and good posture.
- Use caution to avoid overtraining and overuse of limited musculature.
- Encourage regular passive standing in a standing frame. Though it is neither a strength nor an endurance activity, the sustained stretch it provides can attenuate spasticity.

C6

The person with this level of tetraplegia has greater potential for modified independence. Wrist extensors are intact, and the tenodesis grip is useful for certain hand functions. Independent locked-elbow horizontal transfers are usually possible with a transfer board, with or without assistance for management of legs. Manual wheelchair propulsion is usually possible with vertical projections or wrapped rims, though assistance with ramps and uneven terrain is often required. An electric wheelchair facilitates ease and speed of independent wheelchair mobility in many, if not most, individuals with this level of injury.

Fitness recommendations are as follows:

- Focus on multijoint "pull" exercises to emphasize scapular and latissimus dorsi muscles. Work to build rotator cuff and scapular stability that can prevent rounded-shoulder wheelchair posture and shoulder impingement syndromes. Work to increase wrist extension strength and tenodesis grip.

continues

continued

- Encourage endurance wheelchair runs, use of arm-crank ergometers, and use of hand-crank bikes with adapted gloves and cuffs to increase strength and endurance. Trunk stabilization is often required during exercise activities.
- Promote flexibility exercises of shoulders, back, and neck. Daily dressing of the lower extremities can be part of routine flexibility exercise.
- Encourage regular standing time in standing frame.

C7 TO T1

Preservation of triceps in those with C7 levels of injury and partial or complete hand function in those with C8 to T1 motor sparing allow greater independence with these levels of injury. Independence in all ADLs with or without adapted equipment can usually be expected. Lack of hand dexterity in C7 necessitates adaptations to compensate for this. Independent lateral transfers with or without a transfer board are achievable. Overuse syndromes, involving the weight-bearing shoulders in particular, can be observed in this population of individuals simply due to wear and tear during routine independent ADLs that involve multiple transfers and push-up weight shifts and wheelchair propulsion. This holds true for those with paraplegia or injuries below T1 as well. Attention should therefore be directed toward conscientious balancing of exercise activities and instruction in joint-sparing techniques during routine ADLs.

Fitness recommendations are as follows:

- Promote increased strength and endurance of all shoulder girdle muscles for transfers, wheelchair mobility, and driving skills. Those with C7 and sometimes with C8 levels of injury will require hand wrapping or cuff weights for resistance exercises.
- Promote endurance through wheelchair-pushing, arm-crank ergometer, and handcycling activities, using adapted gloves or cuffs as needed. Some individuals may need chest straps or binder-type stabilizers for safety in the chair while performing seated exercise. There is an attenuated heart rate response with endurance activity. Use Borg's Rate of Perceived Exertion Scale for determination of intensity.

T2 TO T6

Upper extremity musculature and shoulder girdle muscles are intact in this population. Partial function of upper back extensor muscles is present. Independence in all ADLs can be expected.

Fitness recommendations are as follows:

- Strengthen all upper extremity muscles, emphasizing multi-joint "pull" exercises to balance back muscles with strong anterior muscles due to wheelchair and crutch mobility.
- The individual may use a variety of equipment for resistance training, including free weights, machines, or a combination. Endurance conditioning may include the use of handcycles, endurance wheelchair runs, and swimming.
- Trunk stabilizers or chest straps may be necessary during certain upright exercise activities.
- Use skin protection measures when exercising out of chair.
- Design exercise routine to limit frequency of transfers. This will reduce wear and tear on shoulders.

T7 TO T12

Independence in all ADLs can be expected. The lower the level of injury, the greater the probability of upright ambulation with long leg braces and gait aids. Ambulation with gait aids and braces, however, requires high levels of energy expenditure and can be very taxing on shoulders and arms. A wheelchair is therefore the principal means of mobility. Upright ambulation can be used for household mobility or for exercise.

Fitness recommendations are as follows:

- Increase strength and endurance of upper extremity and upper body musculature. Include abdominal strengthening and back flexibility exercises for crutch ambulators.
- Note that increases in aerobic endurance are possible at this level and that a central cardiovascular training effect may occur. Heart rate and perceived exertion in combination are recommended for intensity monitoring.

L1 TO S5

For persons with levels of injury between L1 and L3, a wheelchair is usually required for more efficient mobility. Upright ambulation with long leg braces and gait aids is possible for short distances. For those with levels of injury L4 and below, upright ambulation with short leg braces and gait aids is common. A wheelchair may be used for long distances.

Fitness recommendations are as follows:

- Follow strength and endurance program recommendations for other individuals with paraplegia. Concentrate on flexibility of hip flexors by stretching while lying prone. This will aid in upright ambulation activities.
- Balance fitness workouts and functional activities to prevent overuse and injury of shoulders, wrists, and elbows.
- Involve lower extremities as much as possible in cycling, swimming, and walking.

Source: Indira S. Lanig, et al., *A Practical Guide to Health Promotion after Spinal Cord Injury*, Aspen Publishers, Inc., © 1996.

Appendix

Appendix A—Spinal Cord Injury
 Resources 473

Appendix A
Spinal Cord Injury Resources

American Association of SCI Nurses (ASCIN)
c/o Eastern Paralyzed Veterans Association
75-20 Astoria Blvd.
Jackson Heights, NY 11370-1178
718-803-3782
fax: 718-803-0414

American Association of SCI Psychologists and Social Workers
c/o Eastern Paralyzed Veterans Association
75-20 Astoria Blvd.
Jackson Heights, NY 11370-1178
718-803-3782
fax: 718-803-0414

American Paralysis Association (APA)
500 Morris Avenue
Springfield, NJ 07081
800-225-0292
201-379-2690
fax: 201-912-9433
http://www.apa.uci.edu/paralysis

American Paraplegia Society
c/o Eastern Paralyzed Veterans Association
75-20 Astoria Blvd.
Jackson Heights, NY 11370-1178
718-803-3782
fax: 718-803-0414

American Rehabilitation Association
1910 Associate Drive, Suite 200
Reston, VA 20191
703-789-5700
fax: 703-648-0346
e-mail: amrehabexecoff@iarf.org

American Spinal Injury Association (ASIA)
345 East Superior Street, Room 1436
Chicago, IL 60611
312-908-6207
fax: 312-503-0869

Canadian Paraplegic Association Ontario
520 Sutherland Drive
Toronto, Ontario M4G 3V9
Canada
416-422-5644
fax: 416-422-5943

Clearinghouse on Disability Information
Office of Special Education and Rehabilitative Services
Room 3132 Switzer Building
330 C Street, SW
Washington, DC 20202-2524
202-205-8241
fax: 202-401-2608

Eastern Paralyzed Veterans Association
75-20 Astoria Blvd.
Jackson Heights, NY 11370-1178
718-803-3782
fax: 718-803-0414

F.E.S. Information Center
11000 Cedar Avenue, Suite 207
Cleveland, OH 44106-3052
800-666-2353
216-231-3257
fax: 216-231-3258
http://feswww.fes.cwru.edu

Foundation for SCI Prevention
1310 Ford Building
Detroit, MI 48226
800-342-0330

International Medical Society of Paraplegia
The Institute for Rehabilitation and Research
1333 Moursund Avenue
Houston, TX 77225
713-799-5000

Miami Project to Cure Paralysis (MPCP)
1600 NW 10th Avenue, #R-48
Miami, FL 33136
800-782-6387
305-547-6001
fax: 305-243-6017
http://199.227.117.2/mia-proj

National Center for Medical Rehabilitation Research (NCMRR)
6100 Executive Blvd., Room 2A-03
Rockville, MD 20852
301-402-2242
fax: 301-402-0832

National Council on Disability
1331 F Street, NW, Suite 1050
Washington, DC 20004-1107
202-272-2004
fax: 202-272-2022

National Council on SCI
151 Tremont Street
Boston, MA 02111
617-338-7777
fax: 617-451-0962

National Organization on Disability
910 16th Street, NW
Washington, DC 20006-2988
202-293-5960
fax: 202-293-7999
http://www.nod.org

National Rehabilitation Information Center (NARIC)
8455 Colesville Road, Suite 935
Silver Spring, MD 20910-3319
800-346-2742
fax: 301-587-1967
http://www.naric.com/naric

National Spinal Cord Injury Association (NSCIA)
8300 Colesville Road, Suite 551
Silver Spring, MD 20910
301-588-6959
fax: 301-588-9414
NSCIA Hotline: 800-962-9629

National Spinal Cord Injury (PVA) Hotline
2200 N. Forrest Park Avenue
Baltimore, MD 21217
800-526-3456

National Spinal Cord Injury Statistical Center
UAB-Spain Rehabilitation Center, Room 544
1717 6th Avenue South
Birmingham, AL 35233-7330
205-934-5359
fax: 205-934-2709
http://www.spinalcord.uab.edu

Paralyzed Veterans of America (PVA)
801 18th Street, NW
Washington, DC 20006
800-424-8200
202-872-1300

Rehabilitation International
25 East 21st Street
New York, NY 10010
212-420-1500
fax: 212-505-0871

Spina Bifida of America
4590 MacArthur Blvd., NW, Suite 250
Washington, DC 20007-4226
202-944-3285
800-621-3141

Spinal Cord Society
Route 5, Box 22-A, Wendell Road
Fergus Falls, MN 56537
218-739-5252
218-739-5261
fax: 218-739-5262
http://members.aol.com/scsweb/index.htm

The World Institute on Disability (WID)
510 16th Street
Oakland, CA 94612-1500
510-763-4100

ALCOHOL AND SUBSTANCE ABUSE

Alcoholics Anonymous
P.O. Box 459, Grand Central Station
New York, NY 10163
212-870-3400
or
475 Riverside Drive
New York, NY 10115
212-870-3003
fax: 212-870-3199

Families Anonymous, Inc.
P.O. Box 3475
Culver City, CA 90231
818-989-7841

Narcotics Anonymous
World Service Office
P.O. Box 9999
Van Nuys, CA 91409
818-773-9999
fax: 818-700-0700

National Clearinghouse for Alcohol and Drug Information (NCADI)
P.O. Box 2345
Rockville, MD 20847-2345
301-468-2600
fax: 301-468-6433
http://www.health.org

National Institute on Drug Abuse (NIDA)
5600 Fishers Lane, Room 10-A03
Rockville, MD 20857
301-443-4577
fax: 301-443-8908

Substance Abuse Resources for Disabled Individuals (SARDI)
Wright State University School of Medicine
P.O. Box 927
Dayton, OH 45401
937-259-1384
fax: 937-259-1395

U.S. International Center for Disabled Chemical Dependency Services
340 East 24th Street, Room 311
New York, NY 10010
212-481-5780
212-679-0100
fax: 212-889-2440

Toll-Free Information

1-800-COCAINE
Cocaine Helpline

1-800-NCA-CALL
National Council on Alcoholism & Drug Dependence Hope Line

For additional resources, see "What Can I Do about My Drinking?" in Chapter 8.

AMERICANS WITH DISABILITIES ACT (ADA)

ADA Coordination and Review Section
Civil Rights Division
U.S. Department of Justice
P.O. Box 66118
Washington, DC 20035-6118
202-514-0301
800-514-0301
http://www.usdoj.gov/crt/ada/adahom1.htm

Architectural and Transportation Barriers Compliance Board
1331 F Street, NW, Suite 1000
Washington, DC 20004
800-USA-ABLE
202-272-5434
fax: 202-272-5447
http://www.access-board.gov

Council for Disability Rights
176 West Adam Street, Suite 1830
Chicago, IL 60603
312-444-9484
fax: 312-444-1977

Disability Rights Education and Defense Fund, Inc. (DREDF)
2212 6th Street
Berkeley, CA 94710
510-644-2555
800-466-4232 (TDD)
fax: 510-841-8645

ASSISTIVE TECHNOLOGY/ELECTRONIC RESOURCES

ABLEDATA (database of assistive technology information)
National Rehabilitation Information Center (NARIC)
8455 Colesville Road, Suite 935
Silver Spring, MD 20910-3319
800-227-0216
http://www.abledata.com

America On-Line
Disability Forum
Better Health & Medical Forum
8619 Westwood Center Drive
Vienna, VA 22182-2285
703-448-8700

CO-NET
TRACE Research and Development Center
Waisman Center
1500 Highland Avenue
Madison, WI 53705-2280
608-262-6966
fax: 608-262-8848

DRAGNet (Disability Resources Affiliate and Groups Network)
840 12th Avenue, NE
Minneapolis, MN 55401
612-378-9796

National Audiovisual Database of Educational Materials on SCI
Division of Education, Institute for Rehabilitation and Research
1333 Moursund Avenue
Houston, TX 77030
713-797-5945
fax: 713-797-5982
e-mail: lperson@dcm.tmc.edu

Rehabdata
National Rehabilitation Information Center (NARIC)
8455 Colesville Road, Suite 935
Silver Spring, MD 20910-3319
800-346-2742
fax: 301-587-1967
http://www.cais.com/naric

WIDnet (World Institute on Disability)
510 16th Street, Suite 100
Oakland, CA 94612-1500
510-763-4100
fax: 510-763-4109
e-mail: wid@wid.org

HOUSING/HOME MODIFICATIONS

Adaptive Environments Center (AEC)
374 Congress Street, Suite 301
Boston, MA 02210
617-695-1225
fax: 617-482-8099

Barrier Free Environments (BFE)
P.O. Box 30634
Raleigh, NC 27622
919-782-7823
fax: 919-787-1984

Center for Universal Design
North Carolina State University
219 Oberlin Road
Raleigh, NC 27695
or
P.O. Box 8613
Raleigh, NC 27695-8613
919-515-3082
fax: 919-787-1984
e-mail: cahd@ncsu.edu

National Association of Home Builders
NAHB National Research Center
400 Prince Georges Blvd.
Upper Marlboro, MD 20774-8731
301-249-4000
fax: 301-249-0305
http://www.nahb.com/research

National Council on Senior Housing
c/o National Association of Home Builders
1201 15th Street, NW
Washington, DC 20005
202-822-0220
fax: 202-822-0496

National Kitchen and Bath Association
687 Willow Grove Street
Hackettstown, NJ 07840
800-843-6522
fax: 908-852-1695

INDEPENDENT LIVING

Center for Independent Living
2539 Telegraph Avenue
Berkeley, CA 94704
510-841-4776
fax: 510-841-6168

Job Accommodation Network (JAN)
West Virginia University
918 Chestnut Ridge Road, Suite 1
P.O. Box 6080
Morgantown, WV 26506-6080
800-526-7234
fax: 304-293-5407
http://janweb.icdi.wvu.edu

National Council on Independent Living
2111 Wilson Blvd., Suite 405
Arlington, VA 22201
703-525-3406
fax: 703-525-3409
or
4th & Broadway
Troy, NY 12180
518-274-0701
fax: 518-274-7944

The National Rehabilitation Center
Independent Living Research Utilization
2323 South Shepherd, Suite 1000
Houston, TX 77019
800-346-2742
713-520-0232
fax: 713-520-5785
e-mail: ilru@bcm.tmc.edu
http://www.bcm.tmc.edu/ilru/

The Research and Training Center on Independent Living
University of Kansas, Life Span Institute
4089 Dole Building, University of Kansas
Lawrence, KS 66045-2930
913-864-0592
fax: 913-864-5063
e-mail: rtcil@kuhub.cc.ukans.edu
http://www.lsi.ukans.edu/rtcil/rtcbroc.htm

PUBLISHERS OF SCI LITERATURE

Accent on Living
P.O. Box 700
Bloomington, IL 61702
800-787-8444
fax: 309-378-4420
http://www.blvd.com/accent

The Disability Bookshop
P.O. Box 129
Vancouver, WA 98666
800-637-2256
360-694-2462
fax: 360-696-3210

PVA Publications
2111 East Highland Avenue, Suite 180
Phoenix, AZ 85016-4702
602-224-0500
fax: 602-224-0507
e-mail: pvapub@aol.com

Spinal Network
23815 Stuart Road
Malibu, CA 90265
800-338-5412 (ext. 219)

SEXUALITY/REPRODUCTION/WOMEN'S HEALTH

Adoptive Families of America
3333 Highway 100 North
Minneapolis, MN 55422
612-535-4829
fax: 612-535-7808
e-mail: jhauger@mr.net

American Association of Sex Educators, Counselors and Therapists (AASECT)
P.O. Box 238
Mount Vernon, IA 52314-0238
319-895-8407
fax: 319-895-6203

Concerned Persons for Adoption
P.O. Box 179
Whippany, NJ 07981
908-273-5694

Dateable International
35 Wisconsin Circle, Suite 205
Chevy Chase, MD 20815
301-656-8723
fax: 301-657-4327
http://www.dateable.org

Disability, Pregnancy and Parenthood International
Arrowhead Publications
51 Thames Village
London W4 3UF
England

Health Resource Center for Women with Disabilities
Rehabilitation Institute of Chicago
345 East Superior, Suite 106
Chicago, IL 60611
312-908-7997

North American Council on Adoptable Children
970 Raymond Avenue, Suite 106
St. Paul, MN 55114
612-644-3036
fax: 612-644-9848
e-mail: nacac@aol.com

Sex Information and Education Council of the United States (SIECUS)
130 West 42nd Street, Suite 350
New York, NY 10036
212-819-9770
fax: 212-819-9776
http://www.siecus.org

Sexuality and Disability Training Center
Boston University Medical Center
88 E. Newton Street
Boston, MA 02118
617-638-7355

University of Michigan Sex and Disability Unit
Department of Physical Medicine and Rehabilitation
Box 33, Room E3254, University Hospital
Ann Arbor, MI 48109
313-936-7175
fax: 313-764-5335

The Xandria Collection
Special Edition Catalog for Disabled People and Collector's Gold Edition Catalog ($4.00 for both)
P.O. Box 317039
San Francisco, CA 94131
800-242-2823

SPORT AND FITNESS ASSOCIATIONS

Billiards
National Wheelchair Billiards Association
216-234-6922

Certification Organizations
American College of Sports Medicine (ACSM)
P.O. Box 1440
Indianapolis, IN 46206-1440
317-637-9200
fax: 317-634-7817
http://www.acsm.org/sportsmed

Disabled Sports—USA (Formerly National Handicapped Sports)
301-217-0960

IDEA, Inc. (International Dance Educators Associations)
6190 Cornerstone Court East, Suite 204
San Diego, CA 92121-3773
619-535-8979
fax: 619-535-8234
e-mail: ideafit@ix.netcom.com

Golf
Association of Disabled American Golfers
303-220-0921

Handcycling
American Handcycle Association
619-596-1986

Horseback Riding

North American Riding for the Handicapped Association
P.O. Box 33150
Denver, CO 80233
800-369-RIDE
fax: 303-252-4610
http://narha.org

Multisport

Disabled Sports—USA (Formerly National Handicapped Sports)
301-217-0960

Paralyzed Veterans of America, Inc.
1016 N. 32nd Street, Suite 4
Phoenix, AZ 85008
602-244-9168
fax: 602-244-0416

Rick Hansen Centre
W1-67 Van Vliet Complex
University of Alberta
Edmonton, Alberta T6G 2H9
Canada
403-492-9236
fax: 403-492-7161

Wheelchair Sports, USA
3595 E. Fountain Blvd., Suite L-1
Colorado Springs, CO 80910
719-574-1150
fax: 719-574-9840
e-mail: wsusa@aol.com

Outdoor Recreation

Bay Area Outreach and Recreation Program (BORP)
830 Bancroft Way
Berkeley, CA 94710
510-849-4662
fax: 510-849-4616

Breckenridge Outdoor Education Center (BOEC)
P.O. Box 697
Breckenridge, CO 80424
303-453-6422
fax: 303-453-4676
e-mail: boec@colorado.net

Canadian Recreational Canoeing Association
P.O. Box 398, 446 Main Street West
Merrickville, Ontario K0G 1N0
Canada
613-269-2910
fax: 613-269-2908
http://www.crca.ca/
e-mail: staff@crca.ca

Challenge Alaska
P.O. Box 110065
Anchorage, AK 99511-0065
907-563-2658
fax: 907-561-6142

Cooperative Wilderness Handicapped Outdoor Group (C.W. HOG)
Idaho State University
Box 8128 Pond Student Union
Pocatello, ID 83209
208-236-3912
fax: 208-236-4600
http://www.isu.edu/departments/outdoor/cwhog.html

Environmental Traveling Companions
415-474-7662

Horses for the Physically Challenged
503-873-3890

Nantahala Outdoor Center
13077 Highway 19W
Bryson City, NC 28713
704-488-2175
fax: 704-488-0301
http://nocweb.com

National Ability Center
P.O. Box 682799
Park City, UT 84068-2799
801-649-3991
fax: 801-658-3992
e-mail: nac@xmission.com

National Park Service
Division of Accessibility Affairs
P.O. Box 37127
Washington, DC 20013
202-343-7040

Northeast Passage
Chapter of Disabled Sports—USA
P.O. Box 127
Durham, NH 03824-0127
603-862-0070
fax: 603-862-2722

Paraplegics on Independent Nature Trips (POINT)
214-827-7404

Recreational Challenges
208-464-2118

Sierra Club Outings Department
85 2nd Street, Second Floor
San Francisco, CA 94105
415-923-5630
fax: 415-977-5795
http://www.sierraclub.org

Special Populations Learning Outdoor Recreation and Education (S'PLORE)
801-484-4128

Vinland National Center
3675 Ihduhapi Road
P.O. Box 308
Loretto, MN 55357
612-479-3555
fax: 612-479-2605

Wilderness Inquiry
1313 Fifth Street, SE, Box 84
Minneapolis, MN 55414
612-379-3858
800-728-0719
fax: 612-379-5972

Wilderness Institute
28310 Roadside Drive, Suite 152
Agoura Hills, CA 91301
818-991-7327
fax: 818-991-0743
e-mail: info@wildernessinstitute.com
http://www.wildernessinstitute.com

Racquet Sports

National Foundation of Wheelchair Tennis
940 Calle Amanecer, Suite B
San Clemente, CA 92673
714-361-3663
fax: 714-361-6603
e-mail: nfwt@aol.com
http://www.nfwt.org

Skiing

Disabled Sports—USA (Formerly National Handicapped Sports)
301-217-0960

National Sports Center for the Disabled
P.O. Box 36
Winter Park, CO 80482
970-726-5514 (ext. 1740)
fax: 970-892-5823
e-mail: jbuch@csn.net

U.S. Disabled Ski Team
P.O. Box 100
Park City, UT 84060
801-649-9090
fax: 801-649-3613
http://www.usskiteam.com
or
http://www.ussa.org

Softball

National Wheelchair Softball Association
1616 Todd Court
Hastings, MN 55033
612-437-1792

Table Tennis

American Wheelchair Table Tennis
23 Parker Street
Port Chester, NY 10573
914-937-3932
fax: 914-937-3932

Track and Field

Wheelchair Athletics USA
2351 Parkwood Rd.
Snellville, GA 30278
770-972-0763
fax: 770-985-4885
e-mail: bewing@harb.net

Water Sports

Access to Sailing
19744 Beach Blvd., Suite 340
Huntington Beach, CA 92648
714-722-5371

American Canoe Association
7432 Alban Station Blvd., Suite B-226
Springfield, VA 22150
703-451-0141
fax: 703-451-2245
e-mail: acadirect@aol.com
http://www.acapaddler.org

Aquatic Sports Association for the Physically Challenged
619-589-0537

Handicapped Scuba Association
1104 El Prado
San Clemente, CA 92672
714-498-6128

U.S. Rowing Association
201 South Capitol Avenue, Suite 400
Indianapolis, IN 46225
317-237-5656
fax: 317-237-5646
e-mail: usrowing@aol.com
http://www.coxing.com/usrowing

U.S. Wheelchair Swimming
508-946-1964

Weightlifting

U.S. Wheelchair Weightlifting Association
39 Michael Place
Levittown, PA 19057
215-945-1964
fax: 215-946-2574

PROGRAMS FUNDED BY THE NATIONAL INSTITUTE ON DISABILITY AND REHABILITATION RESEARCH (NIDRR)

Model Spinal Cord Injury Systems

Craig Hospital
3425 South Clarkson Street
Englewood, CO 80110
303-789-8220

The Institute for Rehabilitation Research (TIRR)
1333 Moursund Avenue
Houston, TX 77225
713-797-5910

Kessler Institute for Rehabilitation
University of Medicine and Dentistry of New Jersey
1199 Pleasant Valley Way
West Orange, NJ 07052
201-243-6805

Mount Sinai Medical Center
Department of Rehabilitation Medicine
One Gustave L. Levy Place, Box 1674
New York, NY 10029
212-241-5417
fax: 212-423-1225

Northwestern University Acute Spine Injury Center
Northwestern Memorial Hospital
250 East Superior Avenue, Suite 619
Chicago, IL 60611
312-908-3425
fax: 312-908-1819
http://www.nwu.edu/spine

Rancho Los Amigos Medical Center
HB117, 7601 East Imperial Highway
Downey, CA 90242
310-401-7161
fax: 310-803-5876

Rehabilitation Institute of Michigan
261 Mack Boulevard
Detroit, MI 48201
313-745-9770

Santa Clara Valley Medical Center
751 South Bascom Avenue, Suite 2011
P.O. Box 70
San Jose, CA 95128
408-295-9896

Shepherd Center
American Spinal Injury Association
2020 Peachtree Road, NW
Atlanta, GA 30309
404-355-9772
fax: 404-355-1826

Thomas Jefferson University
Jefferson Medical College
132 South 10th Street
375 Main Building
Philadelphia, PA 19107
215-955-6579
fax: 215-955-5152

University of Alabama at Birmingham
Spain Rehabilitation Center
1717 6th Avenue South, Room 506
Birmingham, AL 35233-7330
205-934-3283

University of Michigan/Model Spinal Cord Injury Care System
Department of Physical Medicine and Rehabilitation
300 North Ingalls
Ann Arbor, MI 48109-0491
313-763-0971
fax: 313-936-5492
e-mail: model.sci@umich.edu

University of Washington School of Medicine
Department of Rehabilitation Medicine
Attention: Dr. Diana Cardenas
Box 356490, Health Science Building
Seattle, WA 98195
206-543-8171
fax: 206-685-3244

Rehabilitation Research and Training Centers (RRTCs)

Aging

Craig Hospital
Research Department
3425 South Clarkson Street
Englewood, CO 80110
303-789-8202
fax: 303-789-8441
e-mail: irene@craig-hospital.org

Los Amigos Research and Education Institute, Inc. (LAREI)
Rancho Los Amigos Medical Center
12481 Dahlia Street, Building 306
Downey, CA 90242
310-401-8111
fax: 310-803-5569

Secondary Complications

University of Alabama/Birmingham
Department of Rehabilitation Medicine
RRTC Training Office Spain Rehabilitation Center
1717 6th Avenue South, Room 506
Birmingham, AL 35233-7330
205-934-3283
fax: 205-975-4691
http:www.spinalcord.uab.edu

Community Integration
Baylor College of Medicine
Department of Physical Medicine and Rehabilitation
One Baylor Plaza
Houston, TX 77030
713-797-5910

Rehabilitation Engineering Research Centers (RERCs)

University of Pittsburgh
Rehabilitation Technology Program (RTP)
915 William Pitt Way
Pittsburgh, PA 15238
412-647-1270
fax: 412-647-1277

Children
Rancho Los Amigos Medical Center
Los Amigos Research and Education Institute, Inc. (LAREI)
7503 Bonita Street, Bonita Hall
Downey, CA 90242
310-401-7994
fax: 310-803-6117

Index

A

Abdominal muscles, 47
Accessibility, home, 395–396
Acetic acid solution, 154–155
Acute care hospital location, 24
Adoption, 214–215, 244–245
Aggression, 301–302
Aging, 306–308
　posture and, 90–92
　spasticity and, 87–89
AIDS, 254
Air Carriers Access Act, 377–378
Air conditioning, 393
Air shifts, 59
Air travel tips, 379–380
Al-Anon, 288
Alateen, 288
Alcoholics Anonymous, 288, 289–290
Alcohol intake, 316
　abuse resources, 474–475
　facts about, 283
　skin care, 181
Alcoholism
　definition of, 284
　help for, 286–288
　identification of, 285
Alkaline urine, 152
American Spinal Injury Association, impairment scale, 17

Americans with Disabilities Act, 377
　employment, 381–382
　public accommodations, commercial facilities, 382–383
　public services, 382
　resources, 475
　telecommunications, 383
Aminophylline, 63
Anatomy, 8–10
　arteries, veins, 29
　female sexual, 234
　lungs, 45–46
　male sexual, 221
Anemia, 176
Anesthetic creams, 344
Anger, 299
Ankle stretch, 74
Anterior cord syndrome, 14
Antibiotics, 349
Anticonvulsants, 316
Antidepressants, 316
Arteries, 29
Artificial insemination, 227
Assertion, 301
Assistive technology resources, 475–476. *See also* Equipment
Attending physician, 23
Autogenic training, 322
Automobile driving
　adaptive, 443–445

　car selection, 446–447
　insurance, 376
　trips, 437
　van selection, 447–450
Autonomic dysreflexia, 106–110, 162, 214, 217, 239, 245

B

Baclofen injection therapy, 85, 86, 88, 99–101, 348
Bathroom
　accessibility, 402
　aids, 414–415
　checklist, 391
Bedside drainage bags, 154, 156
Behavior modification, 321
Biofeedback, 321, 326–327
Bipolar disorder, 267–268
Birth control, 235–236, 238
Bisacodyl, 160
Bladder care, 216, 231
　irrigation, 152
　management, 23
　program
　　checklist, 118
　　common problems, 119–121
　　overview, 113–117
　spasms, 150
Bladder stones, 152, 454

Blisters, 192
Body
　image, 242
　stretch, 74
　weight, skin care, 180
Bone
　abnormal formation of, 80–83
　scans, 82
Boots, 411–412
Bowel care, 216, 231
　accidents, 161–162
　nutrition, 453
　medications, 344–346
　program
　　ensuring success of, 160–162
　　overview, 157–159
Breast cancer, 248–249
Breathing, 47–48, 277
　exercises, 31, 51, 58–59
　glossopharyngeal, 63
　quiet technique, 322
　spinal cord injury and, 48
Brown-Sequard syndrome, 14
Bruises, 191
Bulk formers, 344
Burns, 190–191

C

Canes, 417
Car. *See also* Automobile driving
　insurance, 444
　selection, 446–447
Carbohydrates, 458
Cardiac pacing, 102–103
Cardiorespiratory endurance, 464
Caregiver tips, long-term, 309
Cascara, 160
Case manager, 26
Catapres, 348
Catheter, 230
　condom. *See* Condom: catheters
　Foley. *See* Foley catheter
　indwelling. *See* Indwelling catheter
　intermittent. *See* Intermittent catheter
　leakage, 150
Cauda equina syndrome, 11, 14
Central cord syndrome, 14
Central pain, 313–314
Cervical area, 4, 8–9
Cervical caps, 236, 241
Chest physical therapy, 52–55
Children, adoption of, 214–215
Chlamydia, 253
Cimetidine, 349
Circulation
　arteries, veins, 29
　complications of, 32, 33–39
　how works, 30

　maintaining healthy, 31
　skin care and, 175–176
　temperature regulation, 40–41
Clapping, 52, 54–55
Clinical syndromes, 11–12, 14
Clonidine, 348
Closet accessibility, 402
Clothing, 180
　choosing, adapting, 408–412
　mobility and, 417
Commercial facilities, 382–383
Commission on Accreditation of
　Rehabilitation Facilities, 23
Communication, 301–302
　personal assistant, 373–375
　services, 353
　sexuality, 211
Community integration services, 24
Community mental health centers, 287
Condom, 236, 241
　application, 141–143
　　hints about, 149
　　self-adhesive, 144–145
　　two-piece self-adhesive, 146–148
　catheters, 155, 216
Confusion, 300
Congestion, 49–50
Constipation, 161, 165–167. *See also*
　Bowel care
Construction checklist, 389–390. *See
　also* Home modification
Container opening, closing, 404
Contraception, 214, 217, 240–241, 243
Contraceptive sponges, 236, 241
Conus medullaris syndrome, 11, 14
Cooking, 404
Corset, abdominal 63
Coughing, 51, 52
　assisted, 63–64
Coumadin, 349
Counseling, sexuality, 240
Counters, 393
Crede, 115
Crime victims compensation, 376
Culture and sensitivity test, 122
Cupping and vibration, 52
Curb safety, 436
Cutting boards, 403–404
Cystometrics, 123
Cystoscopy, 123
Cytomegalovirus, 253

D

Dantrium, 85, 348
Dantrolene, 85
Deep vein thrombosis (DVT), 32, 36–38
Defecation reflex, 157
Delivery, 244

Dental care, 413
Department of Veterans Affairs, 376
Depo-Provera, 241
Depression, 264–266, 317
　diagnosis of, 267–269
　treatment of, 270–272
Diaphragm, 47, 236, 241
Diaphragmatic assist devices, 62
Diarrhea, 161. *See also* Bowel care
Diazepam, 85, 348
Didronel, 82–83, 349
Diet, circulation and, 31. *See also*
　Nutrition
Dietitian, 26
Digestive tract, 157
Digital stimulation, 158, 160, 163–164
Disabilities, feelings about, 298
Ditropan, 341
Dorsal root entry zone (DREZ), 317
Drainage bag care, leg/bedside, 154
Dressing aids, 410–411
Driver training, 443–444. *See also*
　Automobile driving
Drug allergies, 336
Dulcolax, 158, 160
Dusting, 400–401
Dysesthetic pain, 315

E

Edema, 32, 34–35, 175–176
Ejaculation, 213–214, 218
　electro-, 227
　understanding, 226
Elavil, 347
Elbow exercises, 70–71
Electrical outlets, 393
Electrical stimulation, 317
Electroejaculation, 227
Electronic resources, 475–476
Elevators, 395
Emergency backup care, 370–372
Emotional adjustment, 259–261
Emotional adjustment worksheet, 262
Employer agreement, 368
Employment
　ADA, 381–382
　application, 361–362
Enema, 160, 344–345
　mini, 158
Ephedrine, 341
Equipment, 23–24
　circulation and, 31
　skin injury prevention, 180
Erections (penile), 228, 230
　obtaining, maintaining, 223–225
　types of, 222
Exercise, 278. *See also* Physical fitness
　breathing, 58–59, 63

circulation and, 31
guidelines, 467
muscle relaxation, 325
neck accessory, 59
range of motion, 75–79
relaxation, 324
upper extremity range of motion, 68–72
Exhaling, 48
Ex-Lax, 160
Expiration, 48

F

Family
  education, 24
  reactions, 303–304
Family service agency, 287
Fatigue
  effects of, 275–279
  trouble spots, 280–282
Fat intake, 458
Feelings, 298–300
Female reproductive issues, 240
  gynecologist guidelines, 242–243
  questions about, 238–239
  sexual anatomy, 234
  sexual function, 235–237
Fertility, 235
Fertilization, 227
Fiber, 459
Flaccidity, 11, 85, 115–116
Flexibility, 465
Floor cleaning, 400
Fluid intake, 51, 161, 460
Foley catheter, 134, 156, 219
  insertion, female, 137–138
  insertion, male, 135–136
Follow-up, 24
Food/eating arrangements, 355, 364
Food guide pyramid, 456–457
Food preparation, 403–405
Foot problems, 192
Footwear, 410, 417
Friction burn, 192
Friends' reactions, 303–304
Frostbite, 190
Frustration, 300
Functional chart, 20–22
Functional electrical stimulation, 64, 276
  choice of, 105
  overview, 102–104
Functional independence measure, 13, 17–18

G

Gas, excessive, 162. *See also* Bowel care
Glossopharyngeal breathing, 63

Glycerin, 158
Gonorrhea, 253
Grab bars, 418–419
Gynecologist guidelines, 242–243

H

Hair care, 413
Hamstring stretch, 73–74
Hand exercises, 71–72
Handles, 405
Headaches, 239
Health, general, 51
Health insurance, 376
Heart problems, 454
Heating, 393
Hemorrhoidal suppositories, 345
Hepatitis B, 253
Herpes, 253
Heterotopic ossification, 81–83
Hip exercises, 73
HIV, 254
HIV test, 255–256
Hoists, 395
Home care
  cleaning, 400–401
  storage, 401–402
Home health agencies, 359
Home modification
  accessibility, 395–396
  bathroom checklist, 391
  construction checklist, 389–390
  kitchen checklist, 392
  mechanical checklist, 393–394
  mobility, 416
  resources, 476
  wheelchair user, 387–388
Homemaking needs, 354
Household services, 353
Housekeeping, 355, 364
Human papillomavirus, 253
Humidity, 51
Humor, 299
Hydronephrosis, 121
Hygiene
  female, 172
  general, 170
  male, 171
Hyperreflexia, 106–110, 219
Hypnosis, 320–321
Hytrin, 341

I

Ileo loop drainage, 230
Imagery, 277
  guided, 322
  script, 328–329
Impairment scale, 17

In vitro fertilization, 227
Incontinence, 219
Indwelling catheter, 134, 216, 231
  insertion, female, 137–138
  insertion, male, 135–136
  suprapubic insertion, 139–140
Infertility, 244
Ingrown toenails, 192
Inhalation, 48
Inspiration, 48
Intercostal muscles, 47
Intermittent abdominal pressure ventilator, 62
Intermittent catheter, 124, 216
  cleaning, female, 130–133
  cleaning, male, 125–129
  types of, 155
Interview, personal assistant, 363–365
Intrauterine device, 236, 241
Intravenous pyelogram, 122–123
Inversine, 349

J

Job description
  personal assistant, 357
  worksheet, 358
Joint problems, 96

K

Kidney stones, 120–121, 454
Kitchen
  accessibility, 401
  checklist, 392
Knee exercises, 73
Knobs, 405

L

Labor, 244
Lateral stretch, 58
Laxatives, 160
Leg bags, 154, 155
Lifestyle assessment, 355–356
Lifts, 395
Lighting, 393
Light switches, 393
Lioresal, 85, 86, 348
Lower motor neurons, 4, 10, 157
Lumbar area, 5, 8–9
Lungs
  decreased volume, 49
  diagram of, 45–46
  postural drainage of, 56–57

M

Magnesium citrate, 160
Male reproductive function, 226–227
   sexual anatomy, 221
   sexual concerns, 228–233
   sexual function, 222–225
Manic-depressive disorder, 267–268
Marriage, 213–215
Massage, 323
Mechanical lifts, 395
Mechanical pain, 314
Medicaid, 376
Medical consultation, 24
Medicare, 376
Medication, 63, 216, 278, 349
   bladder, 341–343
   bowel programs and, 159, 344–346
   daily schedule, 340
   instruction sheet, 339
   overview, 335–337
   pain, 316, 347
   safe use of, 338
   self-injection, 223
   spasticity, 85–86, 348
Meditation, 277
Meditation therapy, 320
Menses, 235
Menstruation, 172
Mental imagery. *See* Imagery
Milk of Magnesia, 161
Mindset, 307
Minerals, 459
Minipress, 342
Mobility, 51, 416–419
Mobility services, 353
Motor examination, 15–16, 17
Mucous accidents, 161
Muscle
   relaxation exercises, 325
   strengthening, 67, 465
Music tape, 330

N

Nail care, 414
Nails, ingrown, 192
Narcotics, 316
National Clearinghouse for Alcohol and Drug Information (NCADI), 288
National Council on Alcoholism (NCA), 288
National Institute on Disability and Rehabilitation Research, 480–481
Neck
   accessory exercise, 59
   muscles, 47
Needs inventory, 354
Nerve blocks, 317
Nerve fibers, 3, 8
Nerves, 4
Neuroleptics, 316
Neurological classification, 6–7, 11–12, 19
Neurological examination, 14
   motor, 15–16
   motor scores, 17
   sensory, 15
   sensory scores, 17
Norplant, 236
Norpramin, 347
Number counting, 59
Nutrition
   food guide pyramid, 456–457
   importance of, 453–455
   nutrients needed, 458–460
   skin care, 175
   ventilator support and, 64

O

Obstetrician guidelines, 244–245
Occupational therapist, 25
Oral contraceptives, 236, 241
Oral sex, 231
Orgasm, 211–212, 233, 239
Osteoporosis, 93–95
Outerwear, 409

P

Pain
   dysesthetic, 315
   management
      sources for, 331
      strategies for, 319
   psychological methods for, 320–321
   treatment of, 316–318
   types of, 313–314
Paraplegia, 7, 12, 52–53
Parent, 305
Parking permit, disabled, 444–445
Passivity, 302
Patient education, 24
Peer interaction, 23
Penile implants, 224–225
Percussion, 52
Peristaltic stimulators, 345
Personal assistance services, 353
Personal assistant/attendant
   communications with, 373–375
   emergency backup care, 370–372
   employer agreement, 368
   employment application, 361–362
   finding, 359–360
   interviewing, 363–365
   job description, 357
   job description worksheet, 358
   paying for, 376
   reference information waiver, 367
   reference request, 366
   training guidelines, 369
Personal care, 355, 364
   needs, 354
   routine, 413–415
Personal habits, 355–356, 365
Personal services, 353
Phenolthalein, 160
Phrenic nerve pacing, 62
Physiatrist, 25
Physical fitness
   before starting, 466
   definition of, 464–465
   exercise guidelines, 467
   recommendations, 468–469
   resources, 477–479
Physical therapist, 25
Physical therapy, chest, 52–55
Physiology, 8–10
Pneumonia, 49–50
Positioning, ventilator and, 63
Postpartum concerns, 244
Posttraumatic syringomyelia, 87, 97–98
Postural drainage positions, 56–57
Postural hypotension, 32, 33
Posture, aging and, 90–92
Preeclampsia, 245
Pregnancy, 214, 236–237, 238–239
   baclofen pump and, 100
   obstetrician guidelines, 244–245
Pressure reliefs, 178, 182–185
Pressure ulcers
   care of, 197, 207–208
   helping heal, 198–206
   nutrition and, 454
   overview, 193–196
Pride, 300
Priorities, 308
Probanthine, 342
Problem drinking, 285. *See also* Alcoholism
Progestagen injections, 241
Progestin, 241
Prostaglandin E1, 223
Protein, 458
Psychologist, 25
Psychotherapy, 320
Psyllium hydro-mucilloid, 161
Public accommodations, 382–383
Public services, 382
Publishers, 476–477
Pulmonary embolism (PE), 32, 39

Q–R

Quadriplegia. *See* Tetraplegia
Ramp, 395–399, 436
Range of motion, 67
    additional exercises, 75–79
    exercises for lower extremity, 73–74
    exercises for upper extremity, 68–72
Ranitidine, 349
Rashes, 190
Reaching aids, 416
Recreational therapist, 25
Rectal bleeding, 162
Reference
    information waiver, 367
    request, 366
Referred pain, 314
Reflux, 121
Rehabilitation, center selection for, 23–24
Rehabilitation nurse, 26
Rehabilitation team
    members of, 25–26
    specialization by, 23
Relaxation
    exercise, 274, 324
    techniques, 277–278
    therapy, 320, 322–323
Renal scan, 122
Reproduction resources, 477
Resources, 473–481
Respiratory system
    care for, 51
    complications, 49–50
    how works, 47–48
    lungs, 45–46
Respiratory therapist, 25-26
Rest, 277
    circulation and, 31
    ventilator and, 63
Rocking bed, 62
Root pain, 314

S

Sacral area, 5, 8–9
Sadness, 300
Safe sex, 220
Saturated fats, 458
Scapular retraction, 58
Seat belts, 437
Self-care, 263, 276
Self-esteem, 242–243, 307
Senna, 160
Sensory examination, 15, 17
Sex life, healthy, 251
Sex toys, aids, 223
Sexual counseling, 24
Sexual excitement, 218
Sexuality, 243
    affirmation, 246–247
    marriage, relationships, 213–215
    overview, 211–212
    preparations for, 216–217
    resources, 477
    special concerns, 219–220
Sexually transmitted diseases, 243, 253
Shaving, 414
Shelves, 393
Shoes, 411–412
Shoulder
    exercises, 68–70
    pinches, 58
Side effects, 336
Silverware, 407–408
Skin care, 414
    alcohol and, 181
    body weight and, 180
    breakdown, 189
    checking, 187–188
    circulation, 175–176
    clothing, 180
    feet, 179
    hygiene, 178
    injury prevention, 180–181
    maintaining, 178
    nutrition, 175, 178
    pressure reliefs, 178, 182–185
    problems, 190–192
    spasticity, 181
    stress, 181
    temperature, 180
    tolerance, 186
Smoking, 60, 175, 179
Social workers, 26
Spasms, 216
Spastic bladder phase, 116–117
Spasticity, 67, 84
    aging and, 87–89
    osteoporosis and, 95
    questions about, 85–86
    skin care and, 181
Spastic paralysis, 11
Speech and language pathologist, 25
Spermicidals, 241
Sperm production, transport, 226
Sperm retrieval techniques, 226–227
Sphincter dyssynergia, 121
Spinal cord, 8, 10
Spinal cord injury
    explained, 3–7
    functional chart, 20–22
    level of, 6–7, 11–12
    type of, 6
    understanding, 8–13
Spinal shock, 85
Sport resources, 477–479
Stair safety, 436
State-funded programs, 376
Sterility, 213
Stool softener, 161, 345
Storage accessibility, 401–402
Stress, 181, 273–274, 317–318
Subdermal implants, 241
Substance abuse
    adolescent symptoms of, 291–293
    resources, 474–475
    suggestions to help at home, 296–297
    symptoms of, 294–295
Sudafed, 342
Suppository, 158, 168–169, 345–346
Suprapubic catheter, 134, 139–140, 230
Surgery
    for pain, 317
    posttraumatic syringomyelia and, 97–98
    for spasticity, 86
Swimming pools, 394
Syphilis, 253
Syrinx, 97
Syrinx pain, 314

T

Table setting, 406–407
Tagamet, 349
Tegretol, 347
Telecommunications, ADA, 383
Temperature
    regulation, 40–41
    skin care, 180
Tetraplegia, 7, 12
    breast cancer and, 249–250
    coughing, 52–53
Texas catheters. *See* Condom: application
Thoracic area, 4-5, 8–9
Thought-stopping technique, 323
Thrombophlebitis, 236
Tiedown systems, 445
Toe stretch, 74
Tofranil, 343
Transcutaneous electrical nerve stimulation (TENS), 102–103, 317
Transportation, 353, 364
Travel, 377–380, 437
Tubal ligation, 241

U

Ultrasound, 122
Undergarments, 156
Unsaturated fats, 458
Upper motor neurons, 4, 10, 157
Urecholine, 343
Urinary drainage bag care, 154

Urinary tests, 122–123
Urinary tract infection, 119, 219, 454–455
Urispas, 343
Urodynamics, 122
Urological problems
    catheter leakage, 150
        frequent catheter changes, 151–153
Urological supplies, 155–156

V

Vaginal lubrication, 235
Valium, 85, 230, 348
Valsalva maneuver, 158
Van selection, 447–450
Vascular disease, 176
Vaseline, 231
Veins, 29
Ventilator
    support, types of, 61–62
    weaning, 63–64
Ventilatory dysfunction, 61
Vertebrae, 3–4

Vertebral column, 4, 8
Vibration, 52
Vinegar solution, 154–155
Vitamins, 459
Vocational rehabilitation, 376

W

Walkers, 417
Water intake, 460
Weight gain, 461–463
Weight shifts, circulation and, 31
Wheelchairs
    accessories glossary, 427
    armrests, 422–423, 424, 435
    back posts, 425
    backrests, 424
    brakes, 422, 425, 435
    chair fit, 421
    charging power, 432
    cushions, 421–422, 428–429
    footrests, 421, 422, 435
    frames, 421, 425
    front casters, 426
    home modification for, 387–388
    information sheet, 430
    maintenance, 431
    positioning, 433
    power, 440–442
    ramp construction, 397–399
    rear wheels, 426
    safety, 435–439
    tilting rods, 437–438
    tires, 423, 426
    transfer considerations, 434
    types of, 420–421
Window cleaning, 401
Women for Sobriety, Inc., 288
Women's health resources, 477
Wrist exercises, 71–72

Y–Z

Yoga, 277
Zantac, 349